Ethics in Neurosurgical Practice

Ethics in Neurosurgical Practice

Edited by

Stephen Honeybul, FRCS (SN), FRACS
Sir Charles Gairdner Hospital, Royal Perth and Fiona Stanley Hospitals

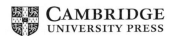
CAMBRIDGE
UNIVERSITY PRESS

CAMBRIDGE
UNIVERSITY PRESS

University Printing House, Cambridge CB2 8BS, United Kingdom

One Liberty Plaza, 20th Floor, New York, NY 10006, USA

477 Williamstown Road, Port Melbourne, VIC 3207, Australia

314–321, 3rd Floor, Plot 3, Splendor Forum, Jasola District Centre,
New Delhi – 110025, India

79 Anson Road, #06–04/06, Singapore 079906

Cambridge University Press is part of the University of Cambridge.

It furthers the University's mission by disseminating knowledge in the pursuit of
education, learning, and research at the highest international levels of excellence.

www.cambridge.org
Information on this title: www.cambridge.org/9781108494120
DOI: 10.1017/9781108643887

First published 2020

Printed in the United Kingdom by TJ International Ltd, Padstow Cornwall

A catalogue record for this publication is available from the British Library.

Library of Congress Cataloging-in-Publication Data
Names: Honeybul, Stephen, editor.
Title: Ethics in neurosurgical practice / edited by Stephen Honeybul.
Description: Cambridge ; New York, NY : Cambridge University Press, 2020. |
Includes bibliographical references and index.
Identifiers: LCCN 2019051669 (print) | LCCN 2019051670 (ebook) | ISBN 9781108494120 (hardback) |
ISBN 9781108643887 (ebook)
Subjects: MESH: Neurosurgery – ethics | Neurosurgical Procedures – ethics
Classification: LCC RD593 (print) | LCC RD593 (ebook) | NLM WL 368 | DDC 174.2/9748–dc23
LC record available at https://lccn.loc.gov/2019051669
LC ebook record available at https://lccn.loc.gov/2019051670

ISBN 978-1-108-49412-0 Hardback

....

Contents

Contributors

Ahmed Ammar, PhD
Department of Neurosurgery, King Fahd University Hospital, Al Khobar, Saudi Arabia

Mario Ammirati, MD, MBA
Center for Biotechnology Department of Biology, College of Science and Technology, Temple University and Sbarro Health Organization at Temple University, Philadelphia, Pennsylvania, USA

Naci Balak, MD
Department of Neurosurgery, Istanbul Medeniyet University, Göztepe Education and Research Hospital, Istanbul, Turkey

Mark Bernstein, MD, MHSc (Bioethics), FRCS (C)
Faculty of Medicine, Department of Surgery, Division of Neurosurgery, Toronto Western Hospital, University Health Network, University of Toronto, Toronto, Canada

Gene Bolles, MD
Department of Neurosurgery, University of Colorado School of Medicine, Denver Health Medical Center, Denver, Colorado, USA

Jannick Brennum, MD, PhD
Copenhagen Neurosurgery, Neuroscience Centre, Rigshospitalet, University of Copenhagen, Copenhagen, Denmark

Marike Broekman, MD, PhD, LLM
Department of Neurosurgery, Leiden University Medical Center, Leiden, Zuid-Holland, and Haaglanden Medical Center, The Hague, The Netherlands, and Department of Neurology, Massachusetts

General Hospital, Boston, Massachusetts, USA

Albert Chiu, FRANZCR, CCINR
Neurological Intervention and Imaging Service of Western Australia, Sir Charles Gairdner, Fiona Stanley and Royal Perth Hospitals, University of Western Australia, Perth, Australia

David Cote, BS
Cushing Neurosurgical Outcomes Center, Department of Neurosurgery, Brigham and Women's Hospital, Harvard Medical School, Boston, Massachusetts, USA

Ignatius Esene, MD, MSc, PhD, MPH
Department of Neurological Surgery, School of Medicine and Public Health, University of Wisconsin–Madison, Madison, Wisconsin, USA

Grant Gillett, FRACS, MPhil
Dunedin Hospital and Otago Bioethics Centre, University of Otago, Dunedin, New Zealand

Kwok Ming Ho, FCICM, PhD
Department of Intensive Care Medicine and Medical School, University of Western Australia, Perth, Australia

Stephen Honeybul, FRCS (SN), FRACS
Department of Neurosurgery, Sir Charles Gairdner Hospital and Royal Perth Hospital, University of Western Australia, Perth, Australia

Alexander Hulsbergen, BS
Department of Neurosurgery, Leiden University Medical Center, Leiden,

Zuid-Holland and Haaglanden Medical Center, The Hague, The Netherlands, and Computational Neuroscience Outcomes Center, Department of Neurosurgery, Brigham and Women's Hospital, Harvard Medical School, Boston, Massachusetts, USA

Eiichi Ishikawa, MD, PhD
Department of Neurosurgery, University of Tsukuba, Ibaraki, Japan

Ian Kerridge, BA, BMed (Hons), MPhil (Cantab), FRACP, FRCPA
Sydney Health Ethics, Sydney Medical School, University of Sydney and Royal North Shore Hospital, Sydney, New South Wales, Australia

Paul A. Komesaroff, MB, BS, BSc (Hons), PhD, FRACP, AM
Faculty of Medicine, Nursing and Health Sciences, Monash University, Melbourne, Australia

Ann Mansur, MD
Faculty of Medicine, Department of Surgery, Division of Neurosurgery, University of Toronto, Toronto, Canada

Tiit Mathiesen, MD, PhD
Department of Neurosurgery, Rigshospitalet, University of Copenhagen, Copenhagen, Denmark, and Department of Clinical Neuroscience, Karolinska Institutet, Stockholm, Sweden

Akira Matsumura, MD, PhD
Department of Neurosurgery, University of Tsukuba, Ibaraki, Japan

Ivar Mendez, MD, PhD, FRCSC, DABNS, FACS, FCAHS
Department of Surgery and Royal University Hospital, University of

Saskatchewan and Saskatchewan Health Authority, Saskatoon, Canada

Lars-Peder Pallesen, MD
Department of Neurology, Dresden Neurovascular Center, University of Technology Dresden, Dresden, Germany

Volker Puetz, MD, FESO
Department of Neurology, Dresden Neurovascular Center, University of Technology Dresden, Dresden, Germany

Jeffery V. Rosenfeld, MS, MD, FRACS, FRCS (Edin), FACS, IFAANS
Department of Neurosurgery, The Alfred Hospital, Melbourne, Department of Surgery, Monash University, Clayton, Australia, and Department of Surgery, F. Edward Hébert School of Medicine, Uniformed Services University of the Health Sciences, Bethesda, Maryland, USA

Nobuyuki Sakai, MD, DMSc
Department of Neurosurgery, Kobe City Medical Center General Hospital, Kobe, Japan

Ulrika Sandvik, MD, PhD
Paediatric Neurosurgery at Astrid Lindgren Children's Hospital, Department of Neurosurgery, Karolinska University Hospital, Stockholm, Sweden

Cara Sedney, MD
Department of Neurosurgery, West Virginia University, Morgantown, West Virginia, USA

George Skowronski, MBBS (Hons), FRCP, FRACP, FCICM, M.Bioeth
St George Hospital, Faculty of Medicine, University of New South Wales and

Sydney Health Ethics, School of Public Health, University of Sydney, Sydney, New South Wales, Australia

Timothy Smith, MD, PhD, MPH
Cushing Neurosurgical Outcomes Center, Department of Neurosurgery, Brigham and Women's Hospital, Harvard Medical School, Boston, Massachusetts, USA

Cameron Stewart, BEc LLB (Hons), GradDipJur, GradDipLegalPrac, PhD, FACLM (Hon)
Sydney Health Law, Sydney Law School, University of Sydney, Sydney, New South Wales, Australia

Magnus Tisell, MD, PhD
Department of Neurosurgery, Sahlgrenska University Hospital, Gothenburg, Sweden

Introduction

Stephen Honeybul

The field of modern-day bioethics is relatively young and continues to constantly evolve in parallel with the ever-increasingly complex nature of contemporary medical practice. These advances present clinicians with an array of therapeutic options that would have not seemed possible only a generation ago. Given these medical advances and the expansion of the academic and medicolegal field of bioethics, one would have thought that clinical decision-making would have become easier. However, paradoxically, this has not proved to be the case. Each advance may provide an answer to a particular clinical question, which is almost immediately replaced by a whole new set of ethical problems that require consideration.

The field of neurosurgery provides a particularly good example of how the ethical landscape has changed over a relatively short period of time. Advances in radiology have seen the grainy appearances of the early CT scans acquired over a 45-minute period replaced with the rapid sequence acquisition, high resolution, whole-body trauma scans of today. The development and refinement of MRI scanning combined with the widespread use of the operative microscope, image-guided technology, and a whole host of other technological advances has led to the development of a field of surgery that would previously have been almost unrecognisable. In addition to these surgical developments, there have been significant advances in intensive care management, oncology treatment, and infection control, to name but a few.

Notwithstanding these developments, there will always come a time when a disease or injury has progressed to a certain point, or a person has reached a certain age where therapy is providing limited benefit and indeed may be becoming overly burdensome. Managing patient expectations and the expectations of families in these circumstances can be ethically challenging.

My own interest in bioethics came about initially because of my experience with long-term outcomes following decompressive craniectomy in the context of severe traumatic brain injury when I moved to Perth, Western Australia, more than 15 years ago. Perth is geographically isolated and has two major neurosurgical centres that service a population of 2.2 million. At around that time, there had been a resurgence of interest in decompressive craniectomy, and a number of studies had demonstrated the successful management of intractable intracranial hypertension and reduction in mortality that could be achieved. However, as demonstrated in subsequent randomised controlled trials, this reduction in mortality comes at the expense of an increase in the number of survivors with severe neurocognitive disability and dependency, and I witnessed firsthand the effect this outcome had on the patients and their families.

I also came across the CRASH (Corticosteroid Randomization after Significant-Head injury) collaborators outcome prediction model. This is a web-based user-friendly outcome prediction model that is based on the CRASH study, which investigated the role of steroids in traumatic brain injury and is described in detail in Chapter 13. The model combines the prognostic significance of certain clinical and radiological features in order to provide a percentage prediction of unfavourable outcome. The use of this model allows patients to be stratified according to injury severity, and comparing the predicted outcome with the *observed* long-term outcome provided an objective assessment of the most likely outcome following surgical decompression for severe traumatic brain injury. Once the percentage prediction reaches a certain level, the most likely outcome is severe dependency, and on initial examination, this would appear to provide clinically useful information. However, as with other surgical advances, it has in many ways made the clinical decision-making and ethical discussion more complex. Once it has been established that the most likely outcome is severe disability, every effort must be made to determine that this would be acceptable to the person on whom the procedure is being performed. This requires the exploration of a number of ethical concepts, such as consent, withholding and withdrawing treatment, adapting to survival with disability, the disability paradox, and the rule of rescue. I went on to collaborate with Grant Gillett and Kwok Ho on a number of publications, and the more I explored these issues in the context of severe traumatic brain injury, the more aware I became of ethical issues in the field of neurosurgery in general. This prompted the project that led to *Ethics in Neurosurgery*.

The book is set out in three sections and is intended as an introduction to practical ethics for all healthcare professionals involved in the management and care of neurosurgical patients. There is a wide variety of contributors from around the world, including clinical ethicists, legal experts, intensive care physicians, and neurosurgeons.

The first section deals with some general principles of bioethics and aims to focus on aspects that are particularly relevant to neurosurgery, such as consent and withholding life-preserving treatment. The second section looks at subspecialty specific fields. The aim is not to cover all aspects of neurosurgery but rather to focus on areas where there are particularly important ethical issues. The final section deals with the future possibilities and covers issues such as surgical innovation, possible application of stem-cell therapies, and the evolving development of brain-machine interface.

I hope the book provides educational benefit as well as general interest, and it may well serve as a stimulus to further explore the field of bioethics, which is an area of increasing importance. I would like to thank all of the contributors, without whom none of this would have been possible.

Introduction to Ethics and Ethical Theory

Ian Kerridge

1.1 Introduction

Clinicians, and their patients, live and practice in a world characterised by illness, sickness, disease, and suffering. Theirs is not an abstract or theoretical world, but a very real one. And in this world their concern is how healthcare can cure, ameliorate, or palliate these symptoms and maladies. For all of these reasons, medicine has been concerned with determining what works and what doesn't, what provides benefit and what is harmful, and what should be done in any given situation. This concern has always been a feature of medicine, even in its pre-scientific manifestations, but over the past 40 years has become a central feature of both evidence-based medicine and personalised medicine.

But while evidence undoubtedly informs decision-making and policy development, it does not, of itself, tell us what we *should* do. This point has been made most eloquently by the Scottish enlightenment philosopher David Hume and by the Austrian philosopher of logic Ludwig Wittgenstein.

Hume articulated this as the 'is-ought' problem, in which he suggested that there is no logical way to go from a statement about how the world *is* to a statement about how it *ought to be*, or what we ought to do to get it there.[1] Wittgenstein agrees, 'You cannot lead people to what is good: you can only lead them to some place or another. The good is outside the space of facts.'[2]

These are important insights because they remind us that data or 'evidence' (which can be loosely defined as data to which we attach value) does not tell us how we *should* act, that decisions are inevitably issues of value and judgement, and that our decisions and actions are influenced as much by our values, perspectives, and our processes of reasoning and reflection as the concepts and ideas we use and the data we draw from.

This does not, however, mean that data are irrelevant to ethical judgements. Indeed, evidence is relevant to ethical thinking and reasoning in at least four ways:

- it can provide descriptive information about ethically fraught issues (e.g., how many people have completed advance care plans, what public support there is for medical assistance in dying, or if patients experience distress if nutrition is discontinued at the end of life);
- it can measure the impact of ethical policies (e.g., the impact of legislation of stem cell research, termination of pregnancy, or organ donor rates);
- it can interrogate the value-laden aspects of medical care, medical 'facts' and medical terms (such as 'quality of life' or 'futility'); and
- it can provide a rich description of an area or domain of experience (e.g., a sociological study of cancer in adolescents or the healthcare experiences of people who survive major brain injury).

The point here is that medicine is inevitably a *moral* exercise – not simply a practical or technical one. It is as much about ethics as it is about evidence.

The other logical error that healthcare providers often make when thinking about how they should act and health services should be organised is to characterise each of these in terms of meeting or fulfilling a patient's preferences or rights. This is particularly problematic because while there is broad recognition that rights are important in healthcare and in society more generally, there is ongoing disagreement regarding what rights are, how they relate to ethics, and whether they are a fundamental part of human existence or only exist when recognised by government.[3]

The idea of universal human rights can be traced back to Plato and Aristotle, and to philosophical doctrines of natural law (particularly the works of John Locke and Immanuel Kant). More contemporary formulations of civil and political rights can be traced to the English Bill of Rights in 1689 and the American Declaration of Independence of 1776, which argued for the right of individuals to be free from arbitrary interference by the state. The modern understanding of human rights, however, really emerged following World War II and the Holocaust, when the international community moved to establish both a collective expression of human conscience and a mechanism for mediating disputes between nations and defusing international crises. The principal international statement of human rights is the Universal Declaration of Human Rights (UDHR), which was approved by the United Nations in 1948. While the UDHR has been the subject of extensive political, ethical, and cultural criticism, there is no question that it has profoundly influenced the way we think about politics, social order, and the meaning and value of rights.

In conceptual terms, rights can be defined as justifiable claims that individuals or groups can make upon society or upon other individuals. They may be expressed as *positive rights* or *negative rights*. A positive right is a right to be provided with a particular good or service by others, whereas a negative right constrains others from interfering with an individual's exercise of that right. Thus the right of liberty is a negative right because it merely suggests that no one should hold one against one's wishes. The right to education is a positive right, as it means that someone must teach. In other words, the concept of 'rights' also entails a definite but often ill-defined notion of associated obligations. For example, if one person possesses a right to life, this imposes an obligation upon others not to deprive that person of life. The extent of this obligation is defined by the specific context and by consideration of the wishes, beliefs, and values of each party. Thus a right to life does not necessarily prevent an individual being killed in war, or by another in self-defence, or an individual contracting with another to assist them to die.

Ethics and rights share much in common. Each are founded on, or express, similar ideas:

- that respect for persons is key to civil society;
- that everyone, and particularly the most vulnerable in society, should be cared for and protected;
- that people should have control over their own futures and should be able to make decisions for themselves;
- that harm should be avoided and ameliorated where possible;
- that privacy and confidentiality should be recognised and respected; and
- that justice and fairness are important.

But ethics and human rights are not identical. Human rights principally establish the obligations of the state (and other institutions) towards people and act through international treaties, declarations, and national laws. Ethics, on the other hand, is principally concerned with the relationships between individuals and communities and acts through personal reflection, conscience, codes of ethics, guidelines, regulations, and law. But despite these differences, ethics and human rights infrequently conflict with each other – more often adding richness and depth to ethical deliberation.

Irrespective of how we understand the relationship between ethics and rights, it is undeniable that the language of rights has been critical to the development of ethics and, at least since WWII, has played a vital role in protecting individuals from the excesses of the state. The question of what role rights should play in defining law, morality, and political organisation, and what role they should play in the design and delivery of healthcare, however, remains controversial.

Thus, even to properly understand the role that rights and evidence play in healthcare, therefore, we must understand something about ethics.

So what then is ethics?

The word 'ethics', which is derived from the ancient Greek *ethikos* – meaning relating to one's character – can refer to several things including the study of how one should live (known as philosophical ethics or moral philosophy) and the human capacity for, interest in and reflection on what it is we value and how we should act or behave. While these two understandings of ethics are often talked of as very distinct things, in fact they are deeply interrelated. The development of philosophical ethics is, for example, not an academic abstraction isolated from the 'real world' but has been shaped by culture, politics, economics, law, religion, and science. In other words, ethics is historically and culturally embedded. Ethical ideas, for example, are present in the poems of Homer (800 BCE), which emphasise heroism and nobility; in Jewish ethics (1300 BCE), which outline ethical duties and processes for ethical analysis; and in Eastern philosophical scriptures, including the Vedas, an ancient Indian religious text (1500 BCE) that identified morally good actions as those that are harmonious with the universe.

In broad terms, therefore, ethics describes both the branch of philosophy and the domain of enquiry concerned with how people should live their lives in order that they, those around them, and society in general should flourish. This means that ethics is concerned with questions surrounding the distinction between right and wrong, virtue and vice, justice and crime, the definition of rights and responsibilities, the means by which we may make good or bad decisions and the means by which we may live a good life.

Ethics is traditionally divided into three areas: metaethics, normative ethics, and practical (or applied) ethics.

- *Metaethics* deals with nature of moral judgement and with the nature and status of moral 'things' and examines what we mean when we say that something is right or wrong.
- *Normative ethics* is concerned with the theoretical and practical means by which we determine a moral course of action.
- *Practical or applied ethics* is concerned with how people should act in particular situations or contexts, such as in healthcare settings, business, law, and so forth.

This chapter will provide a brief introduction to normative approaches to ethics and to ethical principles.

1.2 Ethical Principles

1.2.1 Deontology

One of the major schools of moral philosophy is known as deontology. Deontology embodies the notion that things or actions are right or wrong in and of themselves. For example, a deontological theory might maintain that there is something *intrinsically* wrong with acts of lying, murder, or rape that is independent of outcome or consequences. Many religions are based on deontological theories.

The central theoretical focus of deontological theories is on doing one's duty, which may be expressed by certain universal statements or action guides. These central rules find expression in laws (such as 'Do not kill'); principles (such as respect for human life); institutions (such as the legal system); and 'relational laws' (such as respect for one's parents).

In order to determine what action is required in a particular circumstance, the deontological approach to moral reasoning involves the application of the appropriate universal statement to the specific situation. An example of such reasoning would be: killing is wrong; giving potassium chloride to this patient is killing; therefore this action is wrong.

Exactly where these moral rules or principles come from is a matter of some debate. *Theological* arguments justify rules by appeal to divine revelation, *societal* approaches argue that the correct moral rules are those believed in by most members of society, *intuitionist* approaches suggest that the proper moral rules or actions are those that possess the intrinsic property of 'rightness', while the philosopher Immanuel Kant (1724–1804) argued that the basis of moral rules is *pure reason* (i.e., without the need for empirical observation).

Kant proposes that the moral rules (or imperatives) that we choose to live by should be absolute and binding and that they should be 'univeralisable' – that is, they should be able to be applied to everyone. This is made clear in a series of 'categorical imperatives', which are often familiar even to those who have never studied philosophy. These include:

- 'act in such a way that you treat humanity, whether in your own person or in the person of another, always at the same time as an end and never simply as a means'; and
- 'act as if the maxim of your action were to become through your will a universal law of nature'.

The value of deontological theories is that they remind us of the importance of rationality in moral judgement and of moral standards independent of consequences. They have tremendous appeal for those who seek certainties in life and for institutions (such as the church or government) that have a need to bind together groups of people under some identifiable moral code.

But while deontological theories provide the basis for many moral codes and faith traditions, they are often criticised because the rules and principles are controversial, vague, or difficult to define and may come into conflict. For instance, even if it is accepted that is wrong to kill, or lie, it is not clear whether this means that killing or lying is always wrong in every circumstance. Likewise, where one is contemplating the morality of abortion, what rule takes precedence: the foetus's right to life or the woman's right to bodily autonomy?

1.2.2 Consequentialist Theories and Utilitarianism

Consequentialist theories propose that the rightness or wrongness of an action is based solely on the consequences of performing it and that the nature of the action or the motives and intention of the agent are largely irrelevant.

The most prominent consequentialist theory is utilitarianism, which states that the single fundamental principle of ethics should be the 'principle of utility' – that the morally right action is the action that produces the best possible outcome. Utility is conceived of in different ways by different thinkers. The classical utilitarians, Jeremy Bentham (1748–1832) and John Stuart Mill (1806–73), conceived utility entirely in terms of happiness or pleasure, while others have contended that values other than happiness (such as friendship, health, or autonomy) have intrinsic worth, or that utilitarianism should focus not on happiness but the satisfaction of preferences.

While consequentialist approaches to ethics appear to provide a simple, rational process for moral reasoning, this simplicity is illusory. A number of methodological criticisms have been made of consequentialism.

The first is that it is difficult, if not impossible, to quantify variables such as 'happiness' or 'quality of life' and to compare all the possible outcomes of an action. The second is that it is often unclear as to who are the parties involved in any moral action and what moral significance each of their interests should have. The third is that it is often difficult to predict or to determine outcomes in advance – making ranking or prioritisation of consequences impossible. In medicine, in particular, outcomes are generally not known with any certainty but are expressed as probabilities drawn from epidemiological data and generalised to an individual, and there are certain times that outcomes are not even imaginable at the time that a decision is made or action is taken.

But even if none of these methodological challenges hold true, consequentialist theories are still open to a series of major philosophical criticisms. The first is that consequentialism (by definition) is concerned only with consequences and does not account for certain aspects of ordinary moral thinking (such as the importance of individual rights) in deciding moral issues. The second is that it can lead to actions that would seem morally unacceptable, such as discrimination, imprisonment, torture, or killing if these actions result in the best net balance of good over evil. (This problem is made clear in thought experiments like the famous 'trolley problem'.) And finally, because consequentialism emphasises net satisfaction rather than considerations of justice or equality, consequentialist theories can sanction unjust rules and allow the interests of the majority to override those of the minority.

1.2.3 Virtue Theory

An alternative approach to ethics emphasises not rules, consequences, or principles but moral virtue (i.e., the notion that the rightness or wrongness of an action is derived from the virtues or underlying motives of the person making that action).

The concept of moral virtue derives from ancient philosophical traditions. To Plato, virtue was an intellectual trait synonymous with excellence in living a good life, and it could be attained and maintained by practice. To Aristotle, and later Aquinas, virtue was expressed as a disposition to act in the right way and was the result of a balance between intellect, feeling, and action. Aristotle used the term *ethika arête* to mean 'matters having to do with character', the right character being modelled on a person of virtue or excellence. Aristotle considered happiness, or *eudaemonia*, to be the highest form of goodness and argued that this was gained through excellence of function, which, in man's case, was the capacity to reason. This, in turn, was manifest through a life-long practice of making virtuous choices and acting in virtuous ways. For Aristotle, this involved choosing, and acting between two extremes of vice. (This is known as the rule of the 'Golden Mean'.) Thus, for example, the virtuous person would choose to act in a way that was courageous – as this is the virtue that lies between rashness and cowardice. Such a choice was voluntary and rational and was made possible by the development of *phronesis* (practical wisdom). In other words, virtue was not regarded as an innate capacity but was felt to be a disposition cultivated by proper training, experience, and critical reflection. These notions, particularly the idea that practical wisdom is developed through training and through considered decisions and actions, are often immediately recognisable, and appealing, to those working in the health professions.

Unfortunately, it is not at all clear that virtues are a sufficient basis for decision-making or that consideration of virtues should take precedence over rights, principles, or ethical obligations or considerations of the consequences of one's actions. Virtue ethics is also subject to criticism that it is simplistic and imprecise, does not tell us what we should do or how we should act, relies on circular reasoning (a virtuous person is defined as a person who does good things, and good things are those acts a virtuous person does), and, at least in medicine, emphasises the moral character of the doctor over what is owed to the patient.

1.2.4 Continental Philosophy and Postmodernism in Ethics

'Continental philosophy' is the name given to a large number of philosophies to emerge from Europe since the work of Immanuel Kant at the end of the eighteenth century. In many ways, it is a confusing term because it does not refer to a single philosophical method, style, concern, and tradition, and includes a number of philosophical movements and philosophers, such as Hegel, Kierkegaard, Marx, Nietzsche, Husserl, Heidegger, Merleau-Ponty, Gadamer, Sartre, Adorno, Marcuse, Barthes, Bauman, and Levi-Strauss. A number of these thinkers have had a profound influence on contemporary ethics and medical ethics, including the French philosopher Emmanuel Levinas, who argued that ethics is principally about our responsiveness to the 'other' that we encounter in 'face-to-face' relationships, and Jacques Derrida, who argued the most important feature of ethics is 'hospitality', by which he meant openness to the 'other' (the 'arrivant') and acceptance of the possibility of our own transformation as a consequence of our interaction with others.

The other thinker to have had a major influence on contemporary ethics is the French philosopher, historian, and sociologist Michel Foucault, whose critiques of social institutions, including hospitals, psychiatric facilities, and prisons, and of human experiences, including sexuality and power, undoubtedly enriched our understanding of how ethics 'plays out' in healthcare. The extent of Foucault's influence can be measured by the fact that many of the terms and concepts he coined, such biopolitics, governmentality, state racism, and the 'medical gaze', have become a part of both academic and lay discourse.

Continental philosophy is often confused with postmodernism, which in itself is a term that generates enormous confusion. While the term 'postmodernism' has entered into popular culture, there is very little agreement about what it actually means. Very simply, it describes a philosophical and political movement that arose in the nineteenth and twentieth century that rejected the tenets of the 'modern' societies that developed in Europe and North America following the Enlightenment – notably capitalism (the free market), liberal democracy, secularism, rationalism, humanism, science, industry, and technology.

While postmodern theories and approaches are extraordinarily diverse, they share two common features. First, they reject the idea that truth is discoverable through human reason and scientific method. And second, they reject the idea that there should be a single (best) perspective, system of knowledge, value system, or system of norms. Postmodern ethics, therefore, rejects the ideologies and theoretical traditions of both medicine and ethics, addressing each through a diverse set of new perspectives, new languages, and new paradigms grounded in and formed by their social and clinical context.

1.2.5 Feminist Moral Philosophy

Contemporary feminist philosophers have challenged the inherent ('masculinist') sexism of 'traditional' Western moral philosophy and the historical tendency to devalue women's experiences and lives. While there is enormous variability in the approaches taken by feminist ethicists, most share a number of features, including:

- rejection of the overemphasis on autonomy and individual rights;
- criticism of the philosophical dualisms that have furthered the subordination of women (e.g., mind-body, reason-emotion, objective-subjective, public-private, etc.);
- rejection of the idea that ethics should be value-neutral;
- emphasis of values such as empathy, interdependence, and caring, and the importance of community and solidarity; and
- emphasis on the importance of context and the relevance of politics and power to understanding ethics and healthcare.

Although feminist approaches to ethics do not provide a single moral theory, they have been enormously influential because they have refocused attention on caring and relationships in healthcare, revealed the diverse nature of the oppression of women, and demonstrated how political will is required to reduce inequity and eliminate oppression.

1.3 Ethical Frameworks and Principles in Healthcare

Many philosophers (and clinicians) are sceptical of the ability of any ethical theory to explain or guide behaviour. Instead, they suggest that while ethical theories may provide useful tools or frameworks, ethical decision-making is informed by consideration of many factors – any one of which may assume greater or lesser importance in different situations. These include the ethical probity of the action or decision itself, the consequences that follow that decision or action and the virtues of the 'actor', as well as views about the dignity and rights of persons, the relationships between persons and communities, and the organisation of society. As a result, in recent years the focus of ethics has shifted away from the elaboration of theories to a focus on values (the field of scholarship known as axiology), metaethics, empirical (evidence-based) ethics, and practical (or applied) ethics. This, in turn, has led to the elaboration of many different 'frameworks' for ethical deliberation that emphasise not so much ethical assumptions or rules but a series of ethical principles or concepts or a series of questions that can be used to clarify what is at 'stake'.

Principle-based approaches to ethics begin not with theory but with consideration of the values that we are striving to protect and the principles by which our actions should be guided. The most common formulation of a principle-based approach to ethics in medicine

(Beauchamp & Childress, 2012) assumes that medicine is concerned with 'right' and 'good' actions, decisions, and outcomes, and that this is achieved through attention to six fundamental ethical principles: respect for autonomy, non-maleficence (avoiding harm), beneficence (doing good or providing benefit), justice, veracity (truth-telling), and privacy/confidentiality.[4] Each of these principles have prima facie standing, or worth, and they need to be taken into account, balanced, and specified in any clinical setting.[5]

This process of reflective thinking about principles (rather than simply 'applying' them to a clinical situation in an unsophisticated or unreflective way) is critically important because even if we agree on our moral commitment to these principles, this does not necessarily mean we will agree on their importance, prioritisation, or scope of application. We may, for example, disagree about what, or to whom, we owe moral obligations arising from these principles. For example, we clearly do not owe a duty of beneficence to everyone and everything, so whom or what do we have a moral duty to help, and how much should we help them? And who or what falls within the scope of our obligation to distribute scarce resources fairly and according to the principle of justice?

While a principle-based approach to ethics is not unproblematic and does not generally provide a single or incontrovertible 'answer' to challenging or controversial situations, it does provide a means for systematically working through problems in practice.

1.4 Conclusion: The Value of Ethics to Clinical Practice

Since its origins, medicine has become increasingly complex and increasingly powerful. And there is no reason to believe that this will not continue. At the same time, the world in which illness is experienced, disease defined, and healthcare delivered has become more diverse, with far greater pluralism in faith traditions, culture, and political and social behaviour. It is essential, therefore, that health practitioners understand how ethical ideas, concepts, values, and principles can shape and inform their professional practice. Specifically, this means the following:

- We should understand that medicine is fundamentally an ethical enterprise – concerned with the security and flourishing of individuals and communities, with important ideals, and with concepts like justice.
- We should acknowledge that ethical concepts or values can inform and shape practice. Ideas about efficacy, care, social justices, and reciprocity, for example, underpin the way we organise our healthcare systems, vaccination programmes, and organ donation and transplantation services.
- We should consider how ethical theories and frameworks may help us navigate and think through difficult problems.
- Finally, we should use an ethical 'lens' to consider other ways of seeing the world and other ways of prioritising values. Even if we lack the time, energy, or interest to study the origins and ideas that characterise postcolonial, human rights, disability, or feminist approaches to ethics, we can appreciate the insights they have provided into the impact of power imbalances, discrimination, and inequity on healthcare, health policy, and health outcomes.

Importantly, ethics requires of clinicians both that they appreciate and sensitively respond to difference, but also that they acknowledge that individuals and communities also share many things in common. Chief among these is a desire to have a good life, to achieve one's goals and dreams, to feel secure, to live with others, to nurture and love, and to be treated and to treat others fairly and respectfully. Because clinicians play a major role in the design and delivery of healthcare and have close and often ongoing relationships with patients during their illness experience, they have a profound influence on a patient's experience of illness and healthcare.

Understanding the profoundly ethical nature of healthcare and recognising and respecting the values that are shared by different patients and across different cultures and faith traditions is an important starting point for the delivery of optimal healthcare and for dialogue about goals of treatment.

References

1. Hume D. A *Treatise of Human Nature*. Oxford, Oxford University Press, 1978, 1738–40.

2. Wittgenstein L. *Culture and Values*. Ed. G. von Wright, H. Nyman. Oxford, Blackwell, 1980.

3. Kerridge I., Lowe M., Stewart C. *Ethics and Law for the Health Professions*. 4th ed. Sydney, The Federation Press, 2013.

4. Beauchamp B., Childress J. *Principles of Biomedical Ethics*. 7th ed. Oxford, Oxford University Press, 2012.

5. Gillon R. Medical ethics: four principles plus attention to scope. *BMJ* 1994; **309**: 184–8.

Models and Methods in Ethics

Cara Sedney

2.1 Introduction

A variety of approaches have been developed as a way of engaging in medical ethics. While each model may help illuminate different aspects of ethical cases, each has philosophical or practical limitations that preclude its use in all clinical situations. The methods and approaches are described in what follows, with a brief description of their emphasis and limitations. Each model is illustrated through a basic neurosurgical case and is reiterated with model-specific details to illustrate its important concepts.

> *Case:* A 90-year-old woman is found collapsed and aphasic in her bathroom by her husband. She is immediately transported to a local ER, where she is found to have a left middle cerebral artery stroke. She had recently been taken off warfarin for her history of atrial fibrillation due to bleeding, and current prothrombin time is subtherapeutic but too high for the administration of tPA.

2.1.1 Principlism

Principlism refers to the delineation of fundamental principles by which ethical dilemmas must be resolved. The model as described by Beauchamp and Childress is widely recognized to be the most prominently taught and utilized principlist model of medical ethics. Beauchamp and Childress describe the basic principles to be autonomy, non-maleficence, beneficence, and justice (Figure 2.1).[1] The authors concede that 'prima facie principles do not contain sufficient content to address the nuances of moral problems'.[1] However, these principles are felt by the authors to be both universal and objective, and they are accompanied by a number of further clarifications, including rules, norms, virtues, and so forth, that have been evolving since the initial edition of *Principles of Biomedical Ethics*.[2] The strengths of this method lie in its 'justificatory force', relating specific cases back to universal principles through deliberative methods,[2] while its limitation lies in the difficult nature of resolving ethical dilemmas in which the four principles may be at odds with one another. The four principles have in turn played a formative role in the development of other models and methods in biomedical ethics.

> *Case:* The patient has a known DNR ('do not resuscitate' in the event of a cardiac arrest) order expressing her autonomy. However, this may preclude intubation and stroke intervention, so beneficence may suggest temporarily suspending the order to allow for an interventional procedure.

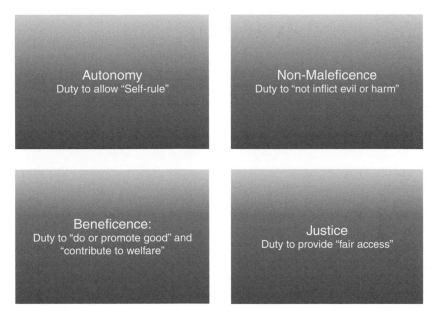

Figure 2.1 Four principles of Beauchamp and Childress (adapted from *Principles of Biomedical Ethics*, 6th ed.)

2.1.2 Utilitarianism

Utilitarianism is a more society-centred approach to medical ethics. Rather than deontological ideals, the outcome dictates the best course of action. This has led to the term 'consequentialist' being used to describe utilitarian ethics. Because the overall good is more broadly construed than for that of an individual patient, at times the best course of action for society may not be the best course of action for the patient. Utilitarianism may be particularly pertinent in societies where the medical cost of care is recognized as a societal burden and finite resource. A complex interplay of cultural norms and health systems models may have an impact on utilitarian concerns.

> *Case*: *A severe storm precludes helicopter transport to the nearest stroke centre, so the patient will need to be transported via ambulance, which will likely take at least two hours. Given the increased time to treatment and the patient's age, the treatment may not be effective and transfer may not be a worthwhile or good use of medical resources.*

2.1.3 Narrative Ethics

Narrative ethics is an approach informed by literary methods and qualitative data regarding the first-person experience of a patient at the centre of an ethical dilemma. The importance of the narrative lies in both the information contained within it as focusing on the 'relational and communicative dimensions of moral situations'[2] – similar to casuistry – and also in its structural elements, such as the narrator, plot, and inclusion/exclusion of narrative details.[2] The strength of the narrative method of ethics is its focus on the patient's life story and the 'social embeddedness' of a moral choice within that historical context.[3] More broadly construed, the narrative method of ethics can incorporate the story not just of the patient but of all those involved in a case or ethical dilemma. The narrative method may be of particular utility in end-of-life decisions. The main criticism of this method lies in its relativism and the difficulty of reaching a resolution when a patient's life story may be inconsistent or fragmented.[2]

> *Case:* The patient's granddaughter calls for an update. When told that her grandmother is currently aphasic, the granddaughter tells stories emphasizing the importance of speech and conversation to her grandmother. She notes that her grandmother was a freelance reporter in her youth when women rarely worked outside the home, wrote eloquent letters to her grandchildren, texted on her smartphone, and enjoyed having family come to 'chew the fat' – an Appalachian colloquialism for chatting. She also relates her grandmother's consistent fear of having a stroke and becoming dependent.

2.1.4 Feminist Ethics

Rosemarie Tong notes that 'all feminist approaches to ethics are filtered through the lens of gender'.[4] This comment can describe a variety of conceptualizations of gender in ethics, including an 'ethics of care', which can be considered a 'feminine' trait, as well as the role of gender within interpersonal relationships and healthcare institutions as part of an ethical dilemma. This model of 'doing' ethics is readily accepted by its proponents not as an independent theory of ethics so much as a 'series of corrective lenses that are meant to improve moral vision'.[5]

> *Case:* The care team is aware of the differential outcomes of female patients after stroke, including worse recovery, higher rate of dependency, and higher rate of depression.[6] Furthermore, since this patient currently serves as the caretaker of her husband, who has mild, early dementia, she may have less social support during recovery.

2.1.5 Communitarian

A communitarian approach to medical ethics recognizes, to varying degrees, the importance of the values and goals of the community in medical decision-making and ethical dilemmas. This can be at odds with individual autonomy in decision-making, which is the main criticism of this approach. However, communitarianism is differentiated from utilitarianism in that individual goals and values are seen as a reflection of communal goals and values, and not necessarily as being at odds with them. Etzioni differentiates between more authoritarian versions of communitarianism (such as that espoused by Cuba in the incarceration of those who contract HIV as a form of disease control) and responsive communitarianism, which recognizes the importance of autonomy but attempts to balance this with the good of the community.[7] Tolerance of a communitarian approach to medical ethics varies based upon the pre-existing values of a particular society and upon the specific medical issues under debate. For instance, Etzioni notes that 'common good' arguments are more acceptable in American society for fatal, highly communicable diseases than with regard to healthcare rationing for chronic diseases.[7]

Case: Given the severity of the storm, the patient's family expresses concern over the delay in ambulance transport to the stroke centre, as they have been waiting in the hospital for an ambulance for nearly three hours. The charge nurse apologizes profusely, noting that an ambulance had been available but was needed to emergently transport a critically ill neonate. The family understands and supports the decision to transport the sick child as a priority.

2.1.6 Casuistry

Casuistry emphasizes the importance of particulars of an ethical dilemma, rather than the use of universal principles to resolve it. After the details of a case are thoroughly reviewed, that case is then compared against other 'paradigm' cases which may point to morally correct action. Casuistry reflects the moral thought of early Catholicism and has been championed by Jonsen as mirroring 'ordinary moral judgment'.[8] However, upon closer study, the reliance on casuistic reasoning in real-world general medical practice has been found to be less prominent than originally asserted by its proponents.[8] However, framing an ethical dilemma in terms of other similar historical cases may be particularly useful for predicting difficulties and understanding legal precedents.

Case: The treating neurologist can reflect on multiple cases in the past of acute strokes in the elderly, in which maximal intervention has been undertaken but proven ultimately ineffective.

2.1.7 Ethics of Virtue

Ethics of virtue reframes the ethical question to be 'What would a virtuous person do?' in particular clinical situations. This refers to virtues with respect to both the physician and the patient.[9] Reframing towards a paradigmatic virtuous clinician is useful in medicine, and perhaps particularly in surgery, given the importance of venerated historical figures within the surgical discipline, as well as the importance of role modelling within surgical training. Osler, Cushing, Dandy, and Penfield, among others, are seen as having various qualities of the 'ideal neurosurgeon'. This may comprise a variety of qualities, of which Gardiner includes compassion, discernment, justice, and trustworthiness.[9] Paul Gardiner describes virtue ethics as 'a framework that focuses on the character of the moral agent rather than the rightness of an action. In considering the relationships, emotional sensitivities, and motivations that are unique to human society it provides a fuller ethical analysis and encourages more flexible and creative solutions than principlism'.[9] Pastura further characterizes virtue ethics as a 'return to professionalism'.[10] Criticisms of this ethical model include its subjectivity, the potential for cultural relativism, and the difficulty in resolving ethical conflicts wherein several or none of the options can be seen as virtuous.[10] Nevertheless, ethics of virtue may have real utility in day-to-day ethical dilemmas for the neurosurgeon.

> *Case: The neurologist on call demonstrates discernment in determining the best course of action for the patient and her family given the weather constraints, all while demonstrating compassion regarding the impact this event will have on the patient and her family.*

2.1.8   Religion and Theology

Both religion and theology have historically had a heavy impact on ethical thought. However, while this can be useful in situations where all parties within an ethical decision share the same religion and values, the limitations of this method of medical ethics are readily apparent when such qualities are not shared among all parties.

> *Case*: *The hospital chaplain visits the patient, asking if she would like to pray together. The patient, although still aphasic, refuses, stating, 'I have my own guru'.*

2.2   Consultation Methods

All of the previously mentioned models of ethics may have clinical utility in real-world cases. As the field of ethics has grown in recent years, a number of best practices have been identified beyond those of pure theoretical models. Such methods are distinct philosophical ethical frameworks and exist in order to assist with real cases in an ethics consultation setting. The American Society of Bioethics and Humanities (ASBH) has worked on a national level within the United States to advocate for standards and best practices in ethics consultation. Such best practices include self-education and external assessment of consult quality, a comprehensive evaluation of all sides and parties within an ethical conflict, and a systematic approach to performing consults.[11]

A variety of methods to ethics consultation have been proposed. Such methods include the 'Four Topics' method (Figure 2.2) and, later, the 'CASES' method (Figure 2.3). Jonsen and colleagues first described the Four Topics method, and it has since been adapted to a variety of clinical settings, including long-term care and psychiatric care.[12] Qualitative analysis of this method by Toh and colleagues revealed it to be useful for a wide variety of clinical ethics questions but also showed that it still relies heavily on clinician judgement regarding ethical issues.[13] This method seeks to identify relevant information that should be taken into account for an ethics consultation.

The CASES method is a systematic process of dealing with ethics consultations advocated by the integrated ethics approach.[14] It is based upon the Four Topics method of Jonsen, but suggests a full ethics consultation process, starting with the intentional construction of an ethical question.[14] This pragmatic method starts first with the question 'Is this an ethics consultation?' and differentiates a clinical ethics question regarding the active care of a patient from some other reasons for which ethics consultants might be erroneously involved, such as legal questions, socio-cultural conflicts, patient care complaints, or the need for spiritual support.[14] Only true clinical ethical questions need to be considered in the full CASES method.

As ethical consultations become more streamlined and standardized, and qualifications of consultants become more stringent, a knowledge of ethical models and methods may be useful for neurosurgeons as they play a variety of roles within ethical dilemmas.

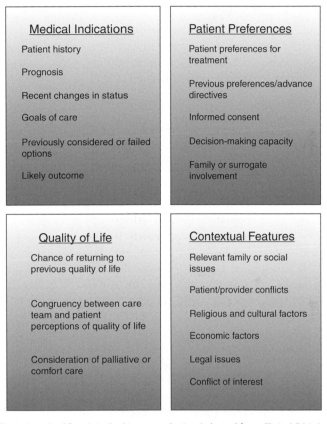

Figure 2.2 'Four Topics' method for clinical ethics consultation (adapted from *Clinical Ethics*)

Case Outcome

  The patient is evaluated by a remote stroke neurologist, who recognizes that the patient is the grandmother of his colleague, a neurosurgeon. The neurologist obtains permission to discuss the case with the patient's granddaughter, and they then discuss the options of no transport and supportive care only (where she would be closer to family), versus ground transport to the nearest stroke centre, given weather-related transportation issues (resulting in increasing transport time, which likely would decrease the efficacy of the intervention and outcome). The neurologist relates medical facts, including that she is currently aphasic and that hypodensity is noted already in the middle cerebral artery distribution of the dominant hemisphere. The granddaughter notes the importance of speech and communication to her grandmother and that she would likely rather pass away than be left aphasic and dependent, but she knows that given age-related brain atrophy in a 90-year-old, an MCA infarction is less likely to be directly fatal due to mass effect. The family and medical team jointly decide that attempting transport for stroke intervention would be most consistent with the patient's preferences and would allow the family to know they had tried whatever possible to avoid an outcome that was specifically known to be unacceptable to the patient. Clot retrieval is successful, but she still suffers an ischemic stroke complicated by haemorrhagic conversion. She makes progress with rehabilitation with respect to hemiparesis and aphasia (Figure 2.4).

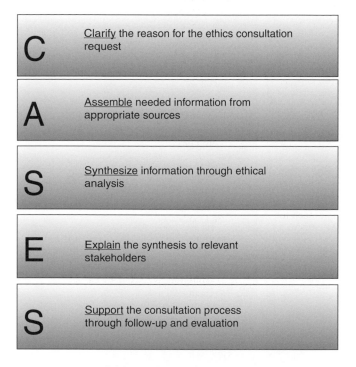

C — Clarify the reason for the ethics consultation request

A — Assemble needed information from appropriate sources

S — Synthesize information through ethical analysis

E — Explain the synthesis to relevant stakeholders

S — Support the consultation process through follow-up and evaluation

Figure 2.3 'CASES' method for clinical ethics consultation (adapted from *Ethics Consultation*, 2nd ed.)

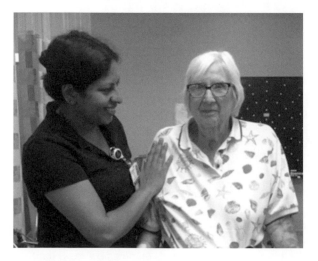

Figure 2.4 Vignette patient participating in post-stroke rehabilitation (used with permission)

References

1. Beauchamp T. L., Childress J. F. *Principles of Biomedical Ethics*. 6th ed. New York, Oxford University Press, 2009.

2. McCarthy J. Principlism or narrative ethics: must we choose between them? *Med. Humanit.* 2003; **29**(2): 65–71.

3. MacIntyre A. *After Virtue: A Study in Moral Theory*. Notre Dame, IN, University of Notre Dame Press, 1981.

4. Tong R. *Feminist Approaches to Bioethics: Theoretical Reflections and Practical Applications*. Boulder, CO, Westview Press, 1997.

5. Tong R. Feminist approaches to bioethics. *Medical Ethics Newsletter* 1999; Winter: 1–8.

6. Persky R. W., Turtzo L. C., McCullough L. D. Stroke in women: disparities and outcomes. *Curr. Cardiol. Rep.* 2010; **12**(1): 6–13.

7. Etzioni A. On a communitarian approach to bioethics. *Theor. Med. Bioeth.* 2011; **32**(5): 363–74.

8. Braunack-Mayer A. Casuistry as a bioethical method: an empirical perspective. *Soc. Sci. Med.* 2001; **53**: 71–81.

9. Gardiner P. A virtue ethics approach to moral dilemmas in medicine. *J. Med. Ethics* 2003; **29**(5): 297–302.

10. Pastura P. S., Land M. G. The perspective of virtue ethics regarding the process of medical decision-making. *Rev. Bioet. (Impr.)* 2016; **24**(2): 243–9.

11. Carrese J. A. and members of the American Society for Bioethics and Humanities Clinical Ethics Consultation Affairs Standing Committee. HCEC pearls and pitfalls: suggested do's and don't's for healthcare ethics consultants. *J. Clin. Ethics* 2012; **23**(3): 234–40.

12. Jonsen A. R., Siegler M., Winslade W. J. *Clinical Ethics: A Practical Approach to Ethical Decisions in Clinical Medicine*. New York, Macmillan, 1982.

13. Toh H. J., Low J. A., Lim Z. U., et al. Jonsen's four topics approach as a framework for clinical ethics consultation. *Asian Bioethics Review* 2018; **10**(1): 37–51.

14. National Center for Ethics in Health Care. *Ethics Consultation: Responding to Ethics Questions in Health Care*. 2nd ed. Washington, DC, US Department of Veterans Affairs, 2015.

Chapter

3

The Concept and Implementation of Values-Based Medicine (VsBM) in Neurosurgery

Ahmed Ammar, Tiit Mathiesen, and Stephen Honeybul

3.1 Introduction

Throughout the history of medicine, the existential backdrop of life and death has formed the basis of clinical practice, and prolongation of life has been the primary aim of care. Life was considered to have 'intrinsic value' (i.e., value *in itself*), not only 'instrumental value' (i.e., as a conditional state in which to experience other values). In recent years, considerable advances in biomedical sciences, combined with numerous technological developments, have changed the fundament of medical values. Technological developments such as the modern-day ventilator have revolutionized the means by which life may be prolonged; however, this will not necessarily provide value, as it may not improve the quality of that life. In addition, the cost of modern-day technology continues to increase, and it is not always possible to allocate resources equitably, which raises the concept of distributive justice.[1] Finally, consideration must be given to the use of technology for prolongation of life in a way that sustains bodily functions in a person who has irreversibly lost the ability to experience and interact with the outer world, because the utility of the prolongation of life in such conditions is doubtful.

In these situations, the scrutiny of values that may be provisional goals is necessary, and it is in this regard that the concept of 'values-based medicine' (VsBM) may be useful.[2] This concept aims to identify a set of intrinsic or instrumental values that are important to a particular individual and to use these values to guide clinical care.

3.2 The Concept of VsBM

VsBM can be defined as 'medical practice that aims at maximizing value, specifically desirable or positive value in every step of a patient's medical management'. This is a wide definition, and it is difficult to disagree with such a benevolent practice. However, disagreements may arise when attempts are made to clarify the concept of value.

Traditionally, medical ethics has focused on values such as benefit, non-maleficence, autonomy, quality of life, dignity, and honesty. Childress and Beauchamp tried to minimize the set of values and base ethical deliberation on the four principles of autonomy, beneficence, non-maleficence, and justice.[3] However, these principles can sometimes be overly abstract and difficult to use in everyday clinical practice. Their application is also not clear when principles come into conflict, such as when a patient's autonomy to receive a particularly expensive therapy may be at odds with the concept of distributive justice, which requires that resources are allocated fairly and equitably in order to maintain a sustainable healthcare system. In these circumstances, there is no theoretical means to choose between the different values. Therefore, the acknowledgment of additional values can be helpful in guiding practice, while a reduction of values is necessary for choosing between conflicting values. In addition, personal values provide another set of preferences that may or may not be compatible with general values.

In response to these limitations, a wider, more expansive model of modern-day bioethics has been proposed that acknowledges an individual's preferences and values. Respect for these values is reflected in the need to consider (a) autonomy, (b) beneficence, (c) non-maleficence, (d) justice, (e) dignity, and (f) truthfulness and honesty (Figure 3.1; Table 3.1).[2]

Table 3.1 The modern-day pillars of bioethics

Values	Description
Autonomy	This can be defined as the right of a patient to make their own decisions without external influence or coercion. This includes the right to refuse management of their medical condition or to discontinue a therapy that has already been commenced. Surgeons must recognize and respect a patient's autonomy and aim to work with the patient as a partner in shared decision-making in order to achieve the desired outcome based on a patient's individual values.
Beneficence	This involves doing what is considered to be good for a patient. This is especially important in the case of neurosurgery, where there is often a need to balance the possible benefits of a procedure against the possible risks.
Non-maleficence	Closely related to beneficence is the need to consider the risk of harm and either avoid a specific procedure or at least minimize the risk of a proposed treatment. Risks of a procedure are especially relevant to neurosurgery, and these must be clearly explained to enable a patient to exercise autonomy and make a truly informed decision regarding consent.
Justice	In the context of medicine, justice can be described as the moral obligation to act on the basis of fair and equitable distribution of healthcare resources within a particular society. This requires that resources are distributed equally and fairly to those in need and includes the distribution of a doctor's time and attention.
Dignity	This implies respect for human beings and requires that patients should be treated as an end, not as a means to realize other goals. Dignity flows in both directions. While the patient is usually a weaker part in a therapeutic situation, they do have a duty to treat the medical team with respect and dignity.
Truthfulness and honesty	The relationship between a patient and the treating surgeon should be based on unconditional honesty. All patient questions should be answered truthfully, and mistakes must be openly disclosed. When a mistake occurs, a surgeon must give a full, truthful account of the incident, not apportion blame to others, apologize, and take personal accountability. Where necessary, steps may be taken to avoid similar incidents in the future.

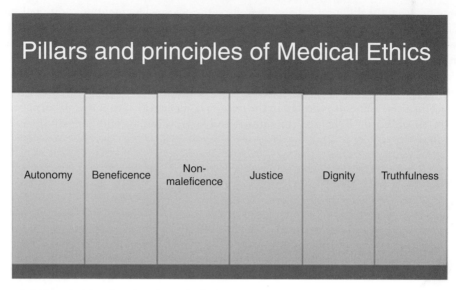

Figure 3.1 The principles of modern-day medical ethics

3.2.1 Ethical Truth and Relativism

The aforementioned values can provide a useful framework through which to consider ethical issues; however, the importance placed on each individual value may vary between societies based on culture, faith, education, and socioeconomic factors. Thus actions that are considered ethically desirable may differ between societies. For this reason, some philosophers have created relativistic ethical theories that either deny that ethical proposals can be made (a moral statement is just an emotional claim of approval or disproval) or propose that ethical truth only reflects what is accepted by an individual or a culture.[4]

This 'ethical relativism' may appear attractive from an anthropological perspective, because it reflects the observation that whether an action is right or wrong depends on the moral norms of the society in which it is practiced. The same action may be morally right in one society but morally wrong in another. However, adopting this position is problematic because not only is it at variance with empirical observations but also it would make meaningful discourse in ethics almost impossible. This relativistic view is also incompatible with the logical axiom 'tertium non datur', a rule attributed to Aristotle whereby a proposition is either right or wrong – but not both right and wrong.

For example, it may be difficult to find the right answer, but it cannot be both right and wrong to take a human life for pleasure. Based on this position, it would be reasonable to determine that all systems of medical ethics would agree that it is wrong to kill a patient for pleasure. Such agreement provides support for a belief that absolute truth may exist in ethics.

There are also other norms that probably reflect universal truth and that are a prerequisite for moral human societies. Two good examples would be not keeping slaves and not torturing people. Hence, cultural differences should not necessarily be taken to indicate ethical differences, and different practices can usually be analyzed in a way where agreement is reached, whether they are derived from basic ethical principles or not; in the latter case, they should probably be abolished. For example, in medicine, there is wide agreement regarding capital punishment and genital mutilation. Ethically correct practices may show variance between societies and cultures; however, such variation should not be confused with ethical relativism because to do so would make discussion and implementation of medical ethics extremely difficult, if not impossible.

Neurosurgeons are obliged to establish ethical and professional relationships with their patients and, to that end, should listen to and be guided by both the patient's medical complaint and their perception of the possible outcomes. It is the duty of neurosurgeons to explain to their patients all stages of investigation, management, surgical procedures, and possible outcomes. Ethical and professional practice thus entails communication, which requires a close professional interaction with a patient and, where relevant, their families. Understanding a patient's culture and beliefs is also important, so that the surgeon can fully comprehend a patient's values and the context in which these values are held. This knowledge and exchange of information will gain a patient's respect, trust, and compliance for the treatment, subsequent follow-up, and in certain circumstances, management of complications. Ethically informed consent requires that the surgeon identifies a patient's individual values in order for those values to be acknowledged, respected, and acted upon.[6]

3.2.2 Conflicting Values

Problems can arise when values conflict. For example, a patient may refuse a procedure that a surgeon feels may prove beneficial. In these circumstances, it is necessary to consider the individual's preconceived ideas and values in order to understand the reasoning behind the decision.

Where there remains clear conflict, coercion, or undue influence to pursue a course of treatment should not be considered ethically justifiable, even if it applies the principle of beneficence at the expense of autonomy, unless of course a profound analysis would support this action as ethically superior. Indeed, applying beneficence at the expense of autonomy may lead to a loss of trust and may cause psychological damage, which in certain cases may be irreparable.

In these situations, an analysis of the values at stake is required. An intrinsic value, a value in itself, is more important to respect than an instrumental value, which is by definition a means to achieve intrinsic value. Some values are probably absolute and universal, while others can be culturally defined or even individual. While all individuals have a personal set of values, it is useful to consider universal values as more 'absolute' and personal values as more 'relative'. Maximization and respect of individual values is possible, as long as they are internally consistent and agree with universal values. When individual values come in conflict with universal values, it is necessary to choose values that are more fundamental, such as absolute values.

For example, adopting this position would support an ethical argument that it is ethically wrong for a psychopath to commit crimes for their own pleasure because committing violent crimes for pleasure is ethically absolutely wrong, even though the psychopath may justify their actions based on their own individual (but no less justifiable) values.

Another example can be seen when considering benefit versus autonomy. 'Good' can be considered an intrinsic value, while autonomy is considered an instrumental value because it usually facilitates the realization of 'good'. This is in part because the autonomous agent usually best understands their own good. If, however, it is possible to objectively realize 'good' by overruling autonomy, then autonomy should be overruled. A typical example is forced care of suicidal patients, where there is a broad agreement that respect for autonomy should not overrule the potential benefit of preserving the patient's life. Reductionism of values to find one more fundamental can be very useful, but it is necessary to consider the possibility that values may exist in parallel without having a common denominator that allows reduction. A useful example of this comes from the myth of Midas, which describes ill-fated reductionism as King Midas reduced all values to gold and found out only too late (when he turned his own daughter into gold) that the possible value of gold is instrumental – not intrinsic.

Where maximum value is concerned, it is possible to consider the total sum of value or use a cost-effective analysis in order to measure value per utilized resource. By using this type of methodology, it is possible to analyze how value is divided among society, thereby ensuring equitable distribution of resources and a degree of distributive justice.[7]

3.2.3   Distribution of Resources: The Patient at the Centre of Care

Distribution of resources concerns the question of how value is equitably applied. Hippocrates described an intimate and central role for the physician-patient relationship, and in modern-day medicine, the patient-physician interaction places the patient at the centre of attention and defines the patient's best interests as a fundamental goal. In the context of an individual consultation, this focus should be self-evident. However, when considering a wider view of a healthcare system, other stakeholders emerge. These may include other professional providers, family and relatives, insurance companies, and other patients with potentially competing interests. In different medical cultures, the relative influence of these secondary stakeholders can vary, and in certain circumstances, patient-centred care can be called into question, especially when it is at odds with the principle of justice that implies care needs to be distributed equitably. Indeed, there may be circumstances where a physician's primary duty to an individual patient may be incompatible with available societal resources.

It has been argued that each patient-physician consultation must serve as a focal point at which resources are distributed fairly and that each physician must consider the risk of allocating too many resources to any one particular individual.[8] However, an alternative viewpoint would argue that societal distribution of resources (which is a necessity) should occur at a government or jurisdiction level, which must be separated from an individual consultation. This ensures that every patient can trust that the physician's duty is to provide or facilitate the best possible care with the resources that are available within that particular healthcare system.

3.3   Evidence-Based Medicine (EBM) and VsBM

Evidence-based medicine (EBM) has been defined as the conscientious, explicit, and judicious use of current best evidence when making decisions about the care of the individual patient. This requires integrating individual clinical expertise with the best available external clinical evidence from systematic research. Over the past 30 years, the use of EBM has been applied across all aspects of medical practice, and during this evolution a well-designed randomized controlled trial, published in a reputable medical journal, has been viewed as the only way to advance clinical practice. Indeed, within the field of neurosurgery, there are notable examples: the International Subarachnoid Trial (ISAT) investigated the role of coiling versus clipping of intracranial aneurysms, the Clifton studies investigated the role of hypothermia in traumatic brain injury (TBI), and the Medical Research Council CRASH (Corticosteroid Randomization after Significant Head Injury) study investigated the role of steroids also in the field of TBI. There is no doubt that the results of these trials have had a significant impact on neurosurgical practice worldwide; however, it is becoming increasingly apparent that there may be some limitations when attempting to apply this approach across all aspects of clinical practice.[9] In addition, it is increasingly recognized that considerable clinical experience is required not only to critically evaluate the quality of the evidence but also to assess the validity of the conclusions that are often presented by investigators. Finally, there are certain limitations when applying information obtained from large data sets to individual patients, because adopting this approach may fail to recognize and acknowledge the diversity of individual values and goals.

3.3.1 EBM and Ethics

If it is accepted that the main goal of EBM is to obtain explicit clinical knowledge in order to guide individual therapeutic decisions, the overarching principle must be that each therapeutic decision should be based on the best possible evidence, and this is usually obtained from randomized controlled trials. This principle is easy to agree with and has been successfully applied across many aspects of clinical medicine. However, problems can arise when applying the evidence (Table 3.2).[10] One of the key issues is the clinician's interpretation of the evidence and the application of that evidence in a manner that recognizes the concept of VsBM. A good example can be seen in the context of decompressive hemicraniectomy for malignant middle cerebral artery infarction. A number of trials have clearly demonstrated that surgical decompression can reduce mortality; however, surgical intervention will not reverse the effects of what by definition, is a very significant ischemic stroke. Notwithstanding the published conclusions that for patients under 60 years of age 'there was an increase in the number of patients with a favourable outcome' or that for patients over 60 years of age 'hemicraniectomy increased survival without severe disability,' many survivors will be left dependent.[11] When considering surgical intervention, the clinician must first make a decision based on their interpretation of the clinical data and then apply that interpretation to the clinical decision such that the most likely outcome would be acceptable to the individual concerned, based on their values and preferences.

Table 3.2 Some of the limitations of EBM – What to do with the data (Dagi 2017)

Limitations
It is ethically important to separate the results of statistical analysis of clinical trials from:
• Statistically significant but clinically irrelevant outcomes
• Judgements about how data about the set should be applied to specific individuals within the set
• The protection of the prerogatives of individual patients in the face of population-based protocols
• The protection of the surgeon's prerogatives in personalizing the treatment of individual patients

For example, for patients older than 60 years of age, most survivors following surgery could not mobilize unaided, could not attend to bodily functions, and had such severe neurocognitive deficits that they could not answer a simple question regarding retrospective consent.[11]

In order to observe the principles of VsBM, the clinical decision to intervene must include a detailed and informed analysis of the evidence and a considered evaluation of an individual's preferences and values (whether previously voiced or documented) in order to be considered truly ethical.

It must be acknowledged that for some individuals, life is valued as sacrosanct and worth preserving at any cost. These values may be rooted in cultural, religious, or individual beliefs and, where possible, these values should be recognized and acted upon. However, for some individuals, survival with severe neurocognitive disability may deemed unacceptable, and for these individuals, caution must be exercised when considering a surgical procedure that increases the risk of an individual surviving with this outcome.

Overall, there can be little doubt that EBM will remain an important tool in the evaluation of clinical practice; however, it is increasingly recognized that the physician needs to apply medically informed specialized knowledge. Some of this will be derived from the hierarchies of EBM; however, this must be analyzed in a framework of individual expertise. This knowledge must be combined with knowledge of the patient's individual medical facts and, importantly, awareness of the patients subjective and absolute values. Only when these are combined appropriately is it possible to make a professionally accountable decision according to VsBM.

Finally, it must be acknowledged that notwithstanding the central focus of the physician-patient relationship, in reality, other stakeholders in the patient's care need to be considered. These may include hospital staff and other physicians, who ideally form a team around each patient. The patient may also have a spouse, family, and friends, whose contributions and rights should be observed. Ideally, the aim should be to create a 'patient–patient's family–doctor complex relationship'. Such a relationship supports patient comfort and well-being and secures future collaboration.

3.3.2 VsBM Professional Ethics and Professionalism

Professionalism describes an attitude and behaviour of a professional body that represents a form of social contract between the profession and the society it serves.[12] Professionals contribute knowledge and skill for the benefit of society in return for trust, power, status, and economic reward. Medical professionalism in this context encompasses all qualities obtained and expressed to conduct or perform tasks and medical duties as described by the organization or hospital to which they belong and as expected by society. Professionals need to be self-regulating, accountable, and successful in delivering expected services in order to uphold the contract. Likewise, society needs to respect their commitments to allow professionals to deliver their service. One of the most important steering mechanisms for professional self-regulation is professional ethics.

3.3.3 Professional Ethics

Professional ethics is the use of knowledge and skills to provide patient care governed by the ethical code of the workplace. This involves moving from abstract values to daily behaviour

The Concept of Values Based Medicine

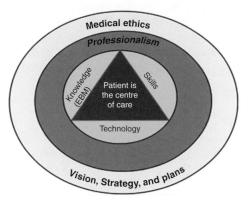

Figure 3.2 Patient's care and interest is the centre of care. This is the main concept of values-based medicine (VsBM).

in the working environment or within professional societies. Professional ethics is one of the fundamental elements of VsBM and requires medical practitioners to maintain a level of values, standards, and behaviour of their medical societies, organizations, and hospitals in which they provide service. Medical professionalism also requires practitioners to maintain and update their knowledge and skills and to maintain familiarity with ongoing medical research, in order to provide contemporary patient care and enhance their career development. The core of professional ethics can be described in many ways, but in this context, the combination of always prioritizing an individual patient within the concept of VsBM is self-evident.

3.4 Conclusion

Modern health systems continue to evolve. Treatments that were once considered extraordinary rapidly become ordinary and then routine, and these developments involve a multitude of stakeholders with a variety of interests. The principles of VsBM may be useful when managing patient expectations and applying the results of EBM in a fair and equitable fashion. While the individual is at the centre of clinical encounters, the protagonists in the social life of patients, in particular relatives and loved ones, need to be involved in medical relationships. At a personal level, formal education and training programmes can raise awareness of the increasingly complex field of bioethics ethics and the duties and accountability of surgeons – especially neurosurgeons, who are uniquely positioned to balance the benefits of rapidly progressive technology with the attendant risks in a surgically complex specialty.

References

1. Devon M. K., Bernstein M. Neurosurgical innovation. *Neurosurgical Ethics in Practice: Value Based Medicine*. Ed. Ammar A., Bernstein M. Dordrecht, Springer, 2014; ch. 15: 171–80.

2. Ammar A. Brief History of Bioethics. *Neurosurgical Ethics in Practice: Value Based Medicine*. Ed. Ammar A., Bernstein M. Dordrecht, Springer, 2014; ch. 1: 3–10.

3. Beauchamp T. L., Childress J. F. *Principles of Biomedical Ethics*, 4th ed. Oxford, Oxford University Press, 1994.

4. Bae J. M. Value-based medicine: concepts and application. *Epidemiol. Health* 2015; 37: e2015014.

5. Brown M. M., Brown G. C. Update on value-based medicine. *Curr. Opin. Ophthalmol.* 2013; **24**: 183–89.

6. Ammar A. Influence of different culture on neurosurgical practice. *Child's Nerv. Syst.* 1997; **13**: 91–94.

7. Stein J. D., Brown M. M., Brwon G. C., Irwin B., Brwon K. S. The comparative effectiveness and cost-effectiveness of vitreoretinal intervention. *Curr. Opin. Ophthalmol.* 2008; **19**: 202–7.

8. Petrova M., Dale J., Fulford B. K. Values-based practice in primary care: easing the tensions between individual values, ethical principles and best evidence. *Br. J. Gen. Pract.* 2006; **56**: 703–9.

9. Honeybul S., Ho K. The role of evidence based medicine in neurotrauma. *J. Clin. Neurosci.* 2015; **22**: 611–16.

10. Dagi T. F. Seven Ethical issues Affecting Neurosurgeons in the context of Health Care system. *Neurosurgery* 2017; **80**(4S): S83–S91.

11. Honeybul S., Ho K. M., Gillett G. R. Long-term outcome following decompressive craniectomy: an inconvenient truth? *Curr. Opin. Crit. Care.* 2018; **24**: 97–104.

12. Cruess R. L., Cruess S. R., Johnston S. E. Renewing professionalism: an opportunity for medicine. *Acad. Med.* 1999; **74**: 878–84.

The Three Functions of Consent in Neurosurgery

Cameron Stewart and Ian Kerridge

4.1 Introduction

Consent is an expression of the therapeutic relationship between health professionals and patients. While we ordinarily relate consent processes to the ethical value of autonomy, the doctrine of consent is also a function of a fundamental respect for persons. In legal discourse, consent functions to protect both autonomy and respect. It does so via two functions. Consent legally performs a *permissive function* requiring patients' permission before any intervention is made to their body. Consent also performs a *risk function*, requiring information to be provided to patients about the risks of having or not having proposed interventions, when those risks are material to the patient. This chapter will analyse both functions of the law of consent from the perspective of common law jurisdictions (such as England and Wales, Australia, Canada, New Zealand, and the United States). It starts with an analysis of the ethical functions of consent and how the values of autonomy and respect are protected by it. The chapter will then look at the legal tests for the permissive and risk functions of consent, as well as the assumptions that underpin consent processes. It will also examine the limits of consent and the particular forms of regulation that affect different types of neurosurgery, including deep brain stimulation and neurosurgery for mental illness. The chapter concludes with the argument that consent also serves a third function – the *relational function* – by providing an environment that fosters relationships of trust between the treating team, the patient, and their family. In neurosurgery, where patients are faced with death and have few, if any, choices open to them beyond surgery, and where surgery is very risky and its outcomes are difficult to predict, we argue that the permissive and risk functions of consent become less important and the relational function comes to the fore.

4.2 The Ethical Values of Consent

In modern Western societies, it is accepted that individuals should ordinarily have the right to make decisions about their own healthcare. Consent is clearly a manifestation of this ethical concern. But respect for autonomy also reflects a deeper respect for the value of personhood – the respect given to patients because they are human beings with their own values, desires, and plans for the future. Consequently, even in cases where patients are unable to make decisions for themselves, respect for patient autonomy and personhood (or human dignity) has the effect of framing the conversations concerning treatment around the topic of consent. For example, in cases of incapacitated patients, discussion shifts to 'substituted' or 'supported decision-making', but consent remains the primary concern.

The primacy of autonomy is not unproblematic. As will be discussed below, many models of patient autonomy are overly simplistic in their assumptions about how individuals want to make decisions and how they actually make them. Simple models of consent presume that patients want to make their own decisions and will do so after rationally considering their own interests. This does not take into account the fact that many patients do not see themselves as autonomous decision-makers but will make decisions in the context of complex social relationships, where the interests of others may be highly important (and may outweigh the patient's own individual concerns).

In difficult cases, such as those where there is a high risk of death in vulnerable populations, it makes more sense to speak of 'relational autonomy', a feminist account of autonomy that focuses on the degree to which autonomy is located socially. Relational autonomy accepts that patients are not atomistic individuals but live interconnected lives and thus are rarely (completely) free to make decisions about their healthcare, as their decisions are dependent on the impact of their condition on their social network of family and friends. Decisions are made in those contexts and according to those values.[1]

4.3 The Underlying Assumptions of Consent

The doctrine of consent in both law and ethics is reliant on a number of assumptions, as explored in the following sections.

4.3.1 Capacity

Consent can only be given by patients with mental capacity – namely, the ability to understand the nature and effects of the treatment being offered to them. If a patient cannot do that, then some form of supported or substitute decision-making process must be employed. Capacity requires an ability to:

(a) understand the information relevant to the decision,

(b) retain that information,

(c) use or weigh that information as part of the process of making the decision, and

(d) communicate the decision. (*Brightwater* v. *Rossiter* (2009) 40 WAR 84)

In common law jurisdictions, adults are presumed to have capacity and concerns about a lack of capacity must be tested. Children are generally presumed to lack capacity but may be able to demonstrate that they fully understand the nature and effects of the treatment being offered. In the United Kingdom, Australia, and New Zealand, this is referred to as 'Gillick competence'(*Gillick* v. *West Norfolk and Wisbech Area Health Authority* [1986] AC 112; *Secretary, Department of Health and Community Services* v. *JWB* (1992) 175 CLR 218; *Moore* v. *Moore* [2015] 2 NZLR 787). In the United States and Canada, this is referred to as the 'mature minor doctrine' (*Smith* v. *Seibly* 431 P 2d 719 (1967); *AC* v. *Manitoba (Director of Child and Family Services)* [2009] 2 SCR 181).

Competent adults have the right to make decisions about their healthcare and even refuse life-sustaining treatments. In most jurisdictions in the United States and Canada, mature minors may also refuse treatment, but in the United Kingdom and Australia, capable children may be forcibly treated when the treatment is in their best interests (*X* v. *The Sydney Children's Hospitals Network* [2013] NSWCA 320).

4.3.2 Substitute Decision-Making

If a patient is unable to make a decision due to incapacity, some form of substitute decision-making needs to be utilised. Different jurisdictions provide different ways for others to act on behalf of patients who are incapable of making decisions, and it is beyond the scope of this chapter to go into detail about these differences. Nevertheless, there are three general classes of decision-makers that are regularly employed: those appointed by tribunals or courts (e.g., guardians, conservators), those who were chosen by the patient prior to incapacity (e.g., health attorneys, enduring guardians), and default decision-makers who are automatically appointed in situations of incapacity (e.g., persons responsible, statutory health attorneys).

Substitute decision-makers often have limits placed on the types of treatment for which they can provide consent. For example, many jurisdictions exclude 'special treatments' from the types of medical treatments for which a substitute may offer consent. These categories include treatments such as sterilisations, abortions, or the long-term use of addictive medicines. In the neurosurgical context, the most relevant categories would be neurosurgery for the treatment of mental illness, which is discussed below.

4.3.3 Voluntariness

Consent must not be unduly influenced by the pressure of others, especially in cases where the patient's ability to decide may be compromised by factors (such as pain and fatigue) and the third-party persuader has a measure of control over the patient. In *Re T (Adult: Refusal of Treatment)* [1993] Fam 95, the patient had refused blood products prior to becoming incapacitated. The patient was not a Jehovah's Witness, but her mother was a member of that denomination. The Court of Appeal found that in this case, evidence supported a finding that the patient was unduly influenced by her mother when she made the decision to refuse treatment, based on the fact that (a) the patient had not previously discussed blood products, (b) the patient was in a great deal of distress at the time she refused treatment, and (c) the patient's mother had a very close relationship with her and was exercising persuasion over the patient at the time of her refusal.

4.3.4 Specificity

Consent should be given for a specific intervention, and consent for one procedure does not cover other procedures. For example, in *Ljubic* v. *Armellin* [2009] ACTSC 21, a patient's consent to the removal of her uterus did not entitle the doctor to also remove her ovaries.

4.3.5 Identity

Consent that is given to one practitioner to perform an intervention may not extend consent to another practitioner to perform the same intervention, unless this has been explained to the patient in the consent process (*Tinnock* v. *Murrumbidgee Local Health District (No 6)* [2017] NSWSC 1003). Consent will also be invalidated if an unqualified person pretends to have qualifications to perform procedures (*R* v. *Maurantonio* (1967) 65 DLR (2d) 674). However, consent may be effective if a deregistered but otherwise qualified person provides treatment (*R* v. *Richardson* [1999] QB 444).

4.3.6 Public Interest

The common law has also placed limits on what can be consented to. In the criminal law of the United Kingdom, Australia, and New Zealand, it is often said that consent is only permitted as a defence to cases of actual bodily harm or grievous bodily harm, when the behaviour being consented to is supported by a recognised public interest. Traditionally, common law has allowed consent to be raised as a defence for harm in contact sports, in ritual body modification (e.g., male circumcision and tattooing), and in the case of rough sexual behaviours, on the basis that these practices are supported by a public interest. However, the common law tends to retreat from consent when the behaviour has a high risk of death or serious injury. For example, consent cannot be raised as a defence for the serious injury or manslaughter of a person caused by choking during sexual intercourse (*R* v. *Emmett* [1999] EWCA Crim 1710; *R* v. *Stein* [2007] VSCA 300). In *R* v. *Brown* [1994] 1 AC 212, a group of consenting sadomasochistic homosexuals were convicted of assault and were unable to plead a defence of consent. It was said that there was no public interest in their behaviour (which was at the extreme end of the spectrum). Lord Mustill stated in this judgment that surgery ('proper medical treatment') was in a special category of its own (at 266F). He did not elaborate further on the nature of 'proper medical treatment'. The concept is nebulous but appears to be based on an underlying concern with a therapeutic outcome.

Performance of surgery in the absence of therapeutic benefit becomes highly problematic under Lord Mustill's dicta. For example, in some forms of cosmetic surgery (where there may be no therapeutic justification at all) or in experimental surgery (where there is no evidence of benefit and the risks of death or serious injury from the surgery are high), it is hard to see how the surgery could be characterised as 'proper medical treatment'. This is not to say that a consent defence could not be supported by public interest in such cases, but it is to say that such a public interest must be of a different kind than that which justifies surgery that is proven to be beneficial and is generally regarded as competent professional practice.

4.4 The Permissive Function of Consent

The common law requires that a person give their permission to be touched, and the 'slightest touching' of another person's body without consent is considered to be a wrongdoing (in tort law, a 'battery' and, in criminal law, an 'assault'; *Collins* v. *Wilcock* [1984] 1 WLR 1172). In both criminal law and tort law, a person can give their permission to be touched only if they understand the broad nature and effects of the touching. For example, in *Reeves* v. *R* (2013) 304 ALR 251, a doctor was convicted of maliciously inflicting grievous bodily harm on a woman after he removed her labia and clitoris during an operation to remove a lesion on her left vulva. The excision of her labia and clitoris was only mentioned to the patient as she was falling unconscious from the anaesthetic in the operating room, and she was never informed of why it was necessary. The court found that the decision was not consensual, as the operation performed was of a vastly different nature than the one she was told would happen.

Fraudulent behaviour on the part of the health professional will usually vitiate or nullify consent because it undercuts the person's understanding of the nature and effects of the intervention (*Papadimitropoulos* v. *The Queen* (1957) 98 CLR 249; *Chatterton* v. *Gerson* [1981] QB 432). This may be proven by an objective assessment of whether the treatment served a therapeutic purpose or was provided solely for some ulterior purpose (such as financial gain; *White* v. *Johnston* [2015] NSWCA 18). For example, in *Dean* v. *Phung* [2012] NSWCA 223, a dentist was found to have battered a patient by providing unnecessary and ineffective treatments totalling more than A\$70,000.

4.5 The Risk Function of Consent

The common law places a duty on a surgeon to provide the patient with information about the material risks of treatment. The test for materiality varies according to the jurisdiction, but in the United Kingdom, Canada, New Zealand, Australia, and some parts of the United States, the materiality of risk is determined by both objective factors (e.g., the known risks that the profession would usually communicate to a patient about a procedure) and subjective factors (e.g., factors that the individual patient may wish to know as being relevant to their concerns). This is often referred to as a 'patient-centred' approach to providing information.

In the Australian case of *Rogers* v. *Whitaker* (1992) 175 CLR 479, a woman with sight in one eye was seeking advice on a cosmetic procedure to correct the appearance of her blind eye. She was very concerned that the sight in her 'good' eye not be exposed to any risk from the procedure. The doctor did not warn the patient of a 1 in 14,000 chance of blindness from sympathetic ophthalmia. The procedure was performed competently, but the risk of sympathetic ophthalmia eventuated and she became blind. While the doctor argued that the (small) risk of blindness would never be communicated to patients by doctors, the High Court found that a patient should be made aware of 'material risks' where:

> a risk is material if, in the circumstances of the particular case, a reasonable person in the patient's position, if warned of the risk, would be likely to attach significance to it or if the medical practitioner is or should reasonably be aware that the particular patient, if warned of the risk, would be likely to attach significance to it. (at [16])

In other jurisdictions (namely, parts of the United States), the only risks that need to be communicated are those that the profession believes should be expressed to the patient. This is referred to as a 'doctor-centred' or 'physician-centred' approach. An example of this standard in action is the case of *Natanson* v. *Kline* 350 P2d 1093 (1960), where the doctor failed to warn the patient of the risk of severe burns from radiation therapy. The patient argued that she had not been properly informed of the risks of treatment. The Supreme Court of Kansas stated that 'the duty of a physician to disclose however, is limited to those disclosures which a reasonable practitioner would make under the same or similar circumstances. How the physician may best discharge his obligation to the patient in this difficult question involves primarily a question of medical judgement' (at 1106).

Both standards are commonly referred to as 'informed consent', but this term is misleading for two main reasons. First, the duty to provide information is based on the materiality of the risk to the patient. Some patients – for example, those who face a high risk of death or serious injury from their conditions – may regard the risks of treatment as irrelevant (because they will die without it). These patients may decide to consent to the treatment without wishing to know or understand the risks because they are faced with the stark choice of either consenting to the treatment or dying. Such a decision is a perfectly valid consent in law, even though it might be described as deliberately uninformed. Second, in those jurisdictions that employ a doctor-centred standard for materiality, the patient is only informed of those risks that the medical professional believes should be communicated. This limits the level of information about risks and may exclude risks that the patient wishes to know, and as such, this can hardly be described as fully informed consent.

4.6 Special Factors Regarding the Consent Process in Neurosurgery

4.6.1 Risks to Personality and Identity Change

It has been argued by some that neurosurgery (and other interventions) presents unique challenges for consent because of the way that these interventions may cause personality and identity changes. The notion of an autonomous consent, according to these arguments, is challenged in cases of identity change as one person (the pre-intervention self) is making decisions for another person (the post-intervention self). Witt has argued the consent process should be adapted so that the patient considers their post-operative life from both their pre-intervention and post-intervention perspectives, where both perspectives on quality of life are weighted equally.[2] Of course, there are severely limiting practical issues with getting patients to attempt this. How can patients weigh and consider factors from a perspective that they do not yet have? This practical barrier seems to be very difficult to overcome. Moreover, it could be argued that all major treatments will affect some form of personality change in patients. The changes wrought by neurosurgical intervention to a patient's personality are arguably only different by degree.

4.6.2 Neurosurgery for Mental Illness

Neurosurgery for mental illness ('psychosurgery' or 'psychiatric surgery') has had a difficult history. It is discussed in greater detail in Chapter 18. In the early history of lobotomy/leucotomy, it was thought that the creation of lesions in the brain would improve a number of conditions, but as the evidence mounted, it became clear that such interventions were highly ineffective and often caused severe adverse outcomes for patients and their families. Moreover, there was clear evidence that neurosurgery had been used inappropriately on vulnerable populations of the mentally ill without proper safeguards or accountability mechanisms.[3]

In recent decades, most Western democracies have either outlawed or severely restricted the use of neurosurgery for the treatment of mental illness. For example, in the state of New South Wales, Australia, psychosurgery has been banned (*Mental Health Act 2007* (NSW), s 83). In England and Wales, neurosurgery for mental illness can only proceed with the patient's consent and with the approval of second doctor and two representatives of either the Care Quality Commission in England or the Healthcare Inspectorate of Wales (*Mental Health Act 2007* (Eng & Wales), s 57). In other jurisdictions, non-consensual neurosurgery for mental illness is allowed with court approval. For example, in the Australian Capital Territory, the Supreme Court may approve of neurosurgery if the patient has a mental illness, lacks capacity, and has not Previously refused surgery, as long as the court finds that the surgery is likely to result in substantial benefit to the patient and all alternative treatments are unlikely to be of benefit (*Mental Health Act 2015* (ACT), s 168).

4.6.3 Innovation, Vulnerability, and the Therapeutic Misconception

Neurosurgery is a discipline in a rapid state of development. Advances in surgical techniques and in emerging diagnostics and therapeutics, such functional brain mapping, deep brain stimulation (DBS), and vagal nerve stimulation, are constantly evolving. Innovations in neurosurgery usually occur in piecemeal ways without undergoing the sorts of processes that one would see in a clinical trial and, consequently, without the consequential oversight mechanisms (for example, human ethics review).[4]

The cost of such high levels of innovation is that patients are commonly exposed to 'experimental' interventions where little is known of the benefits and risks. Additionally, the patients being subject to untested therapies are often those who have run out of standard treatment options, or they may be patients for whom there are no treatment options at all.[5] Such patients may be desperate and vulnerable to the risk of 'therapeutic misconception', where patients believe an intervention will benefit them, even when they have been told about its uncertain and experimental nature.[6] In such cases, ordinary approaches to consent may be inadequate to ensure that the process of deciding whether to treat or not is ethical, and consent needs to be coupled with other mechanisms, such as structured peer review, independent risk assessment, and clinical ethics review.[4]

To illustrate these issues, we will examine DBS. DBS is a neurosurgical intervention that involves the implantation of electrodes in the brain that are used to electrically stimulate precisely targeted brain areas.[7] DBS has been successfully used to treat a range of disorders, including Parkinson's disease, essential tremor, dystonia, and refractory obsessive-compulsive disorder.[7] DBS is considered an experimental treatment for clinical depression, anorexia nervosa, Tourette's syndrome, addiction, anorexia nervosa, schizophrenia, anxiety disorders, and psychopathy.[7,8]

There are a number of factors that increase the risk of therapeutic misconception in the consent process for DBS. First, many of the candidates for DBS have conditions that impact their capacity, so a rigorous investigation of a patient's capacity is a necessary precursor to any attempt at informed consent.[7] Second, DBS is usually the last treatment option for many patients, meaning that many DBS patients will be desperate for some form of relief. This desperation heightens the risk that patients will overestimate the possibility of benefits and underestimate (or ignore) the risks. As Park et al. note:

Desperate patients may also lack the critical faculties to properly interpret what they read in the media about DBS, or misinterpret the nature of the trial. It is thus essential to stress that in such experimental treatment research, there can be no guarantee that a patient will benefit. Rather, it is expected that more general benefits will accrue, such as an improvement in knowledge, or future treatment options. Fully informed consent must involve the recognition of these nuances and the discussion of how DBS should not be regarded as a 'miracle cure.' Researchers must engage in complex discussions with prospective participants about the current situation regarding evidence for DBS, particularly the etiological and outcome uncertainties outlined previously. This is because a failure to appreciate this would almost certainly lead to difficulty in appreciating the underlying principle of equipoise, which governs the ethical approval of clinical research employing DBS. Without this complex understanding, it would be difficult to safely judge that potential participants do indeed possess the capacity to consent to the research.[9]

4.6.4 Therapeutic Ambivalence

One of the features of highly risky medical procedures for critically ill patients is that patients may ignore information about risks altogether. This might be called *therapeutic ambivalence* (in contrast to therapeutic misconception).

We have argued (with Scanlan) that patients undergoing high-risk medical procedures (where the risk of death is certain without treatment and high with it) will often decide to consent to treatment well before they ever even learn about the risks. In high-risk cases, many patients experience the treatment 'choice' as not much of a choice at all, so calculation of risks and benefits becomes irrelevant. In our paper on the experience of patients undergoing bone marrow transplant, we said the following:

> Patients with life-threatening illness did not . . . rationally consider the risks and benefits of BMT [bone marrow treatment] in deciding whether they should undergo it. Rather, their decision-making was, even before they entered the clinic, even before they spoke with their transplant physician, entirely shaped by a desperate hope for a future and a fear that death may come too early. They believed they had no choice but to undergo BMT. In this regard every element of consent – freedom, voluntariness, capacity, understanding and authorisation – was transformed by the lived reality of illness.[10]

Many forms of neurosurgery are very similar to bone marrow transplant in this regard. In one study of patients who were treated with surgery for grade II glioma, patients expressed a desire to leave the decision regarding the surgery to the surgeon, while the surgeons were unanimous in wanting the patients to make the decision.[11] The surgeons struggled with balancing the need for clear information about the disease's progression with leaving room for the patient to still have hope.[11]

Rigorous disclosure of the material risks by the neurosurgeon may satisfy the legal standards, but ensuring an ethical approach to treatment requires a more subtle appreciation of the underlying values at play, such as understanding the investment of trust that patient's make in the neurosurgeon, and the need for them to feel some form of hope. We would argue that in cases where the patients are unable or unwilling to make an assessment of risks and benefits, it is good practice to ensure neurosurgeons are supported with rigorous peer support and have access to guidance through mechanisms such as surgical boards and clinical ethics committees.

4.7 The Relational Function of Consent – Trust, Hope, and Relational Autonomy

We stated at the beginning of the chapter that the classic account of autonomy unrealistically presumes an atomistic form of decision-making that does not often reflect the way that a patient will rely on others (the treatment team, family members, and friends) to make a decision regarding consent. A more rigorous account is that of relational autonomy, which assumes that decisions are made within a web of social relationships, including the relationship of patients with their families, their friends, and the treating team.

The concept of relational autonomy allows for a more complex understanding of decision-making that goes beyond the process of information provision and permission. While the permissive and risk functions of consent are extremely important, it is not sufficient to rely on them as the sole means of understanding the process of consent nor for ensuring its ethical integrity. Instead, we posit a third function for consent: the relational function.

The relational function allows the consent process to provide an environment in which relationships of trust can flourish, where fear can be confronted and hope realistically fostered. As stated above, in cases where patients are out of options and treatment is highly risky, the permissive and risk functions of consent are often ignored by patients, and the relational function of consent comes to the fore. Instead, the consent process creates a space in which the treatment team, the family, and the patient get to listen to each other's expressions of fear about the uncertainty of treatment and negotiate a path forward. The process of negotiation is not just about seeking permission and communicating risk, but it is about building relationships of trust and giving the patient and their family reassurance that, while risky, the treatment was appropriate and had a chance of success.

Once the importance of the relational function of consent is recognised, questions can then be asked about whether the regulation of the legal and ethical aspects of consent is adequate. We would argue that the law has been overly concerned with regulating the permissive and risk functions and that greater attention needs to be given to problems with the relational function. For example, one area of healthcare that is grossly underregulated is that of conflict of interest.[12] Conflicts erode trust and destroy therapeutic relationships and are therefore of paramount importance to the relational function. As such, regulation should be designed to identify conflicts and to manage them, such as through the use of formalised peer support or surgical review panels. These mechanisms to reduce and manage conflicts should strengthen and secure the relational function.

4.8 Conclusion: Consent Is a Necessary, Ethical Component to Neurosurgery

This chapter examined the legal and ethical background of consent to neurosurgery. It has also examined some of the unique challenges that neurosurgery faces in consent. Here, we posited the view that consent has three functions – a permissive function, a risk function, and a relational function. These three functions of consent are equally important, but for high-risk neurosurgical interventions, we have argued that it is the relational function of consent that becomes most salient because of the way that it enables the therapeutic relationship to grow into one of trust and hope. This suggests that the relational function of consent needs not only to be recognised but also strengthened and protected by mechanisms that go beyond the consent process, such as through peer support or surgical review panels.

References

1. Dodds S. M. Choice and control in feminist bioethics. *Relational Autonomy: Feminist Perspectives on Autonomy, Agency, and the Social Self.* Ed. C. Mackenzie, N. Stoljar. New York, Oxford University Press, 2000; 213–35.

2. Witt W. K. Identity change and informed consent. *Journal of Medical Ethics* 2017; **43**: 384–90.

3. Gavrus D. Informed consent and the history of modern neurosurgery. *Handbook of Neuroethics.* Ed. J. Clausen, N. Levy. Dordrecht, Springer, 2015; 505–15.

4. Bell E., Leger P., Sankar T., Racine E. Deep brain stimulation as clinical innovation: an ethical and organisational framework to sustain deliberations about psychiatric deep brain stimulation. *Neurosurgery* 2016; **79**: 3–10.

5. Scanlan C., Stewart C., Kerridge I. Consent in the face of death. *Internal Medicine Journal* 2019; **49**: 108–10.

6. Klein E. Eloquent brain, ethical challenges: functional brain mapping in neurosurgery. *Seminars in Ultrasound CT and MRI* 2015; **36**: 291–5.

7. Mandarelli G., Moretti G., Pasquini M., et al. Informed consent decision-making in deep brain stimulation. *Brain Science* 2018; **8**: E84.

8. Canavero S. Criminal minds: Neuromodulation of the psychopathic brain. *Frontiers of Human Neuroscience* 2014; **8**: 124.

9. Park R. J., Singh I., Pike A. C., et al. Deep brain stimulation in anorexia nervosa: Hope for the hopeless or exploitation of the vulnerable? The oxford neuroethics gold standard framework. *Frontiers in Psychiatry* 2017; **8**: 6.

10. Scanlan C., Stewart C., Kerridge I. Decision making in the shadow of death. *The American Journal of Bioethics* 2016; **16**: 23–4.

11. Brennum J., Maier C. M., Almdal K., Engelmann C. M., Gjerris M. Primo non nocere or maximum survival in grade 2 gliomas? A medical ethical question. *Acta Neurochirurgica* 2015; **157**: 155–64.

12. Lipworth W., Montgomery K. Managing and regulating conflicts of interest in medicine. *Medical Professionals: Conflicts and Quandaries in Medical Practice*, Ed. K. Montgomery and W. Lipworth. New York, Routledge, 2019.

Chapter

5

Withholding and Withdrawing Medical Treatment: Legal, Ethical, and Practical Considerations

Cameron Stewart, Tiit Mathiesen, Ahmed Ammar, and Stephen Honeybul

5.1 Introduction

Over the past 50 years there have been considerable advances across all aspects of medical treatment, especially in the fields of surgery and intensive care. Many of these advances have significantly increased the possibility of patients surviving events that would have previously been fatal. They have also extended patients' lifespans beyond what was previously thought possible, even when patients have significant physical and cognitive impairment. These advances have created new problems for medical decision-making, as considerations have to made regarding withholding or withdrawing life-sustaining treatments. New choices about the most appropriate management of death, have, in turn, created new ethical and legal problems.

These decisions are challenging for healthcare professionals who often feel uncomfortable withholding or withdrawing a life-sustaining therapy and who may feel some degree of responsibility for the patient's eventual death. In addition, there may be considerable pressure from family members who will either ask for treatment to be withheld or withdrawn prematurely or who will 'want everything done', even beyond the point where treatment is serving the best interests of the patient, and it is in these circumstances that the concept of futility must be considered.

This chapter will begin by examining a patient's right to refuse treatment. It will then proceed to examine the legal aspects of treatment decisions for patients who have lost capacity. It will then consider a practical approach to a common neurosurgical scenario where issues of futility and withdrawing life-sustaining treatment need to be considered.

5.2 Refusing Treatment and Advance Directives

Both medical ethics and law supports the notion that mentally capable patients decide whether to consent to medical interventions. Both consent and the value of autonomy which underpins it are discussed in detail in Chapter 4. One of the most famous statements regarding consent and autonomy was made in *Schloendorf* v. *Society of New York Hospital*, 195 NE 92 (1914) at 93 by the American judge Cardozo J: 'Every human being of adult years and sound mind has a right to determine what shall be done with his own body, and a surgeon who performs an operation without his patient's consent commits an assault, for which he is liable in damages.'

Patients are permitted to refuse life-sustaining treatments even in cases where the patient is not terminally ill but still prefers to die without treatment than live with it. In the neurosurgical context, this means that a patient is free to refuse neurosurgical intervention and accept the risk of death, even when that risk is a virtual certainty. In *Re T (An Adult)*

(Consent to Medical Treatment) [1992] 2 Fam 458 at 460, Lord Donaldson said: 'This right of choice is not limited to decisions which others might regard as sensible. It exists notwithstanding that the reasons for making the choice are rational, irrational, unknown or even nonexistent.' There is a large body of case law from the United Kingdom (*Re C (Adult : Refusal of Medical Treatment)* [1994] 1 WLR 290), Canada (*Nancy B* v. *Hotel-Dieu de Quebec* (1992) 86 DLR (4th) 385), New Zealand (*Smith* v. *Auckland Hospital* [1965] NZLR 191), the United States (*Bouvia* v. *Superior Court (Glenchur)* 225 Cal Rptr 297 [1986]), and Australia (*Re JS* [2014] NSWSC 302) that supports this statement.

Decisions to refuse treatment can also be made in advance. Such 'advance directives' are binding when a competent person has made a decision to refuse treatment which was clearly intended to apply in the circumstances that have arisen (*Re T (An Adult) (Consent to Medical Treatment)* [1992] 2 Fam 458; *Hunter and New England Area Health Service* v. *A* (2009) 74 NSWLR 88). Advance care directives may play a significant role in neurosurgical intervention where there is a high risk of an adverse outcome. In such cases, having detailed conversations with the patient regarding their wishes prior to treatment will help strengthen the process of consent and provide guidance in cases where the patient is rendered incapable. Advance directives are often highly regulated, so healthcare professionals need to investigate the particular legal requirements in the jurisdiction in which they practice.

Health professionals who honour competent decisions to refuse treatment are not liable for assisting suicide or for killing the patient, even when they provide assistance, such as through pain-relieving medications or sedation. Decisions to refuse treatment are not considered to be the legal cause of death. In the Canadian case of *Nancy B* v. *Hotel-Dieu de Quebec* (1992) 86 DLR (4th) 385, the patient, who required life-support ventilation and whose mental capacity was unaffected by her condition, wished to refuse treatment. The court found that the woman's right to refuse the treatment was not the cause of her death, but rather the underlying disease was taking its natural course.

Nor are patients who refuse treatment considered to be suicidal. Death is said to be caused by the patient's condition, not by the omission of treatment. In the common law, omissions are not considered to be causes of death unless there was a duty to treat. In cases where a competent patient refuses life-sustaining treatment (either contemporaneously or by advance directive), there is no duty to provide it. In *H Ltd* v. *J* [2010] SASC 176, a 74-year-old South Australian woman with post-polio syndrome and Type 1 diabetes refused her medication and decided to stop eating and drinking. Her nursing home was concerned that it could face liability for assisting a suicide, should it let her die. Kourakis J found that the decision was not suicidal because there is no common law duty to feed oneself. The patient's refusal of food, water, and insulin would not legally be a cause of death, and therefore, it could not be considered suicide.

Illustrative Clinical Case 1

Case 1 is a 32-year-old male. He was involved in a high-speed motor vehicle accident. He sustained multiple injuries, including a severe traumatic brain injury. His pupils were small and unreactive. His initial Glasgow Coma Score was recorded as 3. Following endotracheal intubation, he was transferred to a level one trauma facility, where a CT brain scan confirmed a large left-sided acute subdural haematoma with significant midline shift and obliteration of the basal cisterns. Following the CT scan, his pupils were noted to be fixed and dilated. Family members (brother, sister, and mother) were contacted, and the seriousness of the situation was explained. There was no record of an advance directive. The attending neurosurgeon was reluctant to surgically intervene because it was felt that while surgical intervention would be life-saving, the patient would most likely be left with severe neurocognitive deficits. Following an emotionally charged consultation, the mother and brother were insistent the patient be given the best chance of survival. The sister was less convinced but agreed.

The surgery proceeded uneventfully. The haematoma was evacuated and a primary decompressive craniectomy was performed, as the brain was swollen. The patient was transferred back to the intensive care but made a very poor recovery. At three weeks post-injury, he remained intubated and ventilated, and the only motor function was extensor posturing. His pupils were small and unreactive. He has some respiratory drive, and the intensive care team and the attending neurosurgeon are considering either inserting a tracheostomy or withdrawing therapy. The attending surgeon meets with the brother and mother to discuss the options. When hearing of the prospect of treatment withdrawal, the brother is furious and accuses the surgeon of euthanasia. He is adamant that treatment should continue and threatens legal action against the hospital. The mother takes no part in the discussion but requests time to consider. The neurosurgeon documents the discussion and consults with the hospital administration to determine the legal position.

Two days later, the mother and sister return. It turns out the sister was very close to her brother. He had a close friend who had sustained a severe traumatic brain injury and survived in a nursing home. He had expressed the view on many occasions that he would never want to be left in such a condition. The neurosurgeon asks about the views of her brother. It is revealed that the brothers had been estranged for many years. The neurosurgeon documents the discussion and treatment is withdrawn. The patient dies peacefully three days later.

5.3 Treatment Decisions for Incapacitated Patients: Legal Considerations

5.3.1 Who Is the Decision-Maker?

When patients are incapacitated and have not left an advance directive, decisions must be made for them by others. This is demonstrated in the illustrative case, in which the question arises as to who is the responsible decision-maker.

Understandably, the laws vary widely from jurisdiction to jurisdiction, but it is possible to make some broad observations. Usually any court or tribunal-based decision-maker has primacy in such cases. Superior courts will ordinarily have the power to appoint decision-makers (for example, guardians or conservators), or they may directly exercise power to make decisions for the patient. Alternatively, a patient may have previously appointed a decision-maker via some form of enduring power of attorney (which can be found, for example, in most states of the United States and Australia). Finally, in some jurisdictions, a caregiver, spouse, or close friend or relative may be given the power to consent should there be no formally appointed decision-maker (which is the case in most states of Australia).

Disputes often arise between decision-makers as to who should have the final say in end-of-life cases. For example, in *Schiavo rel Schindler* v. *Schiavo* 403 F3d 1289, Terri Schiavo had suffered a catastrophic brain injury from an anoxic brain injury and was being kept alive with artificial feeding and hydration. Her husband had been appointed as her guardian/conservator by the court system. He had decided to refuse artificial feeding and hydration based on his assessment of what her previous expressly wishes had been. Her parents disagreed with the decision, and there was a protracted legal battle of several years, after which it was held that the husband had made the correct decision.

5.3.2 What Is the Standard for Decision-Making?

Broadly speaking, there are two traditional approaches to decision-making: the best-interests test and substituted judgement. The best-interests test requires a decision-maker to take into account the medical and social data regarding the proposed treatment and make a decision that best serves the interest of the patient. Substituted judgement requires the decision-maker to use whatever is known about the patient's wishes, desires, and values to make a decision that they believe the patient would have made.

Both tests are based on common law tests but historically the best-interests test has had primacy in the United Kingdom, Ireland, New Zealand, Australia, and Canada, whereas substituted judgement has been the primary test in most of the United States. In more recent times, many jurisdictions have combined the tests so that a decision-maker should begin with subjective factors based on the patient's known wishes and interests and then move towards more objective factors regarding the proposed treatment (*Re G* [1997] NZFLR 362).

In 2006 the United Nations created the Convention of the Rights of People with Disabilities, and by 2008, 20 countries had ratified the agreement, bringing it into force. The Convention challenges the traditional capacity-based decision-making models described above. It declares that everyone has equal legal capacity and that states have an obligation to provide support for people with disabilities, to enable them to make decisions based on their will and preferences. The Committee to the Convention has called for the rejection of the common law test of capacity and the abolition of substitute decision-making (Committee on the Rights of Persons with Disabilities, *General Comment No1* (2014) para [25]–[28]). Instead of using functional capacity to determine whether a substitute decision-maker should be appointed, a person with disabilities should be given support to help them make their own decision, even in cases where the person with disabilities is disabled to the degree that he or she unable to contribute towards the making of the decision. Such a decision is described as being one of 'total support'. Australia, Canada, Ireland, New Zealand, and the United Kingdom have ratified the Convention, but none have yet gone so far as to abolish capacity testing or substitute decision-making altogether. Some jurisdictions, like Ireland and the state of Victoria in Australia, have modified their laws by placing the will and preference of the person as the primary factor for decision-making. Nevertheless, these jurisdictions have left capacity testing and substituted judgement as a last resort (*Assisted Decision-Making (Capacity) Act 2015* (Eire); *Medical Treatment Planning and Decisions Act 2016* (Vic)).

5.3.3 When Should Life-Sustaining Treatment Be Withheld or Withdrawn?

In jurisdictions that employ a substituted judgement standard, treatment should be withheld or withdrawn when the decision-maker has made an assessment that the treatment would have been rejected by the patient. In *Matter of Quinlan* 355 A 2d 647 (1976), the father of a severely disabled patient sought to be appointed her guardian so that he could authorize the termination of her respiratory support. It was found that a patient's proxy should exercise his or her best judgement as to whether the patient would have refused treatment in the circumstances that arose. Similarly, in *Superintendent of Belchertown State School* v. *Saikewicz*, 370 NE 2d 417 (1977), a case concerning a man with cancer who had never had mental capacity, it was said that a decision-maker should 'don the mental mantle of the incompetent' and substitute themselves as nearly as possible for the individual in the decision-making process.

Some jurisdictions set a very high level of evidence for substitute judgement, for example, by requiring clear and convincing evidence of the patient's desire to refuse treatment in the circumstances that have arisen. Arguably, such high standards effectively reproduce the requirements for an advance directive and are unfairly restrictive, but in *Cruzan* v. *Director, Missouri Dept of Health* 497 US 261 (1990), the US Supreme Court upheld the right of Missouri to require such exacting standards, when examining the question of whether artificial feeding and hydration should be withdrawn from a woman in a persistent vegetative state.

In jurisdictions that employ a best interests standard, the question of the patient's best interests is determined by factors such as the diagnosis, prognosis, availability of treatment, the patient's prior wishes and values, pain and suffering of both having and not having treatment, and the broad question of the patient's quality of life. A case that illustrates these points is *W* v. *M* [2011] EWHC 2443 (Fam), which involved a woman who was left in a minimally conscious state after contracting viral encephalitis. The patient's family and treatment team believed that it would be in the patient's best interests for artificial feeding and hydration to be ceased, especially given the number of informal statements that the patient had made prior to her illness, indicating that she would not have wished to live in such a condition. The court agreed that the best-interests test should be applied and used the 'balance-sheet' approach, in which the patient's interests are weighed and compared. Ultimately, the judge found in favour of continuing artificial feeding and hydration, as the patient still had some positive experiences, but the judge did agree that a 'do not resuscitate' order was appropriate.

5.3.4 Are Healthcare Professionals Liable for the Patient's Death?

If an appropriate decision has been made to refuse treatment, common law relieves the healthcare professionals of any duty to provide it. The failure to provide treatment is classified as a 'non-culpable omission', meaning not 'a legal cause of death'. For example, in *Barber* v. *Superior Court of the State of California* (1983) 195 Cal Rptr 484, two doctors, who had discontinued the life support of a patient, were found not guilty of murder and conspiracy to murder. The patient in question was in a vegetative state but was not brain dead. The patient had not executed a 'living will' (advance directive) under the Californian statutory scheme. The court found that the removal of artificial nutrition and hydration was an omission to continue futile treatment that provided no benefit to the patient. As the treatments were futile, the physicians had breached no duty in omitting to continue them, and they could not be found to have caused the death of the patient. The leading English case is *Airedale NHS Trust* v. *Bland* [1993] 2 WLR 316. Anthony Bland suffered an anoxic brain injury in the Hillsborough football stadium disaster and was in a persistent vegetative state. Bland's family and treatment team wished to stop artificial feeding and hydration. The House of Lords found that doctors were not bound to provide treatment that has no beneficial effect. Lord Browne-Wilkinson accepted that the physical removal of the feeding tubes from patient's bodies could be classed as an omission. The Lords also said that there was no legal difference between withholding and withdrawing treatment.

5.4 Withholding or Withdrawing Treatment: Practical Considerations

There is no doubt that end-of-life issues will continue to cause considerable conflict in medical decision-making. However, in most cases, recourse to legal action must be seen as a failure in communication that does not necessarily benefit the competing parties. In everyday practical terms, every effort must be made to establish as early as possible areas where there are differences of opinion and to make every effort to explore these issues and mitigate conflict.

These problems are encountered on a regular basis in neurosurgery, and it is important that surgeons are aware of the issues that need to be considered. The illustrative case serves to demonstrate a scenario that is not at all uncommon, and there are a number of key issues that need to be resolved. In the first instance, there is the issue of futility and the intrinsic value attached to life. The second issue is the practical approach to withdrawing life-sustaining treatment.[1]

5.4.1 Medical Futility

Modern medicine has struggled with the concept of futility for many years. Attempts at a clear definition have ranged from doctor-centred definitions such as physiological or quantitative futility to more patient-centred definitions related to contextual futility or qualitative futility (Table 5.1). Each of these definitions has its own advantages and potential applications; however, one of their major limitations is that they seem to imply a level of a certainty that in clinical practice is not only unrealistic but would appear to provide little room for discussion.[2]

A definition that concentrates on the goals of treatment is equally problematic because either the achievement of goals must be retrospectively evaluated (which does not help with the actual clinical decision) or it must be a probabilistic assessment such that the intervention is not likely to achieve the goals of therapy (in which case the argument collapses into the quantitative definition with the associated problems). Further difficulties occur when the goals are not clearly defined or the goals include states that a patient may regard as unacceptable so that it would be ethically unjustified to expose the patient to the risk of the outcome concerned.[2] For example, there is now clear evidence that decompressive craniectomy reduces mortality. However, the reduction in mortality comes at the cost of an increase in the number of survivors with severe neurocognitive disability. Prior to intervening, every attempt must be made to determine that this would be acceptable to the person on whom the procedure is being performed.[2]

It is in this regard that the concepts of 'substantial benefit' and 'risk of unacceptable badness' may be of use. Substantial benefit describes an outcome that the patient would regard as worthwhile either at the present time or in the future. The 'risk of unacceptable badness' is the probability that a patient will end up living in a state that they would describe as intolerable. These terms are intentionally subjective and were described in order to acknowledge that there may be considerable variability regarding an acceptable outcome for a particular individual, which can depend on any number of religious, cultural, or social values. They also highlight the need for a patient-centred approach to any futility assessment.[2]

Table 5.1 Definitions of futility

Type of futility	Description	Example
Physiological futility	This is when the proposed intervention cannot physiologically achieve the desired effect. It is the most objective type of futility judgement	Prescribing antibiotics for viral infection
Qualitative futility	When the proposed intervention, if successful, will probably produce such a poor outcome that it is deemed best not to attempt it	Providing a life-saving intervention such as a decompressive hemicraniectomy for a severe dominant hemisphere stroke that leaves a person with severe neurocognitive deficits
Quantitative futility	When the proposed intervention is highly unlikely to achieve the desired effect	A treatment has only achieved its objectives in a certain probabilistic number of cases
Contextual futility	When the treatment may be effective but the context in which it is provided is inappropriate	Providing cardiopulmonary resuscitation in a patient with end stage cancer who has a very limited time to live
Procedural futility	When a process has been designed to determine whether the treatment is futile, which starts with the treatment team and family members but which may then involve the help of third parties to resolve differences	Using a multidisciplinary team (doctors, nurses, social workers) to work with family members to determine the best course of action for the patient. In cases of dispute, using dispute resolution mechanisms to resolve differences (e.g., using a clinical ethics committee to give advice, involving independent specialists to confirm the prognosis, or going to a legal tribunal to seek resolution)

More recently, the concepts of 'proportionate' and 'disproportionate' have been introduced in order to acknowledge that a specific treatment may not necessarily be futile and therefore useless but may have progressively declining benefit, thus increasing burden in any one particular clinical situation. For a medical treatment to be 'proportionate', the benefits must outweigh the burdens, and this again may vary depending on an individual's values and preferences.[2]

Finally, all of these techniques can be employed in a procedural approach to futility determination (Table 5.1). This approach occurs when medical decision-making is based on clinical consensus, with avenues for appeal and review.[3] A procedural futility determination occurs when the treatment team makes a determination that active treatment has become futile according to the competing futility definitions discussed above. The decision is then shared with the patient and/or their family, including information about having the decision reviewed at a predetermined later date. If the patients' families remain unhappy with that decision, they should be able to have it reviewed by an independent body like a clinical ethics committee. If the clinical ethics committee agrees with the assessment and the patient/family still disagree, then an appeal can be made to a legal body such as a guardianship tribunal or court. These bodies can appoint substitute decision-makers or make their own determinations. Procedural approaches to futility try to enshrine a form a fairness in the deliberation of futility via accountability.

Returning to the illustrative case, it could be argued that the initial surgical intervention was proportionate in that, notwithstanding the risk of dependency and perhaps the neuro-surgeons own personal bias, there may be a small chance of a good outcome, and people can certainly learn to adapt to a level of dependency that they might previously thought to be unacceptable. However, as time goes on, it is becoming increasingly obvious that continued therapy was becoming disproportionate from an outcome perspective and also arguably from the viewpoint of equitable resource allocation. Listening and responding to the family, especially the sister, helped to form a better picture of what the patient would have wanted. The fact that a fair process was engaged made it much easier when making a final clinical judgement and to accept the medical decision of futility.

However, notwithstanding the opinions expressed, the determination of futility rests on the assumption that life has instrumental value only and is a necessary condition either to experience or to perform other activities that provide value. Given that the patient is currently ventilator dependent and showing no signs of awareness, it would appear that he is unlikely to be able to experience activities of any value. However, adopting this position requires clarification.

5.4.2 Assessing Quality of Life: Does Life Have Intrinsic Value?

Given that technology is available that can prolong life in patients who will never regain consciousness, the futility debate rests on the assumption that this in itself provides no intrinsic value. However, a value-based argument rooted in an observer's assessment can be problematic, and it has been argued that the use of quality-of-life criteria in decision-making is dangerous in the way that it allows the decision-maker to decide whether a person's life is worth living, based on a person's disability.[4] This, according to some theorists, offends the principle of the sanctity of life, which holds that every life has an inherent value in the common law, regardless of a person's level of disability.

From a legal perspective, the sanctity of life has been recognized many times by courts. For example, Ward LJ in *Re A (children)(conjoined twins)* [2000] 4 All ER 961 at 1000 said that 'the sanctity of life doctrine compels me to accept is that each life has inherent value in itself and the right to life, being universal, is equal for all of us'. As such, most judges will tend to err on the side of life in difficult cases. However, some judges have been very concerned about using quality of life as a factor in assessing best interests. For example, in the American case of *Matter of Conroy* 486 A 2d 1209 (1985), the court accepted that quality of life could be assessed, but limited that assessment to calculating the effect of the treatment on the patient's level of pain. The court refused to consider wider matters in the calculation of quality of life, as this would put those with disabilities at unacceptable risk. In Australia, in *TS v. Sydney Children's Hospital Network* [2012] NSWSC 1609, Garling J, when discussing the quality of life of a disabled newborn, said that it was 'unhelpful to engage in an ill-defined process which is quintessentially a subjective one for each assessor to determine what Mohammed's quality of life is' (at [70]).

Notwithstanding these rulings, the preponderance of authority from around the common law world supports the view that quality-of-life assessment is necessary and appropriate. In cases where the evidence shows that the patient is suffering, courts have found that the life of the patient is 'intolerable' and that treatment should cease: *Re B (A Minor) (Wardship: Medical Treatment)* [1981] 1 WLR 1421; *Re J (A Minor)(Wardship: Medical Treatment)* [1990] 3 All ER 930. In other cases where the patient may not have the capacity to feel pain (such as in vegetative states or post-coma responsiveness), it will still be open to the courts to say that the life of the patient is not worth living. In the previously mentioned UK court case relating to Tony Bland, Lord Goff wrote: 'I cannot see that medical treatment is appropriate or requisite simply to prolong a patient's life when such treatment has no therapeutic purpose of any kind, as where it is futile because the patient is unconscious and there is no prospect of any improvement in his condition.'

Many people probably share Lord Goff's view; however, this is by no means always the case. In December 2013, a Californian teenage girl, Jahi McMath, suffered a serious life-threatening complication after relatively minor throat surgery. She was resuscitated but sustained profound brain damage. Three days later, Jahi was diagnosed as being brain dead by her physicians, but the family contested the diagnosis. They argued that according to their religious views, she was still alive because her heart was still beating (it was, but because of the intensive care being provided). A Californian court upheld the medical diagnosis of death, but the family continued to object to discontinuation of life support, and they found a medical facility prepared to take over Jahi's care. Jahi body was supported by a mechanical ventilator in New Jersey until she died a second and final time from liver failure in June 2018.

Treating Jahi after brain death was counter to modern-day medical practice because the treatment was clearly futile (on any of the definitions outlined above). However, the family did not share the same values and claimed that their rights to freedom of religion permitted them to reject the existence of brain death as a criterion of futility.

Overall, the value-status of life will continue to provoke powerful emotions and be subject to discordant but strongly held views in different cultures.[5] Monotheistic cultures with Jewish, Christian, or Islamic convictions tend to support intrinsic-value beliefs, although most technologically advanced countries also seem to have a rational attitude to discontinuing prolonged care. Despite the aforementioned rulings, there appears to be an implicit agreement among most medical professionals that life cannot be viewed as intrinsically valuable under all conditions, and even the most pro-life cultures seem to entertain a grey zone where maximum care is not offered or even discontinued if started.

It is here that the second contentious issue is raised, and that is the ethical issues regarding withholding and withdrawing life-sustaining treatment.

5.4.3   Withholding and Withdrawing Life-Sustaining Treatment: Is There a Difference?

A recent paper in a bioethical journal made the following comment: 'The presumption that the distinction between withdrawing and withholding lifesaving treatment carries no moral weight is so commonplace that it is today rarely debated.[6] In addition, policy makers and medical guidelines make it very clear that doctors are under no obligation to provide treatment that they feel is providing no benefit, and they also clearly state that there is no ethical distinction between withholding treatment or withdrawing medical treatment once it has already been started.

However, this position is at odds with the results of studies which have found that up to 50% of physicians felt there was an ethical difference between withholding treatment and withdrawing such treatment once it had been started.

In clinical practice, the ethical tension involved in these decisions increases when the most likely result of treatment withdrawal is the death of a patient, and it is in this regard that the accusation of euthanasia is raised. However, is this a justifiable accusation? In these circumstances a useful analogy can be drawn from the work of the late James Rachels.

5.4.3.1 Acts and Omissions

Rachels used the following thought experiment to defend the morality of euthanasia. Two brothers, Smith and Jones, both stand to inherit a lot of money upon the death of their young nephew, so both want the nephew dead. Smith sneaks into the bathroom one night when his nephew is taking a bath and drowns him. He then arranges things to make it look like an accident. In the second case, Jones sneaks into the bathroom one night when his nephew is taking a bath, prepared to drown him, but the boy slips, hits his head, and drowns all on his own. Jones is ready to push the boy's head back down under the water, but he doesn't have to.

The question arises as to the responsibilities of the uncles, and Rachel's conclusion was: the only difference between the two cases is that one involves killing and the other involves letting die, but what Jones did is just as morally bad as what Smith did, so there's no moral difference between them; thus there's no moral difference between killing and letting die. And if the only relevant difference between active and passive euthanasia is the killing/letting die distinction, then there's no moral difference between active and passive euthanasia.

This argument is highly problematic for the legal explanation of end-of-life decisions outlined above, given that the legal argument rests on the acts and omissions distinction. There are further challenges when the concept of omissions is stretched to include acts (such as removing feeding tubes, sedating the patient, turning off a ventilator), which, if done by a stranger, would constitute active killing. In the Bland case, Lord Mustill said at 388–9:

> The conclusion that the declaration can be upheld depends crucially on a distinction drawn by the criminal law between acts and omissions, and carries with it inescapably a distinction between, on the one hand what is called a 'mercy killing', where active steps are taken in a medical context to terminate the life of a suffering patient, and a situation such as the present where the proposed conduct has the aim for equally humane reasons of terminating the life of Anthony Bland by withholding from him the basic necessities of life. The acute unease that I feel about adopting this way through the legal and ethical maze is I believe due in an important part to the sensation that however much the technologies may differ the ethical status of two courses of action is for all relevant purposes indistinguishable. By dismissing this appeal I feel that your Lordships' House may only emphasise the distortions of a legal structure which is already both morally and intellectually misshapen. Still, the law is there and we must take it as it stands.

In general, contemporary medical practice rejects the ethical importance of the action and omission distinction and judges the appropriateness of medical intervention in relation to purpose and boundaries of medical practice and the professional and ethical integrity of practitioners. In the field of neurosurgery, the act of treatment withdrawal and subsequent death of the patient is commonplace, and neurosurgeons need to be familiar with the ethical distinction between withdrawing life-sustaining treatment and wilfully ending a patient's life. In the illustrative case, the neurosurgeon is being accused of euthanasia.

5.4.4 Withdrawing Treatment: An Illustrative Neurosurgical Case

In order to understand the practical approach to this issue, it is important to consider the two universal indications that must be fulfilled prior to commencing any form of treatment. First, the treatment must be medically indicated and there must be a reasonable chance that the treatment will provide benefit and not harm. Second, the patient (or some form of surrogate decision-maker) must provide consent. If either of these two conditions are not satisfied, then treatment cannot be provided; indeed, knowingly providing treatment that provides no benefit not only violates the ethical principle of non-maleficence but also may constitute a legal charge of battery.

The next stage is considering withdrawing treatment (notwithstanding the clinical result) that is providing no benefit and may indeed be deemed overly burdensome.[7]

One approach to this dilemma is the equivalence thesis, which is a philosophical argument that rests on the assumption that 'all other things being equal, it is permissible to withdraw a medical treatment that a patient is receiving if it would have been permissible to withhold the same treatment (not already provided) and visa versa' (Table 5.2).[7-9]

As previously stated, there are strong ethical arguments to support the equivalence thesis; however, from a practical perspective, it must be recognized that there can be strong psychological and social arguments for non-equivalence (Table 5.2). Many clinicians clearly feel that withdrawing treatment once it has been started in more difficult than not starting that treatment in the first place.

It is important that clinicians acknowledged these differences, in order to avoid perceiving these differences as ethical or legal reasons for non-equivalence, because this might lead to judgements that go against the best interests of the patient.[9] In other words, the psychological reactions of medical personnel involved in the care of the patient can be acknowledged as real, but it must equally acknowledged that these reactions are not relevant and indeed may hamper clinical judgement.[8,9]

In the clinical case described, if the neurosurgeon was concerned that there may come a time when treatment has to be withdrawn, he or she may consider not starting the treatment (surgical decompression) in the first place. Clearly judgement based on this reasoning (i.e., the neurosurgeon's own feelings) cannot be in the best interests of the patient (who may be given the chance to benefit). Likewise, continuing a treatment that a clinician feels is not providing a patient's clinical benefit, notwithstanding the wishes of the family, is clearly not in the patient's best interests.

When the time comes to consider withdrawing ventilatory support, the ethical indications to continue ventilation are the same that were required to initiate ventilation in the first place – namely that the treatment is a medical intervention that is going to provide benefit and the patient continues to provide consent. Notwithstanding the family conflict (which can be a common occurrence in these ethically and emotionally challenging situations), it is now clear that the patient is making a poor recovery, and based on the sister's

Table 5.2 Ethical differences between withholding and withdrawing

Arguments supporting the equivalence thesis	Arguments doubting the equivalence thesis
There is no difference	**There is a difference**
The central argument for ethical equivalence – There are no differences in intentions, consequences, and the ultimate cause of death, and no difference in the moral responsibility	There is a strong psychological and conventional bias for those involved in the care of the patient who may feel responsible for the death of the patient
The vast majority of guideline policy documents state that there is no difference between withholding and withdrawing life support	Almost all surveys report that up to 50% of physicians feel that there is a difference
Healthcare professionals have a cognitive bias against withdrawing treatment (so-called withdrawal aversion) and flawed moral reasoning	Withdrawing treatment is a morally more serious decision than withholding treatment
The perceived differences are psychological and social, not ethical or legal	There is a strong intuitive difference
Withdrawing care and withholding care are just substitution of one form of care for another	It can be better to start a treatment to gain prognostic evidence of benefit and later withdraw that treatment, rather than withhold that treatment
Active treatment is conditional and withdrawing is just postponed withholding	The realities of clinical practice are such that the equivalence thesis is a blunt tool that does not offer much in the way of insight into the moral landscape of withdrawing and withholding lifesaving medical treatment
It is not ethical to continuing treatment that is not providing clinical benefit	Starting treatment can imply crossing an ethical point of no return

viewpoint, it would appear unlikely that the patient would provide consent (based on previously voiced views) for ongoing treatment.

Indeed, a closer examination of this case reveals why withdrawing treatment is a morally more defendable than withholding treatment (although it may not feel that way). It can be argued that notwithstanding the neurosurgeon's initial reservations, an attempt was at least made at saving the patient's life (hoping for a better neurological recovery). Now that it became clear that the treatment had failed to provide the necessary benefit, withdrawal of the treatment was not a new decision but termination of a treatment that had failed.[9]

Based on this reasoning, withdrawing treatment that provides no benefit cannot be compared to the uncle standing by and watching his nephew drown because a physician is not morally obligated to provide treatment that will not provide benefit. Similarly, if a competent patient refuses life-sustaining treatment, the physician has no ethical mandate to provide that treatment, and there can be no case made for passive euthanasia. Indeed, a charge of passive euthanasia can only be made if a physician fails to provide treatment that is medically indicated and for which consent has been obtained. In these circumstances, the physician can be charged with neglect.

The key difference between euthanasia (and patient-assisted suicide) and treatment withdrawal is intent. When a treatment is withdrawn, the intention is to discontinue treatment that is not providing benefit and recognize that the disease process will take its natural course. The patient will die as a result of the severe traumatic brain injury. In euthanasia, the intent is the death of the patient.[10]

5.5 Mitigating Conflict: A Practical and Clinical Approach

The ethical arguments are pervasive and must be recognized; however, as demonstrated by the clinical case, family dynamics can be complicated and these decisions can be challenging for all involved. It is important that the families are not made to feel that they are actually charged with the clinical decision because this is not only unfair but also can promote a sense of guilt; where possible, a process of shared decision-making should be employed.[2] When conflicts develop, every attempt must be made to avoid escalation; however, notwithstanding the aforementioned cases, there continues to be situations where there has been a need to seek recourse to legal action in the courts.

Obviously, there will be regional variation in the legal position that is adopted; however, most courts' rulings have been based on a number of key considerations.[11] These include:

- the medical evidence regarding the person's diagnosis, prognosis, and treatment options;
- the degree to which the treatment may be viewed as overly burdensome;
- the known wishes of the person, be it previously voiced or actually documented (and, interestingly, to a much lesser extent, the views of family members); and
- the quality of life of the person if they receive treatment.

It is important to note that most courts have often stated that organizational interests and availability of resources are *not* relevant to a best-interests assessment.

In additions, in most jurisdictions, courts also consider the process by which the clinicians have decided that ongoing treatment should be withdrawn. These include:

- consultation with other clinicians;
- adherence to clinical guidelines; and
- involvement with surrogate or substitute decision-makers.

When these issues have been adequately addressed, in most cases, the courts have ruled in favour of the clinician's decision, even when there has been strong family opposition. While it must be accepted that there will never be a one-size-fits-all approach to these issues, the position adopted by the courts can act as a useful checklist to mitigate conflict in the first place (Table 5.3).

5.6 Conclusion

There will always come a time when either a disease or an injury has progressed to such an extent that further treatment is providing no further benefit and may actually be overly burdensome. While it is accepted that there is no ethical difference between

Table 5.3 Mitigating conflict when withdrawing or withholding treatment

	Possible mitigating actions
Medical issues	Ensure that the diagnosis is accurate
	Ensure as much as possible that the prognosis for recovery is minimal
	Explore all treatment options and, where relevant, adhere to clinical guidelines
	Obtain second opinions from colleagues involved in management and colleagues who are independent of the case
	Where there appears to be conflicting opinions in any staff members, explore and address the issues involved. Aim for a medical consensus
	Formally document all discussions
Patient issues	Attempt to obtain information regarding a patient's known wishes, either voiced or documented
	If there have been previously expressed wishes, make every attempt to acknowledge and, where possible, act to respect these wishes
	Make every attempt to avoid interventions/outcomes that a patient might previously have deemed unacceptable
Family issues	Explore issues of conflict within the family
	Attempt to address areas of conflict and obtain a consensus opinion
	Explore specific areas of concern and, where possible, address these issues (e.g., is the patient in pain, aware of their surroundings, able to communicate?)
	Where treatments are started in difficult situations, make timelines where a reassessment regarding ongoing therapy or otherwise can be made
	Do not make families feel that they are burdened with making a decision
	Aim for a shared decision-making process based on a patient's best interests
	Make time for repeated discussions
	Document all discussions, even if they seemed congenial

withholding treatment or withdrawing treatment that has already started, it is important to acknowledge that there is a strong intuitive difference that may unconsciously influence clinical decision-making. Families must be involved in a shared patient-centred decision-making process that recognizes cultural, religious, and personal values.

Overall, recourse to legal council must be seen as a failure of communication and a situation that benefits neither clinicians nor the families involved. Paradoxically, both parties may feel that they are acting in the patient's best interests, and clinicians certainly want to avoid the public examination of their clinical judgements, which are not always reported favourably. However, in most jurisdictions, the clinician who acts with clearly stated intentions, having carefully considered the ethical aspects of what they are doing, will not be subject to the 'damned if you do and damned if you don't' mentality that many fear the courts and the media will show in these fraught areas of decision-making. In fact, neither the courts nor ethicists are in the business of making reasonable care more difficult; they are only concerned that it be truly reasonable.

References

1. Gedge E., Giacomini M., Cook D. Withholding and withdrawing life support in critical care settings: ethical issues concerning consent. *J. Med. Ethics* 2007; **33**: 215–18.

2. Honeybul S., Gillett G. R., Ho, K. Futility in neurosurgery: a patient-centered approach. *Neurosurgery* 2013; **73**: 917–22.

3. Stewart C. Futility determination as a process: problems with medical sovereignty, legal issues and the strengths and weakness of the procedural approach. *J. Bioeth. Inq.* 2011; **8**: 155–63.

4. Keown J. The legal revolution: from 'sanctity of life' to 'quality of life' and 'autonomy'. *J. Contemp. Health Law Policy* 1998; **14**: 253–85.

5. Ammar A. Influence of different culture on neurosurgical practice. *Childs Nerv. Syst.* 1997; **13**: 91–4.

6. Emmerich N., Gordjin B. A morally permissible moral mistake? reinterpreting a thought experiment as proof of concept. *J. Bioeth. Inq.* 2018; **15**: 269–78.

7. LØ U. Withholding and withdrawing life-sustaining treatment: ethically equivalent? *Am. J. Bioeth.* 2019; **19**: 10–20.

8. Welie J. V., Ten Have H. A. The ethics of forgoing life-sustaining treatment: theoretical considerations and clinical decision making. *Multidiscip. Respir. Med.* 2014; **9**: 14.

9. Wilkinson D., Savulescu J. A costly separation between withdrawing and withholding treatment in intensive care. *Bioethics* 2014; **28**: 127–37.

10. Schaller C., Kessler M. On the difficulty of neurosurgical end of life decisions. *J. Med. Ethics* 2006; **32**: 65–9.

11. Carrier E. R., Reschovsky J. D., Mello M. M., et al. Physicians' fears of malpractice lawsuits are not assuaged by tort reforms. *Health Aff. (Millwood)* 2010; **29**: 1585–92.

Chapter

6

Surgical Training

Magnus Tisell and Naci Balak

6.1 Introduction

To advance the standard of neurosurgical practice, neurosurgeons who work in teaching institutions have a duty to educate postgraduate trainees or residents in neurosurgery and generously pass on their skills to ensure that future generations will further improve on them.[1] In addition, trainees are expected to respond with finely tuned respect and compassion to the needs and personal integrity of their patients, placing these above their own self-interest.[2] They should also be aware of their responsibilities towards patients, society, and the medical profession and be committed to ongoing professional development. However, there are various factors in the life of neurosurgical residents that compete within education, including research, didactic lectures, applications, teaching, department leadership, family responsibilities, and lifestyles.[3] Ethical dilemmas arise when these obligations come into conflict with each other during surgical training.[3] At this point, educators must seek to achieve a balance between optimal learner education and careful growth of learner autonomy on the one hand and the safety of the patient on the other.[4]

Professionalism is central to all medical education, and the objective of teaching is to internalize the value system of the medical profession to ensure the socially and ethically responsible delivery of care.[5,6] In their future careers, residents will face difficult ethical issues in terms of limitations of resources, inadequate knowledge for decision-making, introduction of new commercial technologies, and a surgical environment that is becoming increasingly institutionalized.[5] Humane and professional care implies responsibility not only to the patients but also to the families of patients and to the team, including attending physicians, fellows, residents, students, nurses, and ancillary staff.[3,6]

6.2 Background Information

Since the time of Hippocrates of Kos (460–370 BC), the profession of medicine has adhered to a code of ethics which underpins practice.[6,7] Medical ethics education has been operating in different forms with the common goals of cultivating virtuous physicians and providing physicians-in-training with the tools to deal with ethical dilemmas they encounter.[2] In 1957 R. K. Merton stated that the task of medical education is to 'shape the novice into the effective practitioner of medicine, to give him the best available knowledge and skills, and to provide him with a professional identity'.[6] M. J. Newton (1986) encouraged ethical education to achieve the analytical skills needed to make ethical judgements when faced with moral ambiguity, where there is no clear-cut right or wrong answer, and where there are limits to rules and codes of morality.[2] In 1994 Frederic Hafferty and Ronald Franks described the teaching of ethics as the 'magic bullet' for the 1990s.[5] This was mainly a response to social controversies surrounding the medical profession, such as radiation experiments performed on children in the 1950s, the view of the patient as a consumer, and information regarding the inmates of concentration camps in World War II.[5] They maintained that 'ethics didactics do little to counter these flaws, lapses, or perversions in ethical behaviour'. Far more effective is the moral culture handed down from physician to resident, the cultural inheritance that they consider to be 'the lynchpin of medical education'.[5]

M. T. Downing et al. (1997) questioned all programme directors of accredited general surgery residencies in the United States.[2,8] They found that 28% offered no formal ethics education, 48% held one teaching event in ethics, and only 24% conducted two or more activities.[2,8] However, it was noteworthy that the majority of them (85%) supported having an ethics curriculum. Medical ethicists were employed in more than half (56%) of programmes at primary teaching hospitals, and in 35% of the programmes at least one member of the surgical faculty had either training or a special interest in ethics.[2] Moral enculturation is an integrated part of the surgical training culture as emphasized by Bosk in 2003.[5] Kodner went further and argued for an ethics curriculum in the training of surgeons throughout 'progressive stages of surgical life', which range from those in surgical training, to experienced surgeons with decades of experience.[2,5] Later, M. A. Escobar and L. B. McCullough (2005) outlined a proposed framework for didactic and practice activity in surgical training.[2,3] They proposed that surgical residency programme leaders should emphasize two nonnegotiable goods for residents (professional formation as a fiduciary physician and achievement of the educational goal of becoming a competent surgeon) and one nonnegotiable good for patients (respect for their autonomy).[2,3]

6.3 Current Evidence

6.3.1 Patient Safety in Neurosurgery

Surgical safety is a global healthcare issue, and teaching about surgical safety is important because unsafe surgical practice results in increased patient mortality and morbidity, legal claims against surgeons, and distrust of physicians.[9] Neurosurgery is one of the most demanding branches of medicine, with high-risk procedures. Therefore, independent practice by trainees is not possible, and supervision must be maintained to ensure patient safety while at the same time providing educational experience for residents.[10] The literature of the results of resident surgery is conflicting. Some studies report outcomes for surgery by residents to be as good as for surgery by the fully trained surgeon, while others show a higher risk of serious complications, reoperation, infection, and longer hospitalization after surgery performed by residents.[2,8]

Requirements of the training programme should include the development of treatment plans and their alternatives, interaction with patients, and participation in surgical procedures as far as trainee ability allows. These should all be carefully graded so that trainees progressively acquire ever greater independence.[10] Furthermore, it must remembered that competency cannot be equated with mastery; rather, it is the ability of an individual trainee to perform all aspects of patient care as well as his or her peers, without endangering the patient.[10] A Joint Committee of the European Union of Medical Specialists (UEMS) and the European Association of Neurosurgical Societies (EANS) published a guidebook titled *Training in Neurosurgery in the Countries of the EU: A Guide to Organize a Training Programme* and described a competent physician as having the knowledge, surgical techniques, and patient management skills adequate to practice independent neurosurgery, being prepared for lifetime learning, and being prepared to mature to expert and master of the field over the next 10 to 20 years.[10]

6.3.2 Professionalism in the Ideal Curriculum

The competent practice of medicine requires certain behavioural patterns, commonly termed professionalism.[10] The Accreditation Council on Graduate Medical Education (ACGME) defines the professionalism of residents as performance of professional responsibilities; observance of ethical principles, including those relating to the provision or withholding of clinical care; sensitivity to patient diversity, including culture, age, gender, and disabilities; confidentiality of patient information; informed consent; and business practice.[2] The ACGME and the American Board of Medical Specialties (ABMS) have prescribed professionalism as one of the six core competencies (medical knowledge, patient care, practice-based learning and improvement, interpersonal and communication skills, professionalism, and system-based practice) that must be attained and sustained by all doctors practicing in the United States, including residents.[7] Subsequently, it is essential to promote an attitude of a high level of professional conduct and ethics within the training programme, including the director, the trainers, and the trainees.[10] Included in professional conduct and ethics are relations with and commitment to patients, relations with peers, the meeting of standards of documentation, personal conduct that does not compromise patient care, and a dedication to lifelong learning. There is clear evidence that students and residents who fail to conform to standards of professional behaviour will commonly go on to experience difficulties in practice and will often be subjected to disciplinary procedures.[10]

The Joint Residency Advisory and Accreditation Committee (JRAAC) provides advice and support to those involved in the organization of neurosurgical education, including teaching in ethics and periodic progress assessment to ensure continuing progress in the trainee's professional conduct and ethics, alongside other knowledge and skills throughout training.[10] An ideal curriculum includes the teaching of professionalism for neurosurgical trainees to become good doctors, good colleagues, and exemplary human beings. This is most commonly done informally through the examples and role models of virtuous mentors; however, many aspects of professionalism can also be taught and discussed in a formal way. Such aspects include the doctor-patient relationship, appropriate conduct of medical research, valid study design and research, responsible medical writing and speech, communication with patients, precise and critical reading and thinking, dealing with conflicts of interest, relations with peers, quality assurance and outcomes assessment, and physician impairment and discipline.[10]

6.3.3 Ethics Training in Neurosurgery

In many countries, surgical residents are facing work-hour restrictions limiting training time, while at the same time, neurosurgical care is becoming more complicated.[2] It is hard to fit all training into the curriculum. Nevertheless, as has been stressed by several authors, continuous ethical training during residency is as important as training in technical clinical skills.[2,3] In order to ensure that graduates have acquired the skills needed to practice safely and independently, trainee performance should be evaluated in a rigorous and consistent manner.[11] Ideally, resident ethics education will provide the tools to handle ethical problems as they arise.[5] Without any previous training, emergence as a fully fledged ethical agent on the day of board certification is highly unlikely. In a strict hierarchic system, there is a risk that residents cannot grasp ethical issues because they just do as they are told. The training environment should be open to ethical discussions; it can even imply a questioning of the clinical decisions of senior surgeons. For this purpose, EANS training courses include ethical discussion groups in all parts of the four-year cycle. For example, it has been decided in Sweden that the oral examination should contain ethical discussions.

There is wide support for professionalism training in the literature, and the need for a formal ethics curriculum has been acknowledged by several surgical societies in Canada, the United States, and the United Kingdom.[2,7,8,12] So-called boot-camp courses in some general surgery and neurosurgery programmes include professionalism training.[7] In spite of these recommendations, thorough skills training and assessment in ethics are not routinely integrated into the didactic curricula in the majority of surgery residencies in many countries, despite the fact that ethics education is almost universally a part of undergraduate medical school curricula.[2] The so-called implicit curriculum and learning through role modelling are common and potentially effective methods of teaching ethics in residency training, but are dependent on the individual teaching physicians and their time, knowledge, and desire to educate residents on ethical issues.[2] The obvious weakness of the implicit or informal curriculum is the lack of structure and evaluation.[2] If, on the other hand, ethics education is systematically integrated into surgical residency curricula, there might be improved knowledge and confidence in handling ethical dilemmas, and subsequently improved patient care.[2] This was the finding of a randomized study into internal medicine at the Johns Hopkins Hospital in 1993, in which residents were randomized to participate in either a lecture-based curriculum, an integrated lecture/case-based curriculum, or a control group that received no specific ethics education. The result of this study demonstrated that the residents who received integrated ethical training performed better.[8]

6.4 Ethical Issues

6.4.1 Surgery by Residents

An operation starts with the indication, and it is a part of ethical training to contemplate the ethical consequences as well as the medical outcome of surgery. It is estimated that throughout the world, between 30% and 70% of surgical operations are unnecessary.[13] The resident might have a tendency to overlook indications in their eagerness to master the technical skills of surgery, but training needs should never constitute a bias towards surgery.[13] Nevertheless, training during neurosurgical care necessarily implies that patients, to varying degrees, will be exposed to less-experienced physicians. If all patients were operated on only by the most-experienced surgeons, the education of future neurosurgeons would be seriously hampered. An inability to pass knowledge on to younger colleagues would, in fact, have negative consequences for future patients. In relation to training, the Hippocratic oath states, 'I will teach them my art without reward or agreement; and I will impart all my acquirement, instructions, and whatever I know, to my master's children, as to my own; and likewise to all my pupils.' However, the mentor has the difficult task of balancing what is best for the surgical trainee against what is best for the individual patient.[14]

Another problem besides the medical outcome is that surgery performed by less-experienced residents is usually more time-consuming, which implies that fewer patients can be treated during the same time period. On the other hand, some patients undergoing less complicated surgery could benefit from greater attention from the trainee than might be received from a preoccupied senior neurosurgeon who is focused on more complicated cases. In fact, the best teaching improves the teacher as well as the students, and there is also a well-recognized cross-fertilization between clinic, research, and education in academic institutions.

The surgical skills of residents can be examined in two ways as technical and non-technical skills. To deal with the ethical dilemma of training, the structure, documentation, and evaluation of both technical and non-technical parts of the surgical training are crucial.[11] Four categories of deficiencies in non-technical skills have been identified: deficiencies in forward planning, self-direction, situation awareness, and patient safety (including judgement).[11] Forward planning is described as 'the ability to anticipate needs, to think ahead and to set up the operative field in an optimum fashion'.[11] Self-direction refers to trainee demeanour. It includes the ability to behave in a professional manner, remain focused and undistracted, and slow down when necessary. Non-technical skills also encompass acceptance of and response to feedback.[11] The shift from routine technical behaviour to analytic, reflective behaviour is taught by modelling, slowing down, or halting the progress of an operation when a critical point arises, so that this behaviour eventually becomes automatic to the trainee.[11] Factors that may impede this shift include fatigue, overconfidence, problems in team management and communication, distractions, and time constraints.[11]

Many studies show that unprofessional behaviours are a contributing factor in medical errors, low patient satisfaction, adverse outcomes, and higher care costs.[11] Furthermore, a failure to address these issues has a negative effect on the morale of trainee colleagues who are expected to cover for the lapses of others. Indeed, these behaviours may have such a detrimental effect on morale that colleagues are pushed to seek new positions in more professional environments.[11] Unprofessional behaviour has been defined as 'behaviour that undermines a culture of safety'. Unfortunately, the evaluation and remediation of such behaviour are frequently hampered by a system that enables and even rewards such actions.[11] For example, staff will often avoid paging uncooperative, hostile trainees, so that bad behaviour is 'rewarded' by the unprofessional individual being left undisturbed.[11] Furthermore, if consultants shout or bully in order to achieve their goals, trainees will understand this to be acceptable professional behaviour.[11]

T. J. Kennedy et al. (2008) identified four factors that influence supervisor perception of trainee trustworthiness: skill and knowledge, awareness of limitations, truthfulness, and conscientiousness.[11] Of these, the least important was knowledge, and yet knowledge is evaluated more often than the other attributes.[11] Identifying problems with professionalism is hindered by a lack of clearly defined standards for achievement and by a 'halo effect' whereby deficiencies in one area are overlooked because of excellence in another.[11] For example, there may be a tolerance of instances of unprofessionalism in a popular, highly technically skilled trainee.[11] Regarding feedback, the insightful individual who recognizes learning opportunities is most likely to benefit and improve, whereas an increasingly argumentative, defensive response is indicative of an inflexible mindset that will be difficult to remediate.[11]

6.4.2 Laboratory Training and Use of Simulators

One strategy to decrease the potential risk of training for the safety of patients is an increased use of simulation and laboratory exercises, including cadavers. However, learning by real-life surgery on humans still dominates neurosurgical training, despite efforts to develop simulators. Moreover, the number of procedures performed as documented in the logbook is still the most common way to estimate competence.[10] In contrast, a pilot in aviation can be fully trained in a simulator and fly the real plane competently on his or her first flight. The evolution of comparable neurosurgical simulators could lead to a major improvement in residency training and patient safety, and be a valuable tool in competency-based assessment.[10,12] Large randomized controlled prospective studies are needed to validate the degree of translation from simulation model to patient.[4] If simulation is shown to be valuable in such studies, it might be unethical not to use them in future training to increase patient safety.[4]

In modern medical training, ethical issues can also be simulated with actors in patient interactions, addressing nontechnical areas as communication, teamwork, judgement, and leadership, corresponding to core competencies that the ACGME has laid out for resident evaluation.[4] Simulation has been integrated into professionalism curricula in various forms and settings.[12] Reviews and guidelines in professional societies advocate a role for simulation in the integration of professionalism into medical education. However, approaches and practical details for the accomplishment of this have not been addressed.[12] Simulations that encompass the ACGME competencies can be done in various ways – for example, using a high-fidelity patient mannequin, using simulated patient emails, through simulation-based courses or workshops.[12] From a patient's perspective, simulation training in the laboratory reduces their exposure to physicians who are less experienced and provides quality care that focuses on their needs and is not compromised by training requirements.[11] While some remediation strategies will be expensive in faculty time commitment, the cost to patients is far greater if they are not implemented and unsafe trainees are allowed to graduate and practice unsupervised.[11]

6.4.3 Informed Consent

Respect for the autonomy of the patient is a nonnegotiable subject, even in the process of education. A cognitive well-functioning patient should choose a planned treatment on the base of information from his/her surgeon. Ideally, this information should not differ from surgeon to surgeon. But high-level evidence often is missing for the decision-making, and it is inevitable that the guidance may be influenced by a non-scientific bias such as the personal experience of the surgeon, the religious and cultural values of the patient, and the economic concerns of all involved parties.[5] In the absence of hard scientific facts, a trainee should learn to be aware of the base of his or her clinical decisions and their ethical implications.[5] According to the American Medical Association's Code of Medical Ethics: 'With the consent of the patient, it is not unethical for the operating surgeon to delegate the performance of certain aspects of the operation to the assistant provided this is done under the surgeon's participatory supervision.'[14]

6.4.4 Technology-Associated Ethical Issues in Training

The rapid technical development of the neurosurgical field involving commercial medical companies also raises new ethical questions.[5] Ethical training might prepare the surgeon for new conflicts of interest.[5] Training per se might contain ethical dilemmas in the balance between learning surgery and the safety of the patient.[5] Scientific evidence of patient benefit from surgical equipment is often much less proven than medical treatment. However, it is critical to consider how to deal with new techniques and their marketing, the role of cadaver training, and the moral obligation to critically evaluate new methods and equipment.[5] M. G. Yaşargil (1999), the father of microneurosurgery, emphasized that to cope with ongoing gratifying and beneficial innovations in scientific technological developments and to successfully apply them, residents should be *officially obliged* to engage in one year of intense, concentrated study, and practice in the laboratory.[15]

6.4.5 Illustrative Cases

A case management format is structured as follows: participants are sequentially presented, starting with the most typical and continuing to the least usual presentations of any specific disease. Diagnostic possibilities are outlined, prognosis is determined, alternative therapies described, and the outcomes of these therapies are presented; where relevant, moral, ethical, and research issues may be addressed.

Illustrative Clinical Case 1

A 73-year-old male presented with a clinical picture of gait deterioration, dementia, and urinary incontinence in the context of enlarged ventricles on neuroimaging, but normal intracranial pressures. The patient had a previous history of hypertension, diabetes mellitus, and cardiac ischemic disease. The patient was diagnosed as having normal pressure hydrocephalus, and a ventriculo-peritoneal shunt insertion was planned. On the day of surgery, a third-year resident wanted to operate on the patient from skin-to-skin without the supervision of the neurosurgeon, because he felt confident and skilled enough to accomplish this surgery alone. However, the consultant neurosurgeon thought that the patient had several co-morbidities and the possible complications of the shunt surgery were many, including infection, shunt blockage, fracture or disconnection, migration, malposition, intracranial haemorrhage, and viscus perforation. Therefore, he was experiencing difficulty in deciding whether to let the resident perform the surgery alone or not.

Comments: This is an example of the risks of surgical training, showing the role of a senior surgeon in reducing those risks. In some institutions, the least experienced surgeon places shunts; in others, it is the most experienced. One study suggested that there is no difference in the risk of revision between experienced and inexperienced surgeons/residents when there is adequate guidance and surgical protocols.[16] Similar results have been reported by some other authors, whereas other studies have found surgeon experience to be important.[16] It may be argued that in an ideal training situation, the risk of complications should not be increased if the operation is performed by junior doctors under the guidance of senior neurological surgeons.[16]

Illustrative Clinical Case 2

A 55-year-old woman presented with sudden severe headache, nausea and vomiting, and transient loss of consciousness. On examination, there was nuchal rigidity, and a computed tomography showed a subarachnoid haemorrhage. A digital subtraction angiography proved that the patient had a ruptured left middle cerebral artery aneurysm. It was decided to perform an emergency pterional craniotomy and clip the aneurysm. A sixth-year resident was keen to perform the surgery because he thought that he was close to completing his training in neurosurgery. However, the attending neurosurgeon was of the opinion that mortality and morbidity following aneurysm surgery are often related to perforator or large vessel occlusion, brain retraction, and cranial nerve traction injury. Furthermore, intraoperative rupture is seen in 15–20% of cases and is associated with increased neurological morbidity and mortality. Therefore, the neurosurgeon decided to perform the operation himself.

Comments: This is another ethical dilemma in training seen in the course of vascular surgery with difficult aneurysms. Competency in neurosurgical training cannot be equated with mastery in every field or an ability to perform all neurosurgery procedures, no matter how difficult. Rather, competency means that individuals can practice independently while being aware of their own limitations and that they are ready for the ongoing education which will finally lead to mastery in the areas of neurosurgery in which they choose to specialise.[10]

6.5 Future Directions

6.5.1 Integrated Lecture/Case-Based Curriculum in Ethics

For surgeons, problems with ethical implications are not likely to diminish; more likely, they will become more numerous in several broad areas. Challenges to professional integrity will be particularly troublesome as bureaucratic intrusions into the practice of medicine intensify.[17]

Modifying the goal of medical education to focus on professional identity formation is essential.[6] The theoretical underpinnings of the teaching of professionalism and the strategies used should be re-examined.[6] Identity formation should be made explicit, and understanding of identity formation and socialization should be expanded.[6] If the aim of medical training is to produce individuals who have assimilated norms and values, the acquisition of professionalism is a gradual educational process, necessitating appropriately staged individual assessment.[6]

Experience of the introduction of professionalism into the medical curriculum suggests that it is essential that faculty understand the cognitive underpinnings of professionalism and the most appropriate methods of teaching and assessment for their own settings.[6] With the evolution of medicine and society, the details of the social contract change, and thus there is an ongoing renegotiation of the definition of the good physician.[6] Teaching professionalism in surgical residency programmes is a relatively recent development.[18] Traditionally, residents are expected to model and assume the behaviour of the senior faculty.[18] Unfortunately, the senior faculty may demonstrate inconsistent and sometimes antithetical attitudes towards colleagues, residents, medical students, and hospital personnel.[18] With patient satisfaction so much to the fore (including financial incentives), in 2002, the ACGME made teaching professionalism and effective communication a mandatory requirement for the continuation of residency accreditation.[18]

6.5.2 Simulators in Training

There is a promising future for simulators in neurosurgery as they become more effectively representative of real surgery.[4] In the past decade, virtual reality (VR) has been progressively adopted as a primary training tool.[4] As a suitable tool for cognitive task analysis and technical skills training, VR has been begun to play a key role in medical and surgical training in particular.[4] The path for the widespread implementation of VR has been smoothed by the continuing rapid development of medical technology, portable electronic devices, and user-friendly software.[4] The immersive experience of VR with haptic feedback comes close to real-world scenarios and situations.[(4)] 3-D printing is another breakthrough technology that promises to enable future simulation practice with high-fidelity, patient-specific models to complement residency surgical learning.[4]

6.6 Conclusions

To advance the standard of neurosurgical practice, neurosurgeons who work in teaching institutions have a duty to educate the postgraduate trainees or residents and generously pass along their skills to ensure that future generations will be better than themselves. The promotion of an attitude of a high level of professional conduct and ethics within the training programme is essential. Good surgical training focuses on surgical safety. Unsafe surgical practice results in increased patient mortality and morbidity, legal claims against surgeons, and distrust of physicians. If ethics education is systematically integrated into surgical residency curricula, there may be improved knowledge and confidence in handling ethical dilemmas, and subsequently improved patient care. Simulation can be integrated into professionalism curricula in various settings and is a valuable tool in resident training and competency-based assessment.

References

1. Umansky F., Black P. L., DiRocco C., et al. Statement of ethics in neurosurgery of the world federation of neurosurgical societies. *World Neurosurg.* 2011; **76**: 239–47.

2. Helft P. R., Eckles R. E., Torbeck L. Ethics education in surgical residency programs: a review of the literature. *J. Surg. Educ.* 2009; **66**: 35–42.

3. Escobar M. A., McCullough, L. B. Responsibly managing ethical challenges of residency training: a guide for surgery residents, educators, and residency program leaders. *J. Am. Coll. Surg.* 2006; **202**: 531–5.

4. Konakondla S., Fong R., Schirmer C. M. Simulation training in neurosurgery: advances in education and practice. *Adv. Med. Educ. Pract.* 2017; **8**: 465–73.

5. Keune J. D., Kodner I. J. The importance of an ethics curriculum in surgical education. *World J. Surg.* 2014; **38**: 1581–6.

6. Cruess R. L., Cruess S. R., Boudreau J. D., et al. Reframing medical education to support professional identity formation. *Acad. Med.* 2014; **89**: 1446–51.

7. de Blacam C., Vercler C. J. Teaching ethics and professionalism in plastic surgery:

a systematic review. *Ann. Plast. Surg.* 2014; **72**: 484–8.

8. Grossman E., Posner M. C., Angelos P. Ethics education in surgical residency: past, present, and future. *Surgery* 2010; **147**: 114–19.

9. Davis C. R., Bates A. S., Toll E. C., et al. Surgical safety training of world health organization initiatives. *Am. J. Med. Qual.* 2014; **29**: 350–6.

10. Reulen H. J. *Training in Neurosurgery in the Countries of the EU: A Guide to Organize a Training Programme*, Vienna, Springer, 2004.

11. Sanfey H. Assessment of surgical training. *Surgeon* 2014; **12**: 350–6.

12. Wali E., Pinto J. M., Cappaert M., et al. Teaching professionalism in graduate medical education: What is the role of simulation? *Surgery* 2016; **160**: 552–64.

13. Tayade M. C., Dalvi S. D. Fundamental ethical issues in unnecessary surgical procedures. *J. Clin. Diagn. Res.* 2016; **10**: JE01–4.

14. Ohye R. G., Jaggers J. J., Sade R. M. Must surgeons in training programs allow residents to operate on their patients to

satisfy board requirements? *Ann. Thorac. Surg.* 2016; **101**: 18–23.

15. Yasargil M. G. A legacy of microneurosurgery: memoirs, lessons, and axioms. *Neurosurgery* 1999; **45**: 1025–92.

16. Farahmand D., Hilmarsson H., Hogfeldt M., et al. Perioperative risk factors for short term shunt revisions in adult hydrocephalus patients. *J. Neurol. Neurosurg. Psychiatry* 2009; **80**: 1248–53.

17. Sade R. M., Kavarana M. N. Surgical ethics: today and tomorrow. *Future Cardiol.* 2017; **13**: 567–78.

18. Hochberg M. S., Berman R. S., Pachter H. L. Professionalism in surgery: crucial skills for attendings and residents. *Adv. Surg.* 2017; **51**: 229–49.

The Aging Surgeon

Stephen Honeybul and Gene Bolles

7.1 Introduction

Over the past 200 years the average global life expectancy has increased from just over 30 years of age to well over 70 years of age. There are many reasons for this, ranging from the eradication of certain diseases, lifestyle changes, and improvements in public health. As people live longer, they also work longer, and this is reflected in the changing demographic of the workforce. However, notwithstanding this increase in life expectancy, the aging process can take its toll in terms of cognitive and functional decline, which may have an impact on the ability of the older person to perform satisfactorily in the workplace. Where this involves physicians and surgeons, there is obvious concern for patient safety.

7.2 Background Information

7.2.1 The Aging Process

In previous years, health-related withdrawal from the workplace was more often as a result of catastrophic life-changing or life-ending events, such as a stroke, myocardial infarct, or a severe infective process. However, as life expectancy has increased, the pattern of aging has changed such that there is a slow, often insidious deterioration of multiple physiological and neurocognitive processes that can have a variable impact on a person's workplace performance.

This decline may at first be merely a reflection of impairment of sensory perception, such as hearing loss, deterioration in visual acuity and depth perception, reduction in tactile sensitivity, loss of strength, and impairment of manual dexterity.[1] It may also be associated with a neurocognitive decline that may reduce the ability to maintain focus over a prolonged period of time and reduce the ability to process and correlate information.

Several studies have demonstrated that as physicians age, crystallized intelligence, which measures knowledge accumulated over time, is relatively well preserved. However, there is a significant decline in fluid intelligence, which involves adaptive thinking, reasoning, and information processing. An example of this would be negotiating a maze or overcoming first impressions of a problem by recognizing that alternative solutions are available.[2] It follows from this that habitual memory (performing a regular task) is better preserved than analytical memory (learning a new task).

The combination of a decrease in cognitive speed and short-term memory function may lead to a reduction in reaction times, and this represents a significant problem for surgeons who are often required to handle unexpected and rapidly evolving situations. Neurocognitive deterioration associated with a decline in motor skills and manual dexterity will decrease the ability to learn new movements and reduce the ability to organize and accommodate new information. All these factors may be compounded by the development of age-related diseases involving the cardiovascular, respiratory, gastrointestinal, mental health, excessive use of alcohol, and drug and substance abuse.

The impact that these changes have on aging medical practitioners has been a source of considerable debate, considering the effect that impaired neurocognitive function may have on clinical decision-making and patient care. For surgeons, there are further considerations given the need for prolonged periods of concentration, combined with complex manual dexterity and neurocognitive requirements to adapt to an evolving surgical environment when unexpected intraoperative surgical problems occur.

However, notwithstanding the results of numerous studies that have investigated these issues among physicians and surgeons, one of the key findings is the great variability in the individual aging process. In addition, there are some aspects of neurocognition that are relatively well preserved, such as semantic memory, which comprises factual knowledge and its application, verbal skills, and long-term memory. It has also been demonstrated that older adults can perform as well as young adults in certain occupationally relevant tasks, such as typing, piano playing, and aviation simulation, despite evidence of age-related decline in basic cognitive, perceptual, and motor abilities. Finally, it has been demonstrated that a cognitively enriched lifestyle (which presumably includes a surgical environment) can influence intellectual development and attenuate cognitive decline.[2]

The impact that all of these issues have on the individual aging surgeon's ability to function satisfactorily in the workplace will obviously vary; however, these are important considerations, given the increasingly aged surgical workforce.

7.2.2 Aging and the Surgical Workforce

Over the past four decades, the number of aged doctors has increased substantially. In the United States, the number of practicing physicians has more than quadrupled, and one-third of surgeons are older than 55 years of age. Twenty-five per cent of surgeons are older than 65 years of age, and in 2014 there were between 99,500 and 100,000 surgeons still practicing into their 70s. In Canada, 17.6% of practicing surgeons are older than 65 years of age, and in Australia, 19% of active surgeons are older than 65 years of age. It is likely that these numbers will increase in the years to come. In fact, it is estimated that in the next 10 years, more than one-third of all active physicians within the United States will be older than 65 years of age.

7.2.3 The Changing Face of Clinical Practice

For many aging surgeons, the clinical practice of today is vastly different from the clinical practice when they were training. Most surgeons in their mid-60s entered solo practice as a consultant more than 30 years ago, and since then many techniques have been considerably modified, abandoned, or replaced. A good example would come from the management of femoral fractures in orthopaedic surgery. These used to be treated with six weeks of traction followed by another six weeks in a plaster cast. This management was replaced with various plating techniques, which were subsequently abandoned with the introduction of intramedullary nailing. In the field of neurosurgery, there have been similar modifications with the instruction of the operating microscope, image guidance techniques, radiological advances, and intraoperative MRI, to name but a few. The development, introduction, and refinement of each technological advance require the older surgeon to learn and incorporate them into their practice, and the neuropsychological changes that come with aging can make this challenging. The increasingly rapid pace of technological advances that are occurring now means that the young surgeon entering clinical practice is likely to face an ever-evolving surgical landscape in the future, and the challenge they face will be keeping up.

7.3 Current Evidence

In the evaluation of clinical outcome, the development of performance metrics has become a central focus across all aspects of medical practice. Anecdotally, many publications on aging and surgical competence have described examples of a surgeon clearly practicing in a situation where their surgical competency is compromised. A historical example of this is that of Ferdinand Sauerbruch (1875–1951).[3] He was a world-renowned surgeon who attracted many students and patients to his clinics and operating theatres at the Charite Hospital in Berlin. In his late 60s, however, he was noted to visibly deteriorate. He 'had sudden changes in mood and periods of forgetfulness'. He 'struck assistants with instruments during operations', and his surgery was performed with 'growing clumsiness, dragging tissues and tearing blood vessels'.

Because he was so famous, his faculty failed to act, and suggestions by friends and colleagues that he should retire were flatly refused. He continued operating with increasing severe complications, and it was only when he was threatened with public humiliation that he relented at the age of 74 and resigned from hospital practice. Even then, he had little insight into the severity of his decline, as he continued to operate at his home with apparently disastrous results.

This type of anecdotal evidence and the fear that there are similar cases in contemporary practice has led many studies to be conducted investigating surgical performance in aging surgeons. The general impression created by many of these studies is that there is a significant neurocognitive decline on the aging surgical workforce, and this is not only measurable but is also leading to worse clinical outcomes and an increase in surgical mortality.[4]

7.3.1 Evidence Supporting Aging Effects on Medical Practice

There is anecdotal evidence and some published evidence that older practitioners can pose a potential risk for patient safety. In the early 2000s a number of studies suggested that more experienced physicians and surgeons may have paradoxically worse clinical outcomes. Hartz et al. found that mortality rates of older surgeons performing coronary artery bypass grafts were higher than younger surgeons.[5] O'Neill et al. found a similar higher mortality in patients having carotid endarterectomy.[6] Waljee et al. examined the Medicare files of a large cohort of surgical patients between 1998 and 1999 and found that mortality for certain procedure (pancreatectomy, coronary artery bypass grafts, and carotid artery arterectomy) was higher among older surgeons, but the difference was small and was limited to surgeons with low procedural volumes.[7] Interestingly, this study found no difference in mortality for oesophagectomy, cystectomy, lung resection, aortic valve replacement, or aortic aneurysm repair. The study concluded that the age of the surgeon was a factor for certain complex procedures with low volume but not for most procedures. In a systematic review of 62 studies, more than half suggested that physician performance for all outcomes declines with increasing age.[4]

Finally, in a larger more recent study by Tsugawa, 736,537 admissions managed by 18,854 hospital physicians were reviewed.[8] Assessments included 30-day mortality rate, re-admissions, and cost of care. They found that physicians under the age of 40 had a 10.8% mortality rate, which increased to 11.1% for patients with physicians in their 40s, 11.3% for physicians in their 50s, and 12.1 for physicians older than the age of 60. These findings were adjusted for patients' illness severity and would seem to confirm that patients treated by older physicians had a higher mortality rate than patients cared for by those who were younger. However, notwithstanding these results, one of the most interesting findings of this study was that although physicians who treated low to medium volumes of patients had higher mortality rates, physicians who treated high volumes of patients had the same mortality across all age groups. The implications of this finding and its relevance to clinical practice are difficult to determine. It could be that treating a high volume of clinical cases is protective of clinical skills; however, it could equally be the case that physicians are treating a large volume of cases because they are maintaining their clinical skills. Likewise, the association between practice volume and clinical skills could be bidirectional. Physicians whose skills are declining might elect or be encouraged to treat progressively fewer patients over time.[8]

The authors of this study stated that the results should be regarded as exploratory and acknowledged that there were some limitations in that this was an observational study which could not fully account for unmeasured confounders. In addition, while mortality can be used as a performance indicator, it is only a surrogate marker for clinical performance.

However, notwithstanding these limitations and acknowledging that there is now good evidence that aging can affect clinical performance, the results of this study serve to high-light that this decline is not uniform and that certain physicians appear to maintain their clinical skills despite their age. The implications for surgical practice are difficult to determine; however, they do help guide the ethical discussion regarding aging and main-tenance of clinical skills.

7.4 Ethical Issues

The findings of the Tsugawa study may in some ways be reassuring, and it would be useful to repeat the study in the surgical workforce. While it was demonstrated that some older physicians are still able to clinically perform safely and effectively into their 60s and 70s, if they maintain a high volume of cases, surgeons are not immune to the aging process. Physical and neurocognitive decline are inevitable, and there will have to come a time when a surgeon must consider either retirement or a significant alteration in their practice.

Overall, there is unlikely to be a simple, one-size-fits-all solution to the complex issue of cessation of a safe surgical practice; however, there appears to be three broad categories that require consideration. The largest group will consist of those surgeons who recognize that they are in some shape or form beginning to struggle with certain aspects of the aging process, and they have insight into the need to either retire or modify their practice accordingly. The second group appears to be a relatively small but significant number of surgeons who appear largely unaffected by the aging process and who continue to practice at a competent level well beyond the time most of their contemporaries have retired. The final group will hopefully be a very small number of surgeons who are aging and losing their capability to practice safely; however, they have limited insight regarding the clinical implications for ongoing practice.

7.4.1 Retirement

The concept of retirement was first introduced in Germany in 1889, and the retirement age was set at 70 years of age. However, in those days, very few people lived long enough to claim the benefit. Today, the statutory retirement age varies considerably around the world, and relatively few professions have mandatory retirement ages. Commercial airline pilots face a mandatory retirement at 60 years of age, and there are mandatory retirement ages in the United States for FBI personnel, fire fighters, national park rangers, air traffic controllers, lighthouse operators, couriers of nuclear materials, and customs/border protection officers. In Britain, surgeons are required to retire from public practice at 65 years of age and from private practice at 70 years of age; however, worldwide there are relatively few countries that mandate retirement from surgical practice based on age. Indeed, notwithstanding the aforementioned examples, in the United States, mandated retirement on age alone is illegal based on the Age Discrimination in Employment Act of 1967.

For surgeons, the decision to retire may be difficult, especially when it is based on an individual's insight into their capacity to continue to participate in a practice that has formed one of the focal points of their adult life. Given the nature of surgical practice, many surgeons come to view their sense of self value in their ability to continue to perform surgery, and this forms an integral part of their self-esteem. The often all-consuming role comes with significant responsibility, and an individual may either not recognize or not want to recognize that they are beginning to fail in their often central role in a particular institution.

For many years, surgeons seemed to manage retirement by removing themselves from the workforce on a gradual basis over a number of years or at a fixed timepoint when they formally withdraw from all clinical activity. It is only in the past two to three decades that there has been a substantial increase in the number of aged surgeons, and in general, contemporary surgeons are poor at planning for retirement. This was demonstrated by a recent survey in Australia indicating that a third of older doctors have made no plans to retire.

Given the enormous amount of planning that is required when entering the surgical workplace (involving initial entry into medical school, specialist training, and ongoing accreditation) and given the relatively recent trend towards later retirement, the time may have come to recognize that a similarly planned approach may be needed to assist surgeons withdrawing from the workforce – hopefully an approach to leaving practice that involves considerably less stress and anxiety than when entering.

In Australia, the Royal Australia College of Surgeons (RACS) has changed its continuing professional development (CPD) regulations to require aging surgeons to have their own GP and to undergo regular health checks. The RACS has also modified the performance requirements for CPD of aging surgeons in order to help identify surgeons who are either performing poorly or, perhaps more importantly, who are at risk of poor performance. The American Medical Association has agreed to recommend guidelines to assess the physical, cognitive, and mental health of older physicians, and there are similar moves in many countries, where it is being increasingly recognized that with aging comes the need to monitor performance.

However, notwithstanding the need for legislation, what is really required is a change in culture among surgeons, such that planning for retirement starts early and takes into account not only financial planning but also recreational and intellectual planning. In general, surgeons are highly motivated and goal orientated, and these characteristics are unlikely to diminish with age. Retirement from surgical practice does not necessarily mean removal from the medical workforce, and there are many avenues available whereby a surgeon can preserve links with their surgical colleagues. Likewise, planning early for retirement will enable surgeons to develop new interests well away from the surgical practice, which is equally important given that currently, many retirees are likely to be alive for a further 20 to 30 years.

7.4.2 The Aging Safe Surgeon and the Aging Unsafe Surgeon

There would appear to be little doubt that some surgeons seem genuinely immune to the aging process and that to mandate a specific retirement age would clearly be a waste of a valuable resource in the surgical workforce. There is also little doubt that surgeons are not immune to the effects of aging, and there will have to come a time when even the most resilient will find that their clinical competency begins to decline. Most older surgeons generally fail or begin to fail as a result of biological decline, rather than wilful misconduct, and this decline tends to occur almost imperceptibly over several years and may manifest in a variety of ways. Unfortunately, these issues often come to the fore up after a patient suffers a disastrous consequence or sentinel event, which may of course be entirely unrelated to a surgeon's age. Complications and their management are an integral part of surgical practice; however, for the aging surgeon, the problem will be defending their position by demonstrating an objective assessment of surgical competence.

Most organizations and hospital policies require surgeons to have some form of continued medical education; however, the requirements for watching and policing are not particularly rigorous. In addition, surgical specialties require varying degrees of recertification, but those processes are usually relatively easy when compared with the initial certification process and seldom involve a physical and cognitive evaluation.

Many healthcare systems have implemented a mandatory protocol to report colleagues who are felt to be impaired in any fashion; however, the peer review process has significant limitations. It has been shown that physicians may report a colleague whose performance was impaired due to substance abuse, but they are far less likely to report a colleague who they felt was showing signs of cognitive decline or psychological impairment.[9] The obvious problem is that these changes are often slow and insidious and may only be observed by those who are close to the subject. They may have known that person for many years and will be understandably reluctant to raise an issue that has potentially career-ending implications.

Several organizations have codes of ethics that relate to the aging surgeon, and a report by the Council of Medical Education stated that 'physicians should be allowed to remain in practice as long as patient safety is not endangered and that, if needed, remediation should be a supportive, ongoing and proactive process'.[10] It is recommended that self-regulation is an important aspect of this; however, this comes back to the essence of the problem in that self-regulation is not dependable and this process will fail precisely those surgeons to whom it should be targeted. This is called *anosognosia*, which is a term that describes a deficit of self-awareness.[11]

If most surgeons fail because of a slow biological decline, of which some may be unaware, measures must be put in place that can detect this decline in order to protect not only the patients and the general public, but also the surgical profession, and this must be the focus of future directions.

7.5 Future Directions

It is being increasingly recognized that some sort of ongoing assessment must be in place not only to protect patients but also to maintain public confidence. Given the increasing age of the surgical workforce, the question of maintaining competence will become increasingly important in order to protect patients, maintain public confidence, and prevent legislation that would mandate retirement at a particular age. In most jurisdictions, the subspecialty boards of the respective surgical colleges are responsible for assessing suitability for entrance into surgical practice; however, they generally have limited impact on the ongoing assessment of surgical practice. There are also national regulatory bodies such as AHPRA (Australian Health Practitioner Regulatory Agency) in Australia, the American Medical Association, and the American Surgical Association, along with many others that address rules and regulations. In the United States, there are 50 state medical boards that are responsible for quality assurance and for discipline or suspension of incompetent physicians. However, each board operates differently, and each are independent of each other.

While these legislative bodies provide useful protection for the public from poorly performing practitioners, they do not provide a uniform means of ongoing assessment of competence that can protect the aging practitioner. What is really needed is some uniform measure of surgical competence that determines a surgeon is cognitively, mentally, and physically able, with the ongoing manual dexterity to perform their craft.

An objective measure of surgical competence may be used to determine that surgeons are at the stage in their career where they should consider either modifying or stopping their practice because the aging process may be beginning to affect their neurocognitive or physical function. This is much kinder approach, rather than waiting for a catastrophic deterioration. Likewise, an objective measure may be used to support ongoing participation in surgery and may protect against unfounded allegations of age-related incompetence in the event of a surgical complication.

Currently there is no specific neurocognitive or physical testing available, although in some jurisdictions there are moves to develop recertification that must be conducted on a regular basis once a surgeon gets beyond a certain age. In Australia there is a move towards revalidation, which is aimed at being complementary to retirement planning. While this is a work in process, the aim of the process would be to involve doctors having to regularly show that they are up to date and fit to practice medicine. This is consistent with the continuing professional development program of the Royal Australasian College of Surgeons, which includes a modified performance requirement for aging surgeons. The aim is to proactively identify doctors who are either poor performers or at risk of poor performance, and this would have the potential to assist older surgeons in gradually stepping down from practice by reducing hours, modifying their responsibilities, and eventually ceasing practice altogether.

In the United States, an alternative to revalidation is the Aging Surgeon programme.[12] This is a two-day comprehensive, multidisciplinary, objective, and confidential evaluation of a surgeon's physical and cognitive function that opened at Sinai Hospital in Baltimore in 2014. The aim of this assessment programme is to protect surgeons from arbitrary or unreliable methods of assessing competence or cognitive capacity; identify treatable or reversible disorders; aid the surgeon in the decision to retire; protect patients from unsafe surgeons; protect surgeons and hospitals from liability risk; and provide objective, comprehensive, unbiased evaluation. The result of the evaluation is sent to the individual who contracted and paid for the programme (likely a chief of surgery or the surgeon themselves), and the report includes only objective findings. Decisions regarding the application of the results to lifestyle changes or retirement are left to those who receive the report. Indications for attending an evaluation are variable but may include surgeons older than 70 years, a recredentialing cycle, a sentinel event, worrisome practice, or at the discretion of the chief of surgery.

The instruction and implementation of these types of programmes will require significant resources and are not without problems. A similar policy initiated at Sandford led to considerable controversy and objection, which resulted in the cognitive part of the programme being removed.

7.5.1 Neurosurgery-Specific Implications for the Aging Surgeon

Notwithstanding these difficulties, it is increasingly apparent that some form of uniform assessment is required if the trend towards later retirement continues. The issues are ever more apparent in the field of neurosurgery because of the significant implications for surgical practice. Performing neurosurgery can be likened to walking along a plank of wood six inches in width – fairly easy. For neurosurgery, that same plank of wood is now 100 metres in the air with no safety net. The implications for failure certainly focus the attention, because in the field of neurosurgery, most procedures are relatively high risk with a very high price to pay for surgical failure.

It is important that the profession is seen to be maintaining due governance in order to prevent blanket legislation that mandates age-related retirement that would not serve public or professional interests.

7.6 Conclusion

There is no doubt that with age comes experience, knowledge, and wisdom in the practice of medicine, both non-operative and operative. However, there is equally little doubt that the effects of aging have been shown to be a reality in some surgeons such that the deterioration of physical, mental, and cognitive functions has a negative effect on patient safety.

As surgeons continue to practice into their later years, some sort of objective evaluation of functional age is becoming increasingly important, in order to balance the dignity of committed surgical practitioners and their ongoing value to society against patient safety and the risk of ending a successful surgical career with a tarnished reputation. It is important that the surgical community develops and implements these assessments in order to make them relevant and reproducible and prevent a mandated retirement based on age.

References

1. Greenfield L. J., Proctor M. C. When should a surgeon retire? *Adv. Surg.* 1999; **32**; 385–93.

2. Eva K. W. The aging physician: changes in cognitive processing and their impact on medical practice. *Acad. Med.* 2002; **77**(10 Suppl): S1–6.

3. Cherian S. M., Nikas K., Lord R. S. Ernst Ferdinand Sauerbruch: rise and fall of the pioneer of thoracic surgery. *World J. Surg.* 2001; **25**: 1012–20.

4. Choudhry N. K., Fletcher R. H., Soumerai S. B. Systematic review: the relationship between clinical experience and quality of health care. *Ann. Intern. Med.* 2005; **142**: 260–73.

5. Hartz A. J., Kuhn E. M., Pulido J. Prestige of training programs and experience of bypass surgeons as factors in adjusted patient mortality rates. *Med. Care* 1999; **37**: 93–103.

6. O'Neill L., Lanska D. J., Hartz A. Surgeon characteristics associated with mortality and morbidity following carotid endarterectomy. *Neurology* 2000; **55**: 773–81.

7. Waljee J. F., Greenfield L. J., Dimick J. B., et al. Surgeon age and operative mortality in the United States. *Ann. Surg.* 2006; **244**: 353–62.

8. Tsugawa Y., Newhouse J. P., Zaslavsky A. M., et al. Physician age and outcomes in elderly patients in hospital in the US: observational study. *BMJ* 2017; **357**; j1797.

9. DesRoches C. M., Rao S. R., Fromson J. A., et al. Physicians' perceptions, preparedness or reporting, and experiences related to impaired and incompetent colleagues. *JAMA* 2010; **304**: 187–93.

10. American Medical Association. Report of the Council of Medical Education, Report 5, Competency and the Aging Physician. 2015. Available at: www.cppph.org/wp-content/uploads/2016/02/AMA-Council-on-Medical-Education-Aging-Physician-Report-2015.pdf.

11. Ries M. L., Jabbar B. M., Schmitz T. W., et al. Anosognosia in mild cognitive impairment: Relationship to activation of cortical midline structures involved in self-appraisal. *J. Int. Neuropsychol. Soc.* 2007; **13**: 450–61.

12. Katlic M. R., Coleman J. The aging surgeon. *Adv. Surg.* 2016; **50**: 93–103.

Healthcare Economics

Naci Balak and Magnus Tisell

8.1 Introduction

Healthcare is an intermediate good that has no intrinsic value itself but has value in its contribution towards the production of health.[1] Therefore, the term *health economics* can be said to be more appropriate than the term *healthcare economics*. However, in practice, these two terms are used interchangeably. The overall cost of medical care is high and creates a major burden for societies and governments. Nevertheless, healthcare economics does not necessarily entail cost reduction but rather is concerned with how to use resources more effectively. When choices are made in the alternative usages of resources, ethical decision-making is mandatory. For this reason, doctors should include budget in their decision-making process and decide if it is worthwhile spending extra money on a minor improvement in individual treatment, rather than spending on health benefits for the whole community. However, there is no definitive determinant between benefit to the patient and social cost, and it may not be easy to achieve balance. Economics as a science is not necessarily related to money but rather is a collection of scientific methods for improving the utilization of resources to achieve different goals. In the financial analysis of healthcare services, which is influenced by patients, community, payers, and providers, a number of factors must be taken into account, including the definition of cost, identification of effectiveness, and utility.

In recent decades, neurosurgery in high-income countries has been characterized by rapid technological development in diagnostics and treatment and widened indications with regard to age and co-morbidity. The increased sophistication of neurosurgical care also implies increased costs. Since the transformation in world politics in the last half of the twentieth century has led to economic crises in many countries, most national health systems struggle with financial constraints. Economics has a direct influence on healthcare, shifting hospitals to profit-making businesses with ethically flawed management. Many academic medical centres are struggling financially, and financial conditions have forced change upon traditional academic mission and training, including reductions in costs or even elimination of certain service lines that are found to be unprofitable.[2]

8.2 Background Information

The cost of healthcare makes up a large portion of Western economies. In the 1990s the Organization for Economic Cooperation and Development reported escalating healthcare costs with unceasing inflation.[3] The reason for this could be an increasingly aged population, advances in technology, increasingly complex services, limited resources, and ignorance regarding the effects that these factors have on the cost burden and health benefit for the population.

The Hippocratic oath states that methods and technologies in medicine should not be taught and exercised in the absence of ethical responsibility. Two main conceptual principles in health services are that the healthcare of the individual patient should not depend on personal wealth and the maximum impact on the health of the whole population should be produced using the resources available. However, resources are always limited; therefore choices must always be made both at the macro level or within the health system, which includes many parties, such as payers, politicians, researchers, providers, and social institutions, and at the micro level, which is at the patient-physician level. From the perspective of physicians, an ethical tension can arise between clinical freedom and social responsibility.

The new hospital reimbursement policies of the 1980s caused turbulence, resulting in changed consumer expectations and new sources of competition.[4] Many developed countries were experiencing the urgency of incentive-based health system reform. In the hospital context, governments expected budget discipline, lower costs, and shorter waiting times for patients.[5] This reform involved continuous increases in efficiency, the use of sophisticated technologies, a labour force disciplined to productivity, clear implementation of the professional management role, continual improvements in quality, emphasis upon devolution and delegation, appropriate information systems, emphasis upon contract and markets, measurement of performance, and increased emphasis on audits and inspection. The term 'new public management' (NPM) has been defined as a movement, as an academic commentary, and as reformed organizational practice in the public sector.[6] Its goal is lessening or removing differences between the public and the private sector and improving public services delivery, and its first principle is managerialism. Many hospitals became profit-making businesses rather than charity institutions, and state spending on healthcare was reduced. The medical profession, which traditionally was associated with deep personal commitment, came under the threat of evolving into an ordinary occupation with fixed working hours, and healthcare institutions became suspected of prioritizing profit over patient care. These changes have affected, in some degree, the self-perception of physicians concerning their functions and duties.[7]

8.3 Current Evidence

The shortage of resources is universal, and this has an effect on all decision-making. In healthcare, too, scarce public resources must be allocated efficiently – in other words, at the least cost with the maximum benefit.[8] Some argue that clinical decisions must be made not only on the basis of strictly medical considerations but also on the basis of economic facts.[8] Healthcare reforms are necessary to balance and rationalize universal healthcare and cost.[9] Others argue that, on the contrary, introducing extraneous factors into medical decisions is likely to cause problems. The question is how to practice: cost-effectively or as safely as possible? Erich Loewy (1980) stated that society has money to spend on luxuries and baubles, and therefore a physician who allows cost rather than purely medical considerations to direct his or her practice is behaving in a disastrously unethical manner.[8] However, even when ethical physicians do not base their practice on the payment abilities of their patients, escalating medical costs can threaten the welfare of society. The advocates of evidence-based medicine insist that choices should be based not only on evidence of effectiveness but also on evidence of cost-effectiveness.[8] If a clinician delivers care that is merely effective, scarce resources will be wasted and some other patients will be deprived of care from which they could otherwise benefit.[8] The rationing of healthcare is based on efficiency, not mere effectiveness. The clinician must be both efficient and ethical when treating patients cost-effectively.

Despite the fact that there has been an ever more rapid increase in the number of economic studies in medical literature, their quality is often less than desirable, and they fail to conform entirely to the Drummond checklist of good practice in economic studies.[8] The evidence currently available shows that there are enormous variations in both clinical practice and the proportion of appropriate use of procedures. The main reasons for this variability are the uncertainty of medical knowledge, the subjectivity of clinical practice, and the relative unpredictability of outcomes. Although according to neoclassical economists a well-functioning market delivers what consumers want, the healthcare market fails to bring about true preferences.[3] When technology, reinforced by regulatory systems, has a commanding influence on society and medicine, there is a risk that patients could be reduced to technological problems and to their diseases per se, while the meaning of illness for patients who just desire their suffering to be stopped is ignored.[3] When technology is considered the only rescuer and the social dimensions of illness are neglected, then the problems of patients may appear resolvable by the consumption of high-cost medical facilities at a continually increasing rate. This tendency fails to recognize the humanity of the patient and results in medical services becoming excessively indulgent in many para-metres, including the number of tests, length of stay at hospital, the number of admissions, diagnosis-related groupings, and quality-adjusted life years.[3] Reducing the patient to an object of numbers creates a vicious circle by intensifying and aggravating the dependence on technological positivism, leading inexorably to a worsening of the situation. In contrast with this, the long-established belief is that medicine is an art and each patient is unique. Moreover, birth, reproduction, and aging cannot be converted into technological phenom-ena. A good clinician must discover both the disease of patient and who the patient is at a particular moment in time. For example, in cancer cases, concern with only the effects of competing interventions on tumour size rather than the effects these treatments on the patients' quality and length of life and their comparative costs could be unethical.[8]

One of the principles of economics is the law of diminishing marginal returns, which means that each successive unit of resource devoted towards a purpose yields progressively less benefit, and finally, the curve is flat where no additional benefit is derived from the sources that are invested.[10] This rule is especially applicable to the utilization of intensive care units, where limiting low-yield care results in significant cost reduction. However, survival estimates at the time of admission are problematic, and even the use of predictive indices such as APACHE fails to determine cost-effectiveness because of uncertainty of prognosis.[10] Therefore, the use of economic analysis to justify rationing of care is debatable. The use of economic analysis to guide patient care is most consistent with the ethical principle of justice, but can be in conflict with the other ethical principle of beneficence.

The NPM, as it has been applied in healthcare systems, might have had a negative influence on the clinical as well as the ethical performance of hospitals. As an organization, per se, hospitals pursue effective care to best serve patients and efficient operation to meet financial measures. To combine these two goals has been extremely challenging due to their inherent contradictions.[4] Indeed, ethical issues are integral to resource allocation decisions, and the failure to align the goal of productivity improvement with ethics and ethical management can cause violations of integrity. In this challenging milieu, healthcare providers can experience moral distress (i.e., stress associated with the ethical dimensions of practice). The difficulties of navigating practice while upholding professional values, responsibilities, and duties can result in a constrained moral response to ethical issues in practice.[11] The manifestations of moral distress include emotional distress (anger, frustration, sadness), moral residue (unresolved moral distress), withdrawal of self from patients, declining quality of patient care, and poor job satisfaction.[11] Profit organizations usually have very little commitment to equity, other than the avoidance of discrimination lawsuits from their employees or clients. By contrast, public organizations often have great commitment to equity; they must provide services to all citizens, regardless of their ability to pay for them, and must ensure equal access to services. Effective productivity improvement requires ethical attitudes.[12] Healthcare professionals who work as organizational employees have been reported to experience considerable uncertainty about managerial support for the enactment of professional values in practice.[11] Blaming and fear of reprisals from supervisors, supervisory reluctance, supervisors' lack of understanding of the situation, and silencing can increase moral distress.[11] Moral distress is a growing concern, and its presence indicates the quality of the healthcare practice environment and the actions required to sustain the healthcare endeavour.[11] Unfortunately, healthcare reform based on the values of corporatization and efficiency can undermine health professionals' attempts to engage ethically with those in their care.[11]

8.4 Ethical Issues

Failure to respect ethical values in the application of NPM in health system will have detrimental effects on healthcare in general and on the practice. First, recentralization benefits top political and top civil servants, as well as a business oligarchy of private clinics, private insurance groups, and consulting firms. Most government corruption occurs at the point of transaction between, on the one hand, officials formally representing government authority and, on the other hand, the use of public money and individuals or organizations seeking money, favour, or influence.[5,12] Corruption diverts money away from investment into training, research, and practice. Second, support of market-based mechanisms, reduced state-ownership, and rising private financing imply more government regulations in the pricing of health services.[5] Both state and private hospitals tend to focus on the most profitable group of patients. In this matter, neurosurgery is one of the most disadvantageous specialties for several reasons, including a shallow or longer learning curve, longer surgery duration, and high risk.

If healthcare provision is considered as a market, it is not a perfect market. In healthcare there is unpredictability of demand, uncertainty about the consequences of decisions, irrationality of provider and consumer decisions, the existence of externalities, and the agency relationship. The patients, so-called consumers, do not usually have the knowledge required to make appropriate choices, so that physicians who have a dual role as provider and agents for patients become key elements in determining the demand for the treatment on behalf of their patients, which is an effect known as *supplier-induced demand*. The elements of marketing (product, place, promotion, and pricing) have been applied to health services. However, in contrast to marketing in traditional business enterprises, which seeks to create demand, health services marketing seeks to meet a demand for its services. Unfortunately, the application of a business marketing approach leads to resources being allocated increasingly in response to profit opportunities rather than to medical need. This can have a negative impact on neurosurgery if unnecessary medical care is provided for profit. It can result in overtreatment or undertreatment, as well as escalating costs.[13] Both private and public hospitals invest greatly in facilities for well-paid procedures that will attract physicians and patients and find it far more cost-effective to shift resources from subspecialists to primary care.

Spending on health could be reduced in several ways, including the substitution of less-expensive services in place of more-expensive services, providing incentives for more efficient delivery of healthcare; elimination of services that do not add value; changing prices directly by regulating the price paid for services; and expansion of cost-effective outpatient care.[14] Operating-room activity drives the margin of any hospital,[2] whereas outpatient office practices of employed physicians seldom return a profit for hospitals.[15] Since inpatient services comprise a large proportion of total healthcare spending, migration of care to outpatient setting is encouraged by hospital managers.[14] At the same time, managers may force physicians to decrease the time spent for each patient in outpatient clinics to a limit that is ethically unacceptable in order to increase the margin of outpatient practice. They may support an increase in ambulatory surgery and a reduction in the length of stay. One consequence of shifting neurosurgeons from the operating room to outpatient activity is a reduction in the opportunity for residents to be well trained in surgical practice. Furthermore, there is no clear evidence to support a move away from hospitalization and towards outpatient care in terms of profitability.

The previously mentioned contradictions can also lead to disparities within neurosurgery, as there is a tendency to focus on profitable neurosurgical procedures to the neglect of others. Although neurosurgery has been found to be one of the most profitable specialties for hospitals, this does not mean necessarily that all types of cranial and spinal procedures are performed.[2] A growing number of neurosurgeons are reluctant to provide trauma coverage, and there is the potential for some neurosurgeons to give up intracranial neurosurgery. This may stem from the application of the relative value system, in which each surgical case generates a different number of relative value units per unit time, depending on case complexity and how the cases are subjectively valued by the system.[2] As a consequence, the busiest surgeon in the hospital may be far from being the biggest generator of margin for the hospital. Similarly, a clinical service may be contributing substantially to the overall hospital margin, but may not cover all types of procedures that are necessary for patients and trainees.

For financial reasons, administrators may want the operating room (OR) to be fully occupied during the workday.[16] Although almost all cases contribute positively to a hospital's finances, optimal operating room utilization differs between surgical specialties. Neurosurgeons deal with many life-threatening, urgent cases and, not infrequently, can only know a day or two in advance which patients have been admitted with an intracranial surgical pathology. This results in suboptimal use of the operating room compared with other surgical specialisms, where scheduling a surgical case months in advance is possible. Additionally, neurosurgery, as a specialty with complex, longer cases, will have a lower utilization rate. Furthermore, the need for certain surgical equipment, such as a microscope, may also limit the number of cases. Another factor affecting utilization is the need to cancel surgery if the intensive care unit will not be able to accommodate a patient post-operatively, which is a common event in neurosurgery.[16] Unfortunately, allocating additional time to subspecialties with negative contribution margins in the hope of expanding those markets does not serve the interests of hospitals unless there is a financial sponsor who is willing to promote that type of medical care.[16] Thus hospital managers may substitute utilization of the OR or block (reserved) time between surgical branches. They may also restrict the number of operating rooms used for neurosurgery, mandate neurosurgeons to share the OR with other surgical specialties, or restrict neurosurgeons to performing specific types of surgery only. Furthermore, a high utilization restricts quick access to the operating room. In other words, the greater the operating room utilization, the less the ability to book cases when desired for surgeons and patients.[17]

Many physicians have experienced a shift from a fixed salary to incentive-driven compensation linked to productivity and clinical behaviour.[15] This approach attempts to maintain productivity levels while encouraging physician behaviours that reduce costs or increase revenues. Again, for financial reasons inherent in the NPM, surgeons may prefer to perform most of the surgical cases themselves to save time and increase the utilization of the operating room for more cases, letting residents do only a limited part of the surgery. With the coding data – the translation of documented clinical activities that is used to calculate payment – being the source of comparisons within and between departments, coding inaccuracies become misleading in regard to departmental activity and subspecialties.[18] For a neurosurgeon, adequate time is vital: time to review a chart, truly listen to and examine a patient, and plan the surgery.[13] The environment of competition for profit resulting from the new public management creates time pressures on physicians, making them more prone to error and leading to the ordering of more tests to compensate for a lack of time. Neurosurgeons, the most likely target for malpractice claims among physicians, are particularly affected.

A significant threat to the future of neurosurgery is posed by reduced government investment in high-risk and high-cost specialist areas and in research and training. Governments are prone to favour primary healthcare, the treatment of more common diseases, and the expansion of outpatient services. Furthermore, primary care is much cheaper care compared to inpatient care. Another issue is economic evaluation in the context of rare diseases. Although investment on primary healthcare is beneficial for society, it should not lead to the neglect of investment into the treatment of complex, rare, severe diseases. A profit-based policy jeopardizes the treatment of high-risk patients with relatively rare neurosurgical disorders that would necessitate costly preventative measures. Patients with rare diseases usually suffer from insufficient medical supply. In these cases, some other approaches, such as the Pearson trade-off or the rule of rescue technique, can be used.[19] The result of an intervention can be expressed in four ways: efficacy, effectiveness, utility, and benefit.[30] Therefore, four types of efficiency analysis can be formulated: cost-efficacy, cost-effectiveness, cost-utility, and cost-benefit. Cost-effectiveness is measured in natural units such as life years saved or admission to hospital prevented, while cost-utility is measured in utilities such as quality-adjusted life years.[10] Consideration of cost is a part of social ethics in the health system; however, the least costly option is not necessarily the most efficient. Efficiency is only one ethical imperative in the provision of healthcare. Equity is another major consideration, and the opportunity for citizens to receive ethical equitable healthcare should ideally be independent of economic, geographical, cultural, or ethnic factors.

As in other specialist areas, there is an autonomy of physician-patient relationship at the centre of neurosurgical service delivery. In neurosurgery, many patients, often at high risk to their physical and mental health, find themselves incapable of understanding their situations enough to be able to make the proper decisions.[20] The treating neurosurgeon may also experience difficulty finding the right choice of treatment. The autonomous relationship between neurosurgeon and patient is under threat from the health service administration in hospitals as they have evolved under the influence of new public management reforms. Due to the vital role of physicians in the healthcare system, the organization must satisfy their needs. In general, there are three types of motivation guiding the actions of people: extrinsic motivation, such as earning payment; intrinsic motivation, such as the pleasure of learning or the development of professional expertise; and transcendent motivation, such as the satisfaction that comes from contributing to another's well-being. The organization plays a significant role in the promotion of these motives, although most health systems offer few incentives to satisfy all three types. If the organization promotes mainly extrinsic motivation, a tie of self-interest develops among its members, whereas the support of intrinsic motivation creates a tie of job attractiveness and the promotion of transcendent motivation fosters the tie of unity in the institution. The failure of the organization to promote enough incentives reduces efficiency and results in the underuse, overuse, or inappropriate use of resources. Physicians are also expected to follow professional ethics. The principles of professional ethics are impartiality, openness, confidentiality, due diligence, fidelity to professional responsibilities, and the avoidance of potential or apparent conflict of interest. The Statement of Ethics in Neurosurgery by the World Federation of Neurosurgical Societies, under the title of 'Good Medical Practice – The Standard of Care' reads: 'When patient care may be compromised by inadequate facilities or equipment, lack of reimbursement for important medical services, or shortages of medical and support staff, we should address the issues to the best of our ability.'[21] The Good Practice guidelines published by the World Federation of Neurosurgical Societies and the European Association of Neurosurgical Societies state under the title of 'Standards of Personal and Professional Life': 'Respect the professionalism of others involved in health care, and do not compete with colleagues for professional and financial gain, to the detriment of those colleagues or patients.'[22] On the other hand, business ethics is the application of general ethical ideas to business behaviour, comprising integrity, impartiality, responsiveness to the public interest, accountability, honesty, and transparency.

It is clear that an intervention that is both more effective and less expensive than a competing strategy should be adopted, whereas a less-effective and more-expensive intervention should be avoided. However, conflicts emerge when an intervention is both more effective and more costly than an alternative, or when it is less costly but less effective.[10] In these situations, careful ethical decision-making is necessary, taking into consideration other factors such as availability, access, or experience. The ratio between costs and effects determines the cost-effectiveness of the healthcare, not the cost per se. Priority should be given to those patients who can benefit the most at the lowest cost, although this is not an easy decision, and economic evaluations in healthcare should always be viewed warily. Striving for efficiency conflicts with the ethical principle of justice. The dangerous consequence of this is that the very sick and helpless could be sacrificed in order to maintain economic savings for the society. The primary goal of healthcare is to aid and not abandon vulnerable patients, such as the elderly, the chronically ill, the handicapped, and those presumed to be at the end stage of life. However, if resources are allocated to patients irrespective of their ability to benefit, other patients who might have benefited more from the same amount of resources can be deprived of treatment. Another issue is that the benefits only become apparent in the long term. Health economists mainly deal with the maximization of health in the population, and this is a utilitarian view. By contrast, an egalitarian view focuses on reducing the variance irrespective of the consequences for the average health of the population. Some argue that obtaining a more equitable distribution of health is possible only at the cost of a lower average level of health. When there is a scarcity of resources, society intentionally choses to prioritize younger patients over older ones. Sometimes it may be reasonable to distribute shares proportionate to the remaining life expectancy of people instead of distributing equal shares. Moral arguments should not become arbitrary and capricious under the cloak of justice.

Management is a significant factor in the cost and quality crisis of current healthcare. Healthcare managers have a legal and moral obligation to ensure a high quality of patient care and to strive to improve care and are in the prime position to mandate policy, systems, procedures, and organizational climates.[23] However, pressure on them to cut costs while increasing both quality and comprehensiveness is encouraging a blame culture and discouraging information sharing. To be a successful hospital administrator, one has to reduce corporate and hospital expenses while simultaneously making efforts to increase both revenue and the quality and comprehensiveness of the services. Such a system may encourage top-down bureaucracies and a culture that seeks to blame clinicians for problems or unmet goals, instead of fostering a problem-solving culture that seeks improvement. Furthermore, information sharing may be seen as more threatening than helpful. These pressures can also lead to the favouring of certain specialties in the allocation of facilities for ease of management and profit motives. Within such an environment, there may be management pressure on neurosurgeons to perform surgery in less than ideal settings. They may be forced either to perform surgery with greater risk to patients in undersupplied settings, to enter into conflicts with hospital administrators by insisting on the provision of ideal neurosurgical facilities, or to apply so-called defensive medicine to avoid malpractice suits. Defensive medicine includes performing unnecessary diagnostic tests and invasive procedures, prescribing unnecessary treatment, and needless hospitalization. Defensive medicine also comprises avoiding risky procedures on patients who could have benefited from them, thereby excluding patients from treatment and hospital admission.[24] All of these scenarios may raise ethical dilemmas. Pressure may take the form of bullying, including constantly belittling the physician's work, persistent unjustified criticism and monitoring of the physician's work, intentional use of discipline procedures, verbal and nonverbal threats, withholding necessary information from the physician, unreasonable refusal of applications for leave/training/promotion, undue pressure to produce work, constant alteration of work targets, circulating negative rumours, and so forth.[25]

The hospital administrator is a moral agent who needs personal ethics for guiding relationships with patients, staff members, institutions (sectarian/non-sectarian), governing bodies, and society. In addition, there is considerable potential for conflict between hospital management and other stakeholders, particularly physicians, policymakers, insurers, and the pharmaceutical industry.[26] It is ethically unacceptable if they benefit at the expense of the organization or patient care; neither can they be negligent in solving patient care problems. Unresolved ethical troubles have a destructive effect on the institution, and the ethical aspects of hospital management need more attention and analysis than ever.[26] Allocating available funds to medical specialties, deciding which clinical services to offer, and ensuring a high quality of service all deserve ethical consideration and scrutiny. Although the decisions of management only indirectly affect patients, hospital managers must integrate ethics into their daily work in order to make responsible decisions and fair and effective use of the available healthcare delivery resources. Thus morally unacceptable conduct cannot be excused because someone was following orders or policy, regardless of their source. Administrators cannot conform to general expectations so as not to disrupt or endanger their sense of security. Nor can they apply any set of values or principles differently and unequally to two or more similar patients, physicians, groups, or situations. When acting in accordance with an ethical code, the manager will not be blindly seduced by productivity indicators or by efficiency in resource management, forgetting that decisions have an impact on the health and well-being of people and on the requirements of fair justice.[27] Administrators, who hold a position of authority, must have a well-developed personal ethic, in addition to an appreciation of biomedical and organizational ethics. Personal ethics refers to the application of values, which are the conception of what an individual or a group regards as desirable, to everything one does. The principles of personal ethics involve concern and respect for the autonomy of others, honesty and the willingness to comply with the law, fairness and the ability not to take undue advantage of others, and benevolence and preventing harm to any creature. Discrimination, nepotism, dishonesty, irresponsibility, selfishness, arrogance, uncooperativeness, and brutality lead to an escalation in medical errors and poor quality healthcare. By contrast, executives should lead with humility, not power. They and all managers in the organization should become students of the work of the hospital, relinquishing their need to seem to have all the answers. Most importantly, they must mentor, coach, and teach. The new leadership role is to help others look for better ways to deliver care – by removing defects, reducing waiting time, and allowing everyone to work at the top of the scope of their licence. Managers are not in control of everything that happens; they should be the facilitators leading change. They can be like catalysts in chemical reactions, having the potential to accelerate the path to achieving a high-quality level of service. So, fears are often expressed that exposing managers to the values of the private sector might cause them to compromise their integrity and lose sight of this possibility.[12]

8.4.1 Illustrative Cases

Ethical Dilemma Case 1

There are extremely limited resources in some regions of Africa, where the choice might be between developing neurosurgery for a few selected cases and using the same resources on the prevention and treatment of widespread infectious diseases hurting a large part of the population, such as malaria, HIV, and tuberculosis. How to choose?

Comment: The use of economic analysis to guide patient care is most consistent with the ethical principle of justice, but can be in conflict with the other ethical principle of beneficence. Although investment on primary healthcare is beneficial for society, it should not lead to the neglect of investment into the treatment of complex, rare, and severe diseases. More efficient healthcare means better care for the individual patient and makes it possible to increase the resources available to improve care for the whole society.

Ethical Dilemma Case 2

Does the financial reward for a procedure make the physicians biased towards certain kinds of surgery? Is more fusion surgery performed if fusion surgery is better reimbursed? If we are paid per operation, do we tend to operate more?

Comment: Unfortunately, there may be a tendency to focus on profitable neurosurgical procedures to the neglect of others. However, surgeons should avoid potential or apparent conflict of interest, and they are obliged to adhere to the principles of beneficence and non-malfeasance. Physicians should not compete with colleagues for professional and financial gain, to the detriment of those colleagues or patients.

8.5 Future Directions

Tremendous developments in neuroscience and neurosurgery have led today to effective and safe surgery for patients with neurosurgical disorders that were once thought to be inoperable or where surgery was extremely risky. Even so, it remains a high-risk specialty. The problem is exacerbated by the rapidly developing technology in neurosurgery, which makes surgery more efficient and safe but also increases the costs. Restrictions on the healthcare of neurosurgical patients may make the future of neurosurgery uncertain. Furthermore, the rapid advances in neurosurgical knowledge and technology have increased the need for the continual, time-consuming, but essential updating of scientific knowledge and skills.[28] Thus neurosurgeons face a very difficult challenge to meet their moral and ethical responsibilities to patients, trainees and colleagues, and society, and to confirm the fundamental and universal principles and values of neurosurgical professionalism.[28] Yaşargil stated: 'The surgical actions and the pre-, peri-, and postoperative observation of the patients are dependent on the steady combination of communication, technology, science, mathematics, philosophy, religion, art and play in the brains of neurosurgeons. The philosophy of art should maintain the dynamic balance between esthetical ethic, and ethical esthetic.'

Despite marked differences in training and professional interests, physicians and hospital managers face similar problems stemming from the unprecedented rate of change in the healthcare delivery system: failure of reimbursement to keep pace with rising costs, new therapeutic modalities, increasing government and managed care regulations, heightened consumerism, and an aging patient population.[29] Raising awareness of the ethical experiences of healthcare providers is the first step to responding effectively to moral distress. Further research and dialogue is required to understand and address the societal (political and economic) and organizational contexts of healthcare so that, ultimately, healthcare professionals can fulfil their fiduciary responsibilities and organizations can enact their missions, in order to promote employee well-being and high quality patient care, within healthcare organizations that are 'morally habitable' and focused on enacting their stated values and fulfilling their missions.[11] It has been reported that 70% to 80% of medical errors are linked to interpersonal interactions in the delivery of care. Despite the tensions created by competition and rapid change, transformation from a blaming to a learning environment may be a key strategic advantage in today's healthcare marketplace.[29]

In medicine and in neurosurgery, there is often no one right answer to an ethical problem. Yet analyzing the problem by a systematic process can reveal all possible viewpoints and approaches and help formulate a solution. The basic causes of most of major health problems derive from value choices, answering questions such as what kind of people we are, what kind of society we want to build for our children and grandchildren, how much individual freedom we want, what kind of life we want, how important our own health and our neighbours' health are to us, and so forth.[8] The physician can play an important role in increasing the efficiency, equity, and the quality of the health system without limiting the delivery of effective services.[30] More efficient healthcare means better care for the individual patient and makes it possible to increase the resources available to improve care for the whole society. Although decisions about health resources are made seemingly by politicians or managers, physicians play a very important role in the use and distribution of resources from both an ethical and economic perspective. Strong management leadership and clinical champions of physicians are required for the successful selection of priorities in healthcare. It should be noted that economics is a positive science, not a normative one, and should be separated from political interpretations of its results. Although society has the moral and ethical imperative to control costs, surgeons are first obliged to adhere to the principles of beneficence and non-malfeasance.

8.6 Conclusions

Hospitals have already become profit-institutions, and all parties, including governing bodies, hospital managers, and insurance companies, have already placed financial gain as the chief goal, contrary to the ongoing nature of medical practice and in breach of ethics. However, neither disparities in the economic or social conditions of countries nor the policies of governments should be used to justify these shortcomings. If businesslike methods are to be introduced into the management of training hospitals, the establishment of practical principles should be ensured in an effective and ethical manner. Training in ethics would facilitate the collaboration between hospital administrators and physicians that is essential for the establishment of the ethical environment needed for appropriate neurosurgery practice. Physicians will increasingly face more clinical guidelines, new administrative programmes, managers/politicians who are under pressure and burdened with urgent business, and more well informed patients. Therefore, they should understand the principles and methods of clinical economics in order to ethically use new information about both the cost and the impact of clinical practice. As far as doctors critically evaluate data on cost and effectiveness, they may be able to preserve their roles not only as advocates of their patients but also as responsible members of hospitals, healthcare organizations, and society in general.

References

1. Edwards R. T. Paradigms and research programmes: is it time to move from health care economics to health economics? *Health Econ.* 2001; **10**: 635–49.

2. Resnick A. S., Corrigan D., Mullen J. L., et al. Surgeon contribution to hospital bottom line: not all are created equal. *Ann. Surg.* 2005; **242**: 530–9.

3. Frankford D. M. Scientism and economism in the regulation of health care. *J. Health Polit. Policy Law* 1994; **19**: 773–99.

4. Kim R. The US Hospital Management from a Strategic Management Viewpoint. *Journal of Hospital & Medical Management* 2016; **2**: 1–7.

5. Simonet D. Assessment of new public management in health care: the French case. *Health Res. Policy Syst.* 2014; **12**: 57.

6. Hood C. The 'New Public Management' in the 1980s: variations on a theme. *Accounting, Organizations and Society* 1995; **20**: 93–109.

7. Stienen M. N., Netuka D., Demetriades A. K., et al. Working time of neurosurgical residents in Europe – results of a multinational survey. *Acta Neurochir (Wien)* 2016; **158**: 17–25.

8. Maynard A. Ethical issues in the economics of rationing healthcare. *Br. J. Urol.* 1995; **76** **Suppl 2**: 59–64.

9. Dagi T. F. Seven ethical issues affecting neurosurgeons in the context of health care reform. *Neurosurg.* 2017; **80**: S83–S91.

10. Wilson K., Cook D. J. Economics and the intensive care unit: a conflict of interests? *J. Crit. Care* 1997; **12**: 147–51.

11. Wall S., Austin W. J., Garros D. Organizational influences on health professionals' experiences of moral distress in PICUs. *HEC Forum* 2016; **28**: 53–67.

12. Kolthoff E., Huberts L., Van den Heuvel H. The ethics of new public management: is integrity at stake? *Public Administration Quarterly* 2006; 399–439.

13. Kuttner R. Market-based failure – a second opinion on US health care costs. *N. Eng. J. Med.* 2008; **358**: 549–51.

14. Goetghebeur M. M., Forrest S., Hay J. W. Understanding the underlying drivers of inpatient cost growth: a literature review. *Am. J. Manag. Care* 2003; **9**: SP3–SP12.

15. Kocher R., Sahni N. R. Hospitals' race to employ physicians – the logic behind a money-losing proposition. *N. Eng. J. Med.* 2011; **364**: 1790–3.

16. Wachtel R. E., Dexter F. Tactical increases in operating room block time for capacity planning should not be based on utilization. *Anesth. Analg.* 2008; **106**: 215–26.

17. Pandit J., Pandit M., Reynard J. Understanding waiting lists as the matching of surgical capacity to demand: are we wasting enough surgical time? *Anaesthesia* 2010; **65**: 625–40.

18. Haliasos N., Rezajooi K., O'neill K., et al. Financial and clinical governance implications of clinical coding accuracy in neurosurgery: a multidisciplinary audit. *Br. J. Neurosurg.* 2010; **24**: 191–5.

19. Silva E. N., Sousa T. R. Economic evaluation in the context of rare diseases: is it possible? *Cad Saude Publica* 2015; **31**: 496–506.

20. Schmitz D., Reinacher P. C. Informed consent in neurosurgery – translating ethical theory into action. *J. Med. Ethics* 2006; **32**: 497–8.

21. Umansky F., Black P. L., DiRocco C., et al. Statement of ethics in neurosurgery of the world federation of neurosurgical societies. *World Neurosurg.* 2011; **76**: 239–47.

22. World Federation of Neurosurgical Societies and European Association of Neurosurgical Societies. Good Practice: A Guide for Neurosurgeons. *Acta Neurochir (Wien)* 1999; **141**: 793–9.

23. Parand A., Dopson S., Renz A., et al. The role of hospital managers in quality and patient safety: a systematic review. *BMJ* 2014; **4**: e005055.

24. Prabhu V. C. Defensive medicine in neurosurgery. *World Neurosurg.* 2016; **95**: 587–9.

25. Quine L. Workplace bullying in junior doctors: questionnaire survey. *BMJ* 2002; **324**: 878–9.

26. Biller-Andorno N., Lenk C., Leititis J. Ethics, EBM, and hospital management. *J. Med. Ethics* 2004; **30**: 136–40.

27. Rego A., Araújo B., Serrão D. The impact of hospital organization in the ethical act of hospital management. *J. Hosp. Admin.* 2015; **4**: 14.

28. Kanat A., Epstein C. R. Challenges to neurosurgical professionalism. *Clin. Neurol. Neurosurg.* 2010; **112**: 839–43.

29. Cohn K. H., Gill S. L., Schwartz R. W. Gaining hospital administrators' attention: ways to improve physician–hospital management dialogue. *Surgery* 2005; **137**: 132–40.

30. Lazaro P, Azcona B. Clinical practice, ethics and economics: the physician at the crossroads. Health Policy. 1996; **37**: 185–98.

Patient Data, Ownership, Storage, and Social Media

David Cote and Timothy Smith

9.1 Introduction

The amount of data associated with healthcare today is massive, ranging from the numerical results of every laboratory test to each image from complex MRIs and CT scans. Today, each healthcare site in the United States has its own repository for the data associated with care provided at that facility. These data include both categorical and numerical data, like patient demographics and the results of laboratory tests, as well as free text data, such as patient progress notes, admission notes, operative notes, and radiology and pathology reports and raw images. The data historically associated with receiving healthcare are protected in the United States under the Health Insurance Portability and Accountability Act of 1996 (HIPAA), which sought to establish security provisions for medical information that is generated and stored in the case of typical clinical care.[1]

Over the past two decades, however, patients have also increased their data production and storage in areas previously unrelated to the healthcare system. This includes data generated by the use of cell phones, such as social connectivity data related to calls and text messages sent and received, global positioning satellite (GPS) data, social media postings and usage, advertising interactivity, and online shopping.[2,3] These data, while historically separated from those generated in the process of receiving healthcare, have increasingly been suggested for use as part of healthcare research and even clinical care.

In this chapter, we will discuss how medical data, such as that generated and stored in a hospital medical record, can be combined with patient-generated data, such as that produced by daily use of a smartphone, in the course of clinical research or patient care. Use of both of these types of data presents ethical dilemmas that we will discuss in detail, with the use of two illustrative cases specific to neurosurgical research and patient care.

9.2 Background

HIPAA was enacted into law in 1996 and at the time was initially considered to be unwieldly and overly complex. It covered only those data generated specifically under 'covered entities', such as clinicians, hospitals and other healthcare facilities, and health insurance plans, yet its rules were complex and difficult to follow, particularly with regard to when hospitals and caregivers were authorized to disclose the information covered under HIPAA's policies.[1] Since its introduction, however, HIPAA, and its amendment in 2009, the Health Information Technology for Economic and Clinical Health Act (HITECH), have largely been effective in protecting patient data that is generated in the course of normal interaction with the healthcare system from unwanted or unknown disclosure. Enacted in 1996, however, HIPAA almost entirely predated the Internet age, and even with amendment in 2009, its criteria for health-related data (i.e., those data generated during interaction with the healthcare or health insurance systems) fall woefully short of data that might currently be considered 'health-related'.

As noted above, increasingly, researchers in the health sciences have been interested in the use of nontraditional health-related data for performing health-services research.[2] These research projects take a variety of forms, but they all rely on the use of data that is typically not collected in a patient's medical record to draw inferences about health-related exposures or outcomes. For example, a researcher investigating outcomes post-hospital discharge could have previously used data from that patient's medical record to evaluate clinical follow-up visits after discharge, such as primary care progress notes or laboratory tests, to draw inferences about how a patient has recovered since hospitalization. Today, researchers are instead proposing to use patient-generated data, in addition to traditional data, to make these inferences. For example, a patient who carries a smartphone produces hundreds of thousands of GPS-data and accelerometer data points per day, which could allow a health-services researcher to determine that patient's overall health status.

The distinction between the latter type of data and the data produced in the healthcare system and protected by HIPAA is key. This latter form of data is increasingly referred to as 'passive data'.[2] Passive data can be distinguished from more traditional forms of data, or active data, by the methods used for collection. Active data are generated by intentional action of either the healthcare provider or the patient, and include all data included in an electronic medical record, such as demographic information, progress notes and physical exams, radiology reports, pathology reports, operative notes, and the results of laboratory tests. In short, each of these types of data are generated by the asking and answering of questions, and each requires active input by a trained professional. Passive data, on the other hand, are collected without any active input from clinician or patient, sometimes without the knowledge of the participant. Examples might include mobile phones that track GPS location, membership cards and scanners that track consumer behaviour, or social media websites that collect and store advertising interactions to provide targeted experiences to their consumers and advertisers. In our example above, researchers can infer the health status of a patient post-discharge by the GPS and accelerometer data generated by their smartphone: a patient who rarely leaves their home and rarely moves may be recovering more slowly than a patient who, immediately after discharge, is able to return to normal levels of physical activity or travel far from their home.

Engagement on social media represents another source of passively collected data, even though it is generated actively by users.[3] A simple Twitter or Facebook search for common health complaints, like 'headache' or 'migraine', yields hundreds of public posts that vary in their content and description of the illness. In some cases, users highlight symptoms (e.g., dizziness, pain, blurry vision, vomiting, etc.) associated with their illness. In others, they highlight potential treatments they are exploring or using (e.g., Tylenol, sleep, etc.). They also sometimes highlight their level of disability (e.g., away from work or school, restricted to bed for the day, etc.). These Twitter and Facebook postings can be collected, cleaned, categorized, and used for analyses.[3]

The use of passive data has many significant advantages over active data. First, it is nearly always high-dimensional. As an example, consider the data generated daily from the use of a smartphone. Most smartphones contain data streams for GPS, Wi-Fi, accelerometer, application usage, phone and text engagement, and screen on/off time. Each of these can be broken down and used to calculate metrics that may be of interest to researchers. GPS data can be used to calculate maximum distance travelled in a day, but can also be used to calculate what proportion of the day an individual spends at home. Call and text data can be used to calculate the maximum number of interactions exchanged in a day, but the metadata of these interactions are also stored, so that researchers can identify how responsive an individual is to text messages versus phone calls, or which individuals a participant may be more or less likely to engage with. Screen on/off time can be used to ascertain how frequently an individual uses their phone, but can also be used to make inferences about a person's duration of sleep each night. Taken together, these data streams result in the production of at least millions of data points per participant per week – far more than that generated in a week for even the most active traditional hospital medical record of an intensive care unit patient.

Further, passive data are not actively collected, which reduces the risk of some forms of bias. If a physician were to ask their patients if they exercised at every clinic visit, the average response in clinic would be biased upwards, with more patients reporting regular exercise. With the use of the accelerometer data on a smartphone, researchers can directly ascertain how active an individual is over the course of a study period based directly on the number of steps they have taken. Personal heart rate monitors, such as those included in many smartwatches, can make such inferences even more accurate and effective. Additionally, passive data collection methods are low-cost and non-invasive. In 2015 more than 77% of US adults owned smartphones, a number that is only expected to grow.[4] The amount of data generated by these devices that could be used for health-services research is astounding.

Passive data of course have several important limitations that must be discussed. First, passive data often have a relatively high degree of limitations. Some individuals do not keep their phones with them all the time, and when phones are powered off, either intentionally or due to battery exhaustion, data cannot be collected. These limitations are addressed through the imputation of important data streams based on a patient's historical behaviour and other data streams, but this can lead to bias. Additionally, passive data may lead to ethical issues with data collection, ownership, storage, and use – the key focus of this chapter.

9.3 Current Evidence

Passive data are already being collected from patients, whether they know it or not. Recent news stories have highlighted the use of data collected from internet activity, social media postings, and advertising interactivity by companies like Google, Facebook, and Amazon to sell targeted advertising.[5] By categorizing individuals based on the websites they visit, the individuals they interact with on social media sites, and the products they buy, these companies have succeeded in allowing advertisers to target the users that are most likely to respond positively to their advertisement. The use of social media in particular encourages users to identify their interests and likes and dislikes, allowing direct ascertainment of their preferences for the use of corporations and advertisers.[3] While users of these websites nominally consent to these methods by accepting the user agreements of each website, rarely do individuals realize the extent to which their data are being collected, stored, and used by each website.

In a more controlled setting, passive data are also currently being used for health-services research. Published research includes the use of digital phenotyping – defined as the 'moment-by-moment quantification of the individual-level human phenotype in-situ using data from personal digital devices' – for research in psychiatry and neurosurgery.[6] In one study by Staples et al., researchers used passive data collection to determine the correlation between smartphone-estimated sleep duration with patient self-reported sleep quality, finding moderate correlation (r = 0.69, 95%CI: 0.23–0.90).[7]

In our own research, we have enrolled a cohort of more than 100 adult neurosurgical patients with spine disease for participation in a passive data study that also actively assesses, by way of smartphone questionnaire, daily Visual Analog Scale (VAS) pain. Each enrollee has installed an application on their personal smartphone that collects data from a variety of streams (Figure 9.1), and our aim is to correlate data from those streams with the VAS pain score in this cohort of patients. Each patient generates hundreds of thousands of data points daily, with GPS sampling occurring for one minute every five minutes (i.e., 17% of the time), and accelerometer sampling occurring for 10 seconds every 10 seconds (i.e., 50% of the time).

The benefits of passive data in these settings are immediately apparent. Clinic-based assessments of pain, mobility, psychiatric symptoms, and other important health metrics are expensive (requiring trained research assistants or administrators), time-consuming, and biased. They require patients to return to clinic and self-report their experience, but the goal often is not clear. When a patient is asked to report their pain on a clinic survey, is it their current pain? The maximum pain they experienced since their last visit? The average pain since their last visit? Asking patients or research participants to make these distinctions is difficult.

Passive data collection, on the other hand, is inexpensive and easy to implement. Adding active questionnaires to the application is also easy, allowing immediate and regular querying of participants at discrete moments in time. As these data become more accessible to health-services researchers, research projects focused on the use of passive data for medical research will continue to expand.

9.4 Ethical Issues

The use of passive data on the scale referenced above does produce ethical issues that must be addressed. These issues can be categorized into four main groups: (1) issues of data collection, (2) issues of data ownership, (3) issues of data storage, and (4) issues of data use. Below, we discuss each in turn.

9.4.1 Data Collection

The collection of high-dimensional modern data highlights important issues in informed consent and data privacy.[8] Smartphone-based collection methods result in the collection of a great deal of sensitive data, some of which may not be intended for collection by the participant. Collection of data from a participant's daily life, rather than that which they decide to share during a clinic visit, is inherently more sensitive and private, leading to higher stakes in protection of that data.

Most experts agree that current informed consent standards for the collection of passive data are insufficient. As highlighted above, many individuals already consent to such collection through the use of websites like Facebook, Google, and Amazon, without realizing the extent to which they have surrendered their control over their own data.[5,9,10] Consent forms in an electronic format are often long and tedious, and many users simply agree to them reflexively, without truly weighing their options. In health-services research,

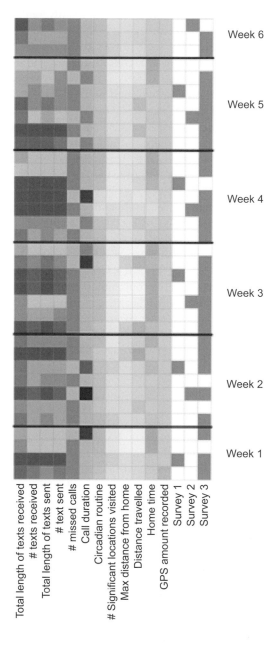

Figure 9.1 Visual display of daily summary statistics collected for a patient. Surveys are represented in orange. Measures of mobility obtained from smartphone GPS are shown in purple. Measures from call logs are in blue and measures from text logs are in green. Measures are calculated from raw smartphone data on a daily basis. Only a smaller representative sample of the total set of measures both collected and calculated are displayed. Darker colour represents a larger quantity/amount of the measure on a given day. Each column represents one day of data collection, with vertical black lines representing division between weeks.

on the other hand, informed consent procedures have historically attempted to ensure that adequate care has been taken so that research participants have fully weighed their options.

In the context of passive data, informed consent is even more difficult. While researchers can highlight the data streams they plan to tap into, they can never fully predict what the use of that data will reveal. Therefore, informed consent procedures will inherently under-represent the true use of the data being collected. A further complication is that an individual's use of smartphones often involves interaction with third parties – such as those they exchange text messages or calls with – who may not fully consent to participating in the research at hand.

To address these issues, experts have argued that informed consent procedures for the use of passive data should be dynamic and flexible. If researchers discover a new way to use the data being collected, consent should be actively sought by researchers and reasserted by the participant. Further, researchers should always collect the minimum amount of data necessary to answer the question being considered. If the study will focus only on GPS data, social connectivity data should not be collected, even though it may be easy or inexpensive to do so.

For social media data, the collection and use of data is even more complicated.[3] Many individuals who post publicly on their personal social media pages about their symptoms of illness, possible treatments, or medication side effects may not consent to use of that data for research purposes. While the benefits of such research include wide representation and direct interaction with patients, the limitations are many. Research using social media postings will not be representative of the population at large, but rather representative only of social media users who are willing to post about their health conditions online, resulting in significant selection bias. Social media can, however, be an effective means of reaching possible participants. For example, researchers engaging in a study and hoping to use social media may market their study to support groups or user pages dedicated to the health outcome being studied, or may reach out directly to users who post publicly about their illness to ascertain their willingness to participate.[3]

9.4.2 Data Ownership

The ownership of passively collected data is also controversial. Patients, researchers, corporations, and academic institutions could all lay claim to some ownership of passive data. Patients generate the data in their daily lives for the purposes of research, and are also most at risk from inappropriate disclosure of the information. Researchers often plan the collection of the data and perform analysis with it, thereby increasing its potential value both to the participants and to society as a whole. Corporations provide the technical means necessary for collection of the data through the generation of hardware and software used in smartphones and other personal digital devices, and also may serve to benefit the most financially from the use of passive data. Lastly, academic institutions often sponsor and fund the ongoing research, particularly in the medical context.[10]

Due to the size of passive data collection programmes, the complexity of the data generated, and the potential value of the data, if properly applied, ownership of passive data is an issue that may not be easily settled. In general, because of these many complications and the aforementioned sensitivity of the data generated in the process of passive data collection, most experts agree that ownership should err on the side of giving patients more control over the data.[10] An ownership structure that places control over the data in the hands of corporations, researchers, or academic institutions may prioritize financial or societal incentives over the protection of the individual participants, whereas concentrating power in the hands of the individuals who generated the data will generally help ensure adequate protection.

To allow this, some authors have advocated for ownership discussions to occur during the informed consent process, before individuals agree to become participants. Further, some authors have suggested that participants should have the option to specify a data expiration date, after which researchers would have to destroy the data, rather than storing it indefinitely.

9.4.3 Data Storage

As highlighted above, data collected passively from smartphone and personal digital devices can be particularly sensitive. Despite best efforts at data deidentification in medical research, passively collected data often cannot be truly deidentified. For example, a passive data study that collects GPS data may include no information about a person's name, date of birth, or address; nevertheless, individuals in the study may be easily identified simply by using GPS data to determine the location where they spend the hours of midnight to 6:00 a.m. every night. Ostensibly, this would be their address, and cross-referencing with additional information collected in the process of passive data collection or other publicly available records may allow easy identification of the participants in a particular study.

As a result, the storage of data collected passively requires specific protections.[9] First, if data are collected from personal digital devices, data should never be stored in an accessible format on those devices. Smartphones and other personal digital devices are rarely secured and can be lost or stolen easily. Once collected, these data should be deidentified to the greatest extent possible, but given the aforementioned difficulty in ensuring this, all storage and analysis of data should take place in an encrypted setting behind a firewall. Participants in the research study at hand should always be given complete access to their own data upon personal request, and should also be given the option to exit a study and have their data destroyed at any point.

9.4.4 Data Use

The use of passively collected data may lead to ethical complications in both research and clinical settings.[9] Passive data may require the ownership and use of a smartphone, and therefore research using passive data may bias towards a younger population being studied. Further, it is important to remember that the use of passive data to answer research questions is a relatively new endeavour and is not easily summarized in the traditional setting of hypothesis testing. With such a large amount of data, dozens or hundreds of hypotheses could be tested with regard to a single outcome, increasing the possibility of false positive findings.

In the clinical setting, the use of passive data for normal clinical care, such as the evaluation of how physically active a patient has been, highlights a few important ethical issues. First, use of such data may lead to stigmatization or unconscious bias. If an obese patient is shown to be physically inactive by passively collected data, the attending clinician may assume that they are lazy or unwilling to engage actively in their own health, rather than coming up with ways to encourage a healthier lifestyle.

Further, the use of passive data may disrupt the doctor-patient relationship. Some patients would inevitably be uncomfortable with the idea of being 'tracked' and may not like the idea that their physician has a wealth of personal information about them and their daily behaviour. Among elderly patients in particular, the emphasis on technology and data may highlight the replacement of human interaction with technological innovation, increasing feelings of social isolation or depersonalization in the medical system. Additionally, clinical applications of passive data would likely lead to incidental findings. Accelerometer data, for example, may detect a Parkinsonian tremor in an otherwise healthy patient.

To address these concerns, researchers using passively collected data must have reasonable a priori hypotheses to avoid the generation of false positives. Studies that evaluate many hypotheses should further adjust for multiple hypothesis testing by an appropriate procedure to control the rate of false positives from these high-dimensional data. Populations included for research should be highlighted, and researchers should make special effort to recruit individuals who may be less likely to participate, such as the elderly, as appropriate. In the clinical setting, there must be plans put in place regarding the disclosure of incidental findings, to ensure appropriate disclosure and adequate quality of life for patients. Further, important metrics for clinical decision-making should be stated prior to implementation to avoid the introduction of unconscious bias.

9.5 Illustrative Cases

Illustrative Clinical Case 1: Depressive Symptoms after Glioma Surgery

This first case concerns a hypothetical research study on the presence of depressive symptoms after glioma surgery among a cohort of adult neurosurgical patients. Researchers have hypothesized that depressive symptoms are common after glioma resection and are more common among individuals who have low social interactivity. To assess this hypothesis, they designed a study using passively collected data from personal smartphones to ascertain social interactivity after glioma surgery. Through the same application, they administer Patient Health Questionnaire (PHQ-9) surveys every other day. Using this data, they hope to illustrate that individuals who are more active socially, in terms of their interactivity by text messages and phone calls, will have a lower frequency of depressive symptoms.

Ethically, such a study should focus first on informed consent. Participants in this study should be told exactly which data will be collected (i.e., PHQ-9 surveys every other day, text message and phone call logs) and the purposes for that data (i.e., the study hypothesis). It should be clear to them that participation in this study will not serve to benefit them, other than through the increased screening for depressive symptoms they will undergo. Further, they should be told exactly how the data will be protected and safely stored. This consent process should include a discussion about data ownership and should highlight ways that individuals can exit the study should they change their mind about consenting to the research process.

In designing the study, the responsible researchers must focus on collecting the bare minimum data necessary (i.e., patient demographics, phone and text logs, PHQ-9 surveys), disabling collection of all other passive data that is unrelated to the project (i.e., GPS data, accelerometer data). They should also highlight an intended number of patients to enroll and period of data collection (i.e., one year after survey versus one month), as well as an expected project time frame to report their findings.

Illustrative Clinical Case 2: Passive Data in Clinical Assessment of Spine Patients

Symptoms of spine disease are notoriously difficult to assess, and often rely on patient-reported outcome measures (PROMs) as a way to assess a patient's symptomatic burden. This hypothetical scenario represents a new clinical approach to the diagnosis and treatment of spine disease that relies on traditional clinical assessment augmented by a one month period of passive and active data collection, which takes place during the pre-surgical period during which patients may seek conservative treatment. Clinicians in this scenario will use GPS and accelerometer passive data, as well as daily VAS pain scores and weekly PROMIS-10 surveys, to determine whether or not individuals with spine disease are good surgical candidates.

This study brings about ethical issues that are largely distinct from Case 1, because this scenario focuses on the application of passive data collection to clinical care rather than research only. In this setting, issues of informed consent for patients as well as adequate data protection and storage remain important, but there are additional issues related to the use of these data in the course of clinical care. Clinicians in this setting should decide a priori on criteria for assessing whether a patient is a good surgical candidate before observing any of the data, to avoid unconscious bias. For example, an individual who is physically inactive and reports high daily pain may be a good surgical candidate, because it may be that their high degree of pain is causing their physical inactivity. On the other hand, a patient with low pain who is physically inactive may be a poor surgical candidate, because their symptoms are less severe and they may benefit from more conservative management like physical therapy. Trends can also be assessed by passive data collection, and patients whose symptoms appear to be worsening with conservative therapy may be better surgical candidates than patients whose symptoms improve with conservative therapy.

Further, clinicians in this setting must maintain the historical standard of care via clinic assessments and face-to-face doctor-patient interactions, to avoid allowing digital data collection to replace clinical assessment. Particularly, while passive data collection and the methods used for analysis are in their nascent stages, it is important that clinicians avoid overemphasizing the importance of passive data in clinical decision-making. Lastly, the clinic assessment process should be set up to allow patients to opt out of passive data collection and still receive full clinical care. Particularly this is necessary for patients who may not be able to participate in passive data collection, such as those who do not have smartphones or who are unwilling to consent to collection.

9.6 Future Directions

The use of passively collected data in medical research and clinical care will continue to expand as the devices used for such collection become more ubiquitous and more researchers and clinicians develop the analytical tools necessary to make use of these data. Consideration of the ethical issues highlighted in this chapter – including issues of data collection, data ownership, data storage, and data use – can help ensure adequate protection of participants and patients, while allowing this massive expansion of data to inform research and clinical decision-making.

Funding: National Institutes of Health (NIH) Training Grant T32 CA 009001 (DJC).

References

1. Cohen I. G., Mello M. M. HIPAA and protecting health information in the 21st century. *JAMA* 2018; **320**: 231–2.

2. Onnela J. P., Rauch S. L. Harnessing smartphone-based digital phenotyping to enhance behavioral and mental health. *Neuropsychopharmacology* 2016; **41**: 1691–6.

3. Mikal J., Hurst S., Conway M. Ethical issues in using Twitter for population-level depression monitoring: a qualitative study. *BMC Medical Ethics* 2016; **17**: 22.

4. Smith A. *U.S. Smartphone Use in 2015*. Pew Research Center. 2015.

5. Singer N. 'Weaponized ad technology': Facebook's moneymaker gets a critical eye. *New York Times*, 16 August 2018.

6. Torous J., Staples P., Onnela J. P. Realizing the potential of mobile mental health: new methods for new data in psychiatry. *Current Psychiatry Reports* 2015; **17**: 602.

7. Staples P., Torous J., Barnett I., et al. A comparison of passive and active estimates of sleep in a cohort with schizophrenia. *NPJ Schizophrenia* 2017; **3**: 37.

8. O'Doherty K. C., Christofides E., Yen J., et al. If you build it, they will come: unintended future uses of organised health data collections. *BMC Medical Ethics* 2016; **17**: 54.

9. Bietz M. J., Bloss C. S., Calvert S., et al. Opportunities and challenges in the use of personal health data for health research. *JAMA* 2016; **23**: e42–8.

10. Godard B., Schmidtke J., Cassiman J. J., et al. Data storage and DNA banking for biomedical research: informed consent, confidentiality, quality issues, ownership, return of benefits. A professional perspective. *Eur. J. Hum. Genet.* 2003; **11 Suppl 2**: S88–122.

10

A Historical Overview of Ethics in Neurosurgery

Cara Sedney

10.1 Introduction

Current medical ethics and bioethics, as well as neurosurgical ethics in particular, are derived from a number of historical sources. Early medical ethics became increasingly deontological, and transformed into bioethics with increasing societal impact. Neurosurgeons have been involved in ethical issues since the inception of the field.

10.2 Medical Ethics

The history of neurosurgical ethics begins with that of medical ethics. The earliest recorded origins of medical ethics in Western civilization are from a variety of Hellenic texts, some of which are attributed to Hippocrates but which were likely written by a variety of authors over centuries, in which physicians are exhorted to 'help and not to harm'.[1] It may be noted that this exhortation was mainly with respect to prognostication rather than treatment, given the limited treatment modalities available in that era.[1] The culmination of such texts, and still relevant and recited by medical trainees today, is the Hippocratic oath, again originally attributed to Hippocrates. In spite of the broad influence of such sources, Jonsen notes that the guidance offered in these early Hellenic texts focuses mainly on the relationship between the individual physician and patient and what might be termed decorum rather than deontology, while furthermore not commenting on the broader role or responsibility of the physician in society.[1]

The Medieval period saw the development of further conceptualization of medical ethics principles and integration with religious thought, as care of the sick was embraced by the Abrahamic religions. Jonsen notes that a deontological tone arose within Christian and Islamic medical ethics during this time, as well as the societal responsibility of the physician to care for the poor. Ishaq Ibn ʿAli al-Ruhawi penned an ethical treatise wherein he noted the physician's responsibility to care for their own physical and spiritual health, the importance of confidentiality, and the need to be just in caring for all patients regardless of ability to pay or differences of beliefs or backgrounds.[1] The Talmudic scholar Maimonides furthermore expounded on the responsibilities and ideal qualities of physicians. These deontological principles contrasted what Jonsen terms a 'guild ethics' of Medieval medicine as physicians and surgeons organized into professional social groups.[1] This so-called guild ethics tended to be more self-interest focused.

At the same time, Indian and Chinese medical ethics were developing and had similarities with respect to duties of physician to patient, while again the duty of the physician in society is overlooked.[1] The Sanskrit text *Charaka Samhita* is felt to be comparable in some respects to the Hippocratic oath, stating 'Day and night, however you may be engaged, you shall strive for the relief of the patient with all your heart and soul. You shall not desert or injure your patient even for the sake of your life or living'.[1]

As medical, anatomical, and physiological knowledge increased in the Renaissance and beyond, the importance of the physician within society as well as the importance of ability or competence became more prominent in medical ethical thought.[1] Classical texts were rediscovered and read by physicians, and theological thought regarding medical issues became more refined. Catholic theologians distinguished between the preservation of life through 'ordinary' and 'extraordinary' means.[1] Various writers of the time noted the immorality of practicing medicine without sufficient knowledge or failing to recognize one's limitations, overcharging or abandoning patients, being prideful, or lacking 'fidelity' to patients.[1] The decorum-based ethic of the early classical texts was carried forward and refined as the medical profession became more subspecialized and integrated, while simultaneously becoming more organized and more self-regulated.

Thomas Percival wrote the text *Medical Ethics*, which borrowed heavily from classical concepts but also reframed the responsibility of the physician to society rather than simply individual patients.[1] This text in turn was heavily utilized by the American Medical Association (AMA) in crafting its own 'Code of Ethics'. While Paul Starr has postulated that a variety of socioeconomic pressures were the impetus underlying the 'Code of Ethics',[2] it nevertheless encompassed the myriad ethical aspects of medicine from previous eras and placed a particular emphasis on competence and training, while the very existence of the AMA promulgated the importance of professional organizations in the determination of ethical issues. Work product from an AMA committee regarding the controversy of anaesthetic use in surgery contained the first mention of risk/benefit analysis with respect to medical decision-making.[1]

Scientific advances in the eighteenth and nineteenth centuries saw refinement of medical ethics away from simple exhortations on professional etiquette and towards an 'ethic of competence' and scientific basis for care, as espoused by physician and philosopher Richard Cabot.[1] Role model–based ethics was similarly important within the medical profession at this time, wherein the behaviours modelled by beloved clinicians such as William Osler were extolled within medical practice and training.[1]

10.3 Early Neurosurgical Virtue Ethics

It is at this time that the early neurosurgeons had a similarly profound impact on the ethics of the nascent neurosurgical field. What might currently be called the 'virtue ethics', or role model–based ethics, of these early pioneers and mentors of others in neurosurgery can be gleaned from historical accounts and their own writings. Ethicist Rosa Lynn Pinkus has termed the influence of the early founders of neurosurgery as illustrations of the 'tacit component' of neurosurgical ethics.[3] She further notes that, upon study of early published clinical cases by the founders of neurosurgery, 'ethical issues were not bracketed from the technical aspects of practice but were integral to them. Specifically, they document awareness and resolution of moral dilemmas intrinsic to concepts that today are labelled brain death, informed consent, competency, paternalism, and coercion', as well as innovation.[3] Don Long notes that 'if we examine the characteristics of neurosurgical behaviour and think about the styles of the two great neurosurgeons whom we all emulate, we can outline a rudimentary structure for a philosophy of neurosurgery'.[4] Samuel Greenblatt, noted neurosurgical historian, has recounted that such ideals are still present in the field today and include manual or technical competence, scientific rigour, and humanistic interest.[5]

The contributions of Harvey Cushing to the current neurosurgical ethic modelled through his own example include his adoption and development of new technologies, his role as a clinician scientist, and his prolific surgical career. His ethic of competence included qualities such as those of being 'careful, precise, and methodical'.[4] Don Long wrote, 'To this day neurosurgeons maintain this heritage, honoring prolific surgeons who write about their experiences, and innovative surgeons who develop new techniques'.[4] Robert Harbaugh furthermore expounded on the essential seven founding principles of neurosurgery, all modelled by Cushing, in his 2015 AANS presidential address.[6]

Walter Dandy similarly influenced the ethics of the field with particular emphasis on surgical excellence and courage in dealing with difficult clinical problems or scientific questions, with a goal of cure or mastery. Both men implicitly demonstrated the ethic of competence with a consistent pursuit to improve care and surgical technique. This can be seen in the ethic of neurosurgery today, as in the words of Donald Quest: 'We can all commit ourselves to improving our judgement and our operative techniques . . . each one of us can contribute by our commitment to increasing our knowledge of the nervous system and its disorders'.[7] Both Cushing and Dandy furthermore inculcated an ethic of hard work through their enormous clinical productivity, which remains a common ideal within the neurosurgical ethic today.

Both early surgeons demonstrated an implicit emphasis on patient-centredness that is still heavily emphasized in the field. Maxwell gives an exceptionalist argument for patient-centredness in the ethics of neurosurgery, stating that 'the neurosurgeons' concept of patient-centred care is consistent with those of other health care providers, but the emphasis is likely to be at a more intimate and personal level' due to the serious nature of neurosurgical conditions.[7] Issam Awad notes that 'Our patient-centered mission imposes a moral dimension on our work, including our methods, tools, and objectives'.[8]

10.4 Societal Issues and Early Bioethics

Neurosurgery intersected with broader ethics and social opinion in an unfortunate fashion with regard to the early treatment of psychiatric diseases. The lobotomy, pioneered for neuropsychiatric disorders by Egas Moniz and popularized by Walter Freeman and James Watts, experienced extreme popularity in the mid-twentieth century.[9] It is believed that more than 60,000 lobotomies were done in various settings for psychiatric reasons in the United States alone. Caruso and Sheehan have investigated the ethical considerations of the events surrounding the popularity of, and eventual public outcry over, both the procedure and the conduct of Walter Freeman.[10] The ethical issues contributing to the overall social pressure against lobotomy included poor outcomes, consent issues, lack of scientific publications in support of the procedure, and the use of the procedure as a form of control over institutionalized patients.[10] In contrast, more nuanced objections regarding the permanent alteration of the intrinsic personhood of the patient were also expressed by contemporaries such as Siegfried Haddenbrock, who stated that a lobotomy represented 'definitive destruction of the self-confident and free personality of the human being'.[11] Disturbingly, Caruso and Sheehan relate an account of the very first patient to undergo a lobotomy, who decided at the last minute to withdraw her consent, but that her refusal was not accepted: 'On the day of the operation she continued to resist, and she struggled while she underwent sedation and general anesthesia'.[10] It should be noted that Walter Freeman was not a neurosurgeon by training, and was instead a neurologist; however, the lessons learned from, and stigma associated with, these historical events have profoundly influenced later attempts to reintroduce neurosurgical procedures for psychiatric diagnoses.

One of the new developments in ethics in the twentieth century is the synergistic effect of media and public opinion upon social issues, such that individual neurosurgeons themselves are not always the final arbiters of neurosurgical ethics questions. Furthermore, the societal uneasiness regarding science, research, consent, and the human mind relate to broader questions on the nature of scientific progress in society. It is in this realm that still other neurosurgeons have made substantive contributions in what would come to be known as 'bioethics'.

According to Jonsen, 'bioethics' refers to a more interdisciplinary discourse to address increasingly complex problems: 'Bioethics was born inheriting some of the ideas and values of the old medical ethics but encountering unprecedented problems, evolving through unique styles of analysis and embracing many more participants than the old medical ethics ever had'.[12] This field was formed organically through a number of broadly attended conferences airing issues including medical and scientific progress, along with interdisciplinary centres such as the Hastings Center and Kennedy Institute, which weighed in on ethical matters in current events in an interdisciplinary fashion.[12]

Wilder Penfield demonstrated thought that was grounded in traditional medical ethics but recognized the limitations of traditional medical ethics, as twentieth century medical interventions had more far-reaching consequences.[13] He recognized the broader implications of his own work and invited an interdisciplinary process as well as public participation in the discussion of advances in neuroscience.[13] He furthermore directly participated in the interdisciplinary discourse that created the modern discipline of bioethics.[13] He stated in the Dartmouth Convocation on Great Issues of Conscience in Modern Medicine, held in 1960, that 'the code of medical ethics and the conscience thus created is not enough to guide the race of man, now moving so swiftly in the stream of social evolution'.[14] He then called for an interdisciplinary discussion regarding scientific advances, including philosophical and religious thinkers.[13] He furthermore went on to create such discourse, taking on what he termed a 'social-philosopher' role through his writings and wide-ranging sociopolitical interactions.[15] Penfield modelled in his clinical and scientific practice a balance between progress and ethics, and noted ethicist Joseph Fins has remarked that Penfield demonstrated a 'pragmatic' ethic, 'which advanced, rather than feared, incremental therapeutic engagement'.[16]

10.5 Modern Ethical Contributions

Several individual neurosurgeons were similarly involved in societal debates regarding ethical issues, particularly regarding brain death. William Sweet served as a neurosurgical member of the Harvard Medical School Ad Hoc Committee to Examine the Definition of Brain Death.[17] Robert White was an advisor to the pope regarding brain death as well as in vitro fertilization.[18] Such involvement on an individual level ensures that neurosurgeons continue to have a voice in continuing ethical debates.

Ethics has also been a point of concentration for several neurosurgical organizations throughout the past 30 years. The American Association of Neurological Surgeons convened a Committee on Ethics to delineate a neurosurgical code of ethics, spearheaded by

Bruce Sorensen.[19] This code evokes previous decorum-focused codes of ethics as well as deontological exhortations. It instructs members of the organization to effect an ethic of competency, act in patient's best interest, work productively within the healthcare team, disclose conflicts of interest, and not misrepresent themselves professionally. Importantly, it concludes with the stipulation that 'the AANS Member, in addition to providing patient care, has a social obligation to be involved in the community and world activities, especially those matters affecting health'.[20]

Later efforts by the World Federation of Neurosurgical Societies, headed by Felix Umansky, similarly produced a statement on ethics.[21] This broader document describes more completely the duty of competence in patient care, including the responsibility to keep accurate and timely operative reports and try to avoid travel in the immediate post-operative period. Patient competency issues in neurosurgical conditions are described in detail, as are not starting versus withholding treatment. Additionally, broad societal responsibilities are described in detail. The duty to care for patients who cannot pay as well as prisoners is described. Reflecting events in the early twentieth century, the statement on ethics further directs 'we should not be a party to torture, or to any form of physical or psychological punishment'.[21] Furthermore, the duty to society over a patient's right to confidentiality is described. Additional broader topics such as research ethics and the duty to assist peers in the developing world are also addressed. Overall, these two examples of organizational codes of ethics represent the efforts by professional specialty societies to define and influence the ethical behaviour of their members.

10.6 Conclusion

The history of medical ethics and bioethics, as well as neurosurgical ethics in particular, create a complex landscape for neurosurgeons of today. While neurosurgeons may not always be the final arbiters of societal ethics issues, the historical and organizational precedent of involvement and advocacy places neurosurgical ethics firmly within the purview of the field.

References

1. Jonsen A. R. *A Short History of Medical Ethics*. New York, Oxford, 2000.

2. Starr P. *The Social Transformation of American Medicine*. New York, Basic/Perseus, 1984.

3. Pinkus R. L. Politics, paternalism, and the rise of the neurosurgeon: the evolution of moral reasoning. *Med. Humanit. Rev.* 1996; **Fall**: 20–44.

4. Long D. M. The founding philosophy of neurosurgery. In *Philosophy of Neurological Surgery*. I. Awad, ed. Park Ridge, AANS, 1995.

5. Greenblatt S. H. Neurosurgery's ideals in historical perspective. In *Philosophy of Neurological Surgery*. I. Awad, ed. Park Ridge, AANS, 1995.

6. Harbaugh R. E. Neurosurgery's founding principles: the 2015 AANS presidential address. *J. Neurosurg.* 2015; **123**: 1351–7.

7. Maxwell, R. E. Patient-centered neurosurgery. In *Philosophy of Neurological Surgery*. I. Awad, ed. Park Ridge, AANS, 1995.

8. Awad I. A. Conceptual synthesis: elements of a philosophy of neurological surgery. In *Philosophy of Neurological Surgery*. I. Awad, ed. Park Ridge, AANS, 1995.

9. Agarwal P., Sarris C. E, Herschman Y., Agaral N., et al. Schizophrenia and neurosurgery: a dark past with hope of a brighter future. *J. Clin. Neurosci.* 2016; **34**: 53–8.

10. Caruso J. P., Sheehan J. P. Psychosurgery, ethics, and media: a history of Walter

Freeman and the lobotomy. *Neurosurg. Focus* 2017; **43**(3): E6.

11. Gross D., Schafer G. Egas Moniz (1874–1955) and the 'invention' of modern psychosurgery: a historical and ethical reanalysis under special consideration of Portuguese original sources. *Neurosurg. Focus* 2011; **30**(2): E8.

12. Jonsen A. R. *The birth of bioethics.* New York, Oxford, 1998.

13. Sedney C. L., Bernstein M. Wilder Penfield – bioethicist. *Can. J. Neurol. Sci.* 2014; **41**: 177–81.

14. Proceedings: Dartmouth Convocation on Great Issues of Conscience in Modern Medicine. The Dartmouth Convocation in Hanover. 8–10 September 1960.

15. Lewis J. *Something Hidden: A Biography of Wilder Penfield.* Garden City, Doubleday, 1981.

16. Fins J. J. A leg to stand on: Sir William Osler and Wilder Penfield's 'neuroethics'. *Am. J. Bioeth.* 2008; **8**(1): 37–46.

17. Ad Hoc Committee of the Harvard Medical School to Examine the Definition of Brain Death. A definition of irreversible coma. *JAMA* 1968; **205**(6): 337–40.

18. Malchesky P. S., Robert J. White: renowned neurosurgeon, author, bioethicist, medical adviser to popes. A man for all seasons. *Artificial Organs.* 2011; **35**(1): 1–3.

19. Patterson R. H. A code of ethics; the 1986 AANS presidential address. *J. Neurosurg.* 1986; **65**: 271–77.

20. AANS Board of Directors. AANS Code of Ethics. Revised 2014. Available at: www .aans.org/-/media/Images/AANS/Header/ Govenance/AANS_Code_of_Ethics_11–22 -2014.ashx?la=en&hash=124B159D6B41A CF78DFB0110EB55B10E68D5D3DD.

21. WFNS Committee for Ethics and Medico-Legal Affairs. Statement of Ethics in Neurosurgery. Revised 2007. Available at: www.wfns.org/WFNSData/Document/Stat ement_of_Ethics_in_Neurosurgery.pdf.

Evidence-Based Neurosurgery: Principles, Applicability, and Challenges

Chapter 11

Ignatius Esene

11.1 Introduction

Evidence for optimal patient care is usually derived from research designs that might be descriptive, analytic, or integrative, and ranked into 'levels of evidence', evaluated for quality and graded into 'strength of recommendation'. Sources of evidence range from expert opinions via randomized control trials (RCT) to systematic reviews and meta-analyses. The conscientious, explicit, and judicious use of the best available evidence in making decisions related to individual patient care defines the concept of evidence-based medicine. Herein, the principles, methodology, application, and challenges of the concept of evidence-based neurosurgery are discussed.

11.2 The Concept of Evidence-Based Neurosurgery

Evidence-based medicine (EBM) has become one of the linchpins of modern neurosurgery. Advancements in research methods and information technology led to the emergence of the concept of EBM. Sackett defined evidence-based medicine (EBM) as 'the conscientious, explicit, and judicious use of current best evidence in making decisions about the care of individual patients'.[1] When applied to the field of neurosurgery, it is termed 'evidence-based neurosurgery' (EBN). EBN is a paradigm of practicing neurosurgery that integrates the best available research evidence; surgical expertise, experience, and judgement; patient values, expectations, and preferences; and clinical circumstances to provide a framework for optimal patient care.[2–4] These constitute the pillars of EBN (Figure 11.1).

In a domain as old as neurosurgery, other kinds of 'evidence', such as traditional paradigms based on pathophysiology and surgical experience, have been and are practiced in place of EBN, with considerable influence on decision-making. These parodies, which are less reliable alternatives, are inadequate guides for practice[3] and are very weak substitutes for research evidence, although they can be very compelling at the emotional level because they can provide a convenient way of coping with uncertainty.[5]

The techniques of evidence-based medicine are relevant in neurosurgery and should guide decision-making as far as possible. To optimize the translation of evidence into practice requires an understanding of the basics of 'research methods'.

11.3 Overview of Research Designs in Neuroepidemiology

A sound knowledge of the different types of research designs in clinical neuroepidemiology is the initial step to understanding the concept of EBN (Figure 11.2).

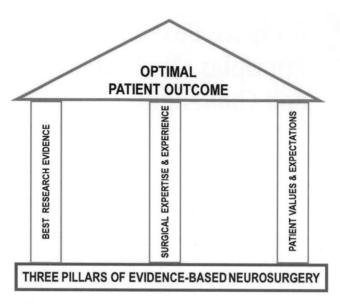

Figure 11.1 Three pillars of evidence-based neurosurgery

Clinical research is broadly categorized into primary and secondary research. Primary involves conducting 'de novo research', while secondary research makes use of existing data, summarizing them to answer specific, clinical questions.

Primary research designs can be descriptive (without a comparison group) and/or analytic (with a comparison group). Descriptive studies include case reports, case series, and descriptive cohorts. Analytical studies can be observational (investigators does not assign the exposures/intervention) or experimental (investigator assigns the exposures/intervention). Observational studies include cross sectional, case-control, or cohort studies. Experimental studies include clinical, laboratory, or field trials.

Descriptive studies are useful primarily for describing the pattern of disease occurrences and hypothesis formulation, while analytic studies are mainly used to test research hypotheses.[6]

Secondary (integrative) studies pool data from primary studies to draw conclusions and include traditional reviews and systematic reviews with/without meta-analyses.

Each research design is suited for answering specific clinical questions.[4] The RCT is excellent for studying therapeutic interventions; the cohort study is suitable for common outcomes, while the case-control design is the most appropriate research tool for studying complications of interventions. Case series and case reports remain superior for communicating new, unique, rare, or strange observations, whereas anatomic studies remain the 'gold standard' for developing new surgical approaches and techniques. The design tree shown in Figure 11.2, although inexhaustive, covers most basics quantitative designs seen in routine neurosurgical practice.

11.4 Methodology of Evidence-Based Neurosurgery

Evidence-based neurosurgery is a tool of considerable value that provides a secure base for high-quality and safe neurosurgical practice.[4,7] The process of EBN involves several steps that include using experience to identify knowledge gaps and information needs,

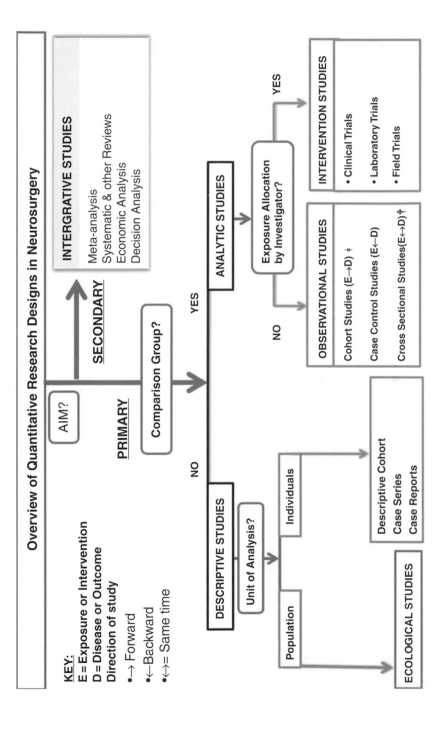

Figure 11.2 Overview of common quantitative research designs in neurosurgery (Courtesy of Esene I. N. et al.[8])

Table 11.1 Five basic steps to taking an evidence-based approach

1. ASK: Formulate a focused, clinically pertinent question from a patient's problem. A strategy for formulating specific questions is the P.I.C.O.T.S. acronym:
   - Patient (person presenting with the problem, or the Problem itself; e.g., post-traumatic IC-HTN)
   - Intervention (action taken in response to the problem; e.g., decompressive craniectomy)
   - Comparison (benchmark against which the intervention is measured; e.g., standard medical treatment)
   - Outcome (anticipated result of the intervention; e.g., Glasgow Outcome Score)
   - Time frame
   - Settings

2. ACQUIRE: Searching for and retrieving of appropriate literature (best-available research evidence)

3. APPRAISE: Critically review and grading of this literature (critically evaluating and appraising the evidence for its validity and usefulness)

4. APPLY: Summarizing and formulating recommendations from the best available evidence

5. ACT: Recommendations from step 4 are integrated with the physician's experience and patient factors to determine optimal care (that is, implementing the findings in clinical practice)

formulating answerable questions, identifying potentially relevant research, assessing the validity of evidence and results, developing clinical policies that align research evidence and clinical circumstances, and applying research evidence to individual patients with their specific expectations and values.[3] These steps are summarized as the 'five basic steps of evidence-based neurosurgery' (Table 11.1).[8]

Practicing EBN is an onerous task, as practitioners must know how to frame an answerable clinical question to facilitate the use of literature in its resolution. Using the 'PICOTS' format, a question should include the population/problem, the intervention, comparison group, relevant outcome measures, as well as the timing and setting because the determinants of a disease also depend on time and place. Thus the patient's concern/problem can be transformed into an answerable clinical question (Table 11.1).[8,9]

Next, the acquisition of literature is done from electronic databases (Medline, Embase, trial registries such as Cochrane Databases, and other specialized registers; e.g., CINAHL) and searching other resources (bibliographies, hand searches of journals, personal communications, conference presentations, grey literature: unpublished studies, theses, non-peer-reviewed journals). Other restrictions might include the language (e.g., English literature) and a specific time frame. Data acquisition is followed by its 'appraisal' using the undermentioned appraisal tools (Table 11.2). The application of the obtained results (research evidence) on individual patients ought to integrate the surgeon's experience and patient's values via the process of 'clinical decision-making'.

11.5 Clinical Decision-Making and Evidence-Based Neurosurgery

Evidence-based neurosurgical decision-making is the process of delivering evidence-based neurosurgery (EBN). Proponents of EBN often consult original texts, including the

Table 11.2 Common critical appraisal tools and reporting guidelines for specific study designs

Study design	Initiative	Meaning	Link or Source
Meta-analysis and systematic reviews	**PRISMA** (Replaced QUOROM)	Preferred Reporting Items for Systematic Reviews and Meta-analyses	www.prisma-statement.org/
	AMSTAR	Assessment of Multiple Systematic Reviews	www.biomedcentral.com/content/pdf/1471-2288-7-10.pdf
Meta-analysis of observational studies	**MOOSE**	Meta-analysis of Observational Studies in Epidemiology	www.editorialmanager.com/jognn/account/MOOSE.pdf
Randomized clinical trials	**CONSORT**	Consolidated Standards of Reporting Trials	www.consort-statement.org/downloads
Observational studies	**STROBE**	Strengthening the Reporting of Observational Studies in Epidemiology	www.strobe-statement.org/
Studies of diagnostic test accuracy	**STARD**	Standards for the Reporting of Diagnostic Accuracy Studies	www.stard-statement.org/
Other resources			
EQUATOR		Enhancing the Quality and Transparency of Health Research	www.equator-network.org/reporting-guidelines/stard/

'methods', 'results', and 'discussion' sections of research articles – not just the 'introduction' and 'conclusion' section as many traditional practitioners will do.[3]

The process of searching for evidence usually leads to an avalanche of clinical evidence, with many of the studies yielding mixed results. Obviously, not all conclusions can be correct. Thus clinicians should know what kind of evidence to look for to answer specific questions.[4] An EBN approach to sorting through the confusion involves ranking of the evidence from clinical studies according to the type of study design and the methodological rigour followed in each individual study.[5] This has led to the notion of a hierarchy of evidence, where some study designs are ranked as more powerful than others in their ability to answer specific research questions.

The sorts of questions that research addresses may be etiologic, diagnostic, therapeutic, prognostic, or economic/decision analysis,[2] and different schemes for levels of hierarchy exist for these different types of research questions. Common to these schemes are 'meta-analyses of RCTs' at the top and 'expert opinions' at the base of the hierarchical pyramids. This implies that as one ascends from the base to the top of the pyramid, the research design becomes more rigorous, the quality of evidence increases, and the chance for bias decreases.[3]

Since neurosurgery is an intervention-oriented specialty, the sections that follow will focus on the hierarchy of evidence for clinical decision regarding 'therapy' (intervention).

11.6 Evaluation of the Level/Class of Evidence

Evidence-based neurosurgery emphasizes a hierarchy of evidence consisting of levels of evidence and grades of recommendation in the clinical decision-making process. Study design dictates the level/class of evidence that in turn determines the strength of recommendation. The level of evidence is defined using commonly accepted standards in the literature, such as the likelihood that the methodology of the study would control bias,[10] as diagrammed in Figure 11.3.

A reorganization of the 'five-tiered classification' (Figure 11.3) provides the 'three-class system' of evidence hierarchy for making clinical decisions. This distinction is relevant when translating the level of evidence into a grade of recommendations. The five-tiered strategy, as in the NASS scheme[11] (Figure 11.3), assigns separate levels to 'case series' and 'expert opinion', while the three-tiered combines all lower levels of evidence.[12,13] The hierarchy implies that in searching for evidence on the effectiveness of interventions or treatments, properly conducted systematic reviews of RCTs, with(out) meta-analysis or properly conducted RCTs, will provide the most powerful form of evidence.[14] However, less than 4% of the neurosurgical literature is Level 1 evidence.[2]

If a systematic review or individual RCTs are not available, the evidence-based practitioners will look for high-quality observational studies of relevant treatment strategies. If

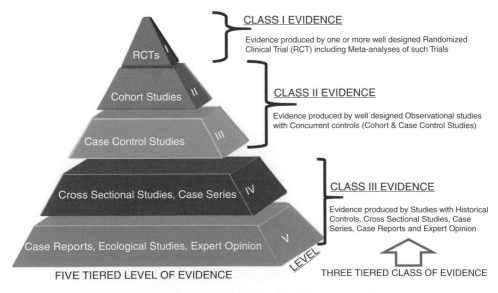

Figure 11.3 Hierarchy for the level and class of evidence for clinical decision regarding therapy

unable to get the desired evidence from the above searches, they will fall back on the underlying biology and pathophysiology and resort to their own or their colleague's clinical experience.[3] The strength of evidence is strongly determined by the quality of the study design.

11.7 Evaluation of the Quality of Evidence

The basis for evidence-based practice rests on the meticulous evaluation of the quality of research evidence.[11] Studies are usually evaluated for quality and graded into recommendations.

Numerous guidelines/checklists/scales exist for the assessment of the quality of evidence obtained from studies, such as the methods delineated by Sackett that carefully assess the methodology of each study according to its relevant category of diagnosis, therapy, prognosis, or harm.[1] Other criteria for quality assessment commonly used by neurosurgeons are as in the methodology used in developing the AANS/CNS[13] and the Brain Trauma Foundation guidelines.[12,15]

However, in recent years, the EQUATOR (Enhancing the Quality and Transparency of Health Research) guidelines[16] have provided the most popular, validated, accepted, and respected criteria for the assessment of quality of evidence in medicine.[17] EQUATOR guidelines are used for both quality assessment and critical appraisal (details at www .equator-network.org/reporting-guidelines/stard/; see Table 11.2).

11.8 Grading of the Strength of Recommendation

Each study is usually described in terms of 'level' and 'class' of evidence and summarized into 'strength' of recommendation.[18] The level/class of evidence assigned to each study is based on study design alone (i.e., Level I–V or Class I–III), while the strength of the recommendations (i.e., Level I–III) takes into account aspects of study quality,[13] consideration of applicability,[15] and not just study design. Terminologies often used synonymously with 'recommendations' are 'practice parameters', 'practice guideline' or 'consensus statements'.[19,20]

Three levels of recommendations, Level I, II, III, are derived from their respective class of evidence (Class I, II, and III).[12,13] The Brain Trauma Foundation methods grade recommendations into Level I, II A, II B, or Level III,[15] another rating scheme into Levels A, B, C, and D,[21] while the North American Spine Society (NASS) strategy scheme grades the recommendations into A (good evidence), B (fair evidence), C (poor evidence), and 'I' (insufficient evidence for recommendation).[11] Table 11.3 summarizes all the aforementioned rating schemes commonly seen in neurosurgical literature.

Class I evidence from well-designed RCTs is used to support recommendations of the strongest type, defined as Level I recommendations, indicating a high degree of clinical certainty. Class II evidence support recommendations defined as Level II (reflecting a moderate degree of clinical certainty). Other evidence such as case series and expert opinion, as well as RCTs with flaws so serious that the conclusions of the study are truly in doubt, are considered Class III evidence and support Level III recommendations, reflecting unclear clinical certainty.[13]

Some neurosurgical literature use the terms 'standards', 'guidelines', and 'options', respectively, for Classes I, II, and III of recommendations of scientific evidence, but these are used less frequently.[22] Two other systems for evaluating levels of evidence and grading

Table 11.3 Strength of recommendation for decision-making regarding therapy

STRENGTH OF RECOMMENDATION			
LEVEL*	STRENGTH	LEVEL**	DESCRIPTION
LEVEL I High Degree of Certainty	Standards	A	Based on consistent CLASS I EVIDENCE (well-designed RCT)
		B	Single Class I study or consistent CLASS II EVIDENCE (especially when circumstances preclude RCTs)
LEVEL II Moderate Degree of Certainty	Guidelines	C	CLASS II EVIDENCE (less well- designed RCT or one or more observational study) or a preponderance of CLASS III EVIDENCE
LEVEL III Unclear Degree of Certainty	Options	D (or 'I')	CLASS III EVIDENCE (case series, case reports, and expert opinion)

I = Insufficient evidence for recommendation
*AANS/CNS levels of recommendation ** North American Spine Society (NASS) grade of recommendation

recommendations increasing seen in neuroscience literature are the 'Oxford Centre for Evidence-Based Medicine' system (www.cebm.net) and GRADE Frame (Grading of Recommendations, Assessment, Development and Evaluation; www.gradeworkinggroup.org /publications/JCE_series.htm).[23] Limitations of both systems are that they are detailed and may appear complex to those not familiar with the field. It is worth noting that because judgements about evidence are complex, no single classification is universally accepted.

11.9 Critical Appraisal

Critical appraisal is the systematic assessment of evidence by reviewing its relevance, validity, and the applicability of its results to specific situations.[24] The process of critical appraisal requires a meticulous reading of the whole article, especially the methodology and not just the 'easy' bits like the introduction and conclusion sections. The ability to critically analyze is a fundamental skill of the physician to enhance the appropriate incorporation of new clinical knowledge into practice and enable the distinction of real advances from fads or over-enthusiastic promotions.[10] Critical analysis helps identify the strengths and limitations of the study; enables an understanding of the research process, to judge its trustworthiness, its value, and contextual relevance;[24] and avoids taking the author's conclusions at face value.[10]

Several critical appraisal tools are available for the evaluation of quality of methods and reporting of different study designs.[16] The most common are the Oxford Centre for Evidence Based Medicine (CEBM) criteria and EQUATOR checklists[16] (see Table 11.2). Critical appraisal methods form a central part of the systematic review process. They are used in evidence-based healthcare training to assist clinical decision-making and are increasingly used in evidence-based social care and education provision.[16]

11.10 Challenges of Evidence-Based Neurosurgery

Evidence-based neurosurgery is a tool of considerable value for neurosurgical practice, albeit not without inherent drawbacks and challenges.[7] EBM/EBN aims to address the persistent problem of clinical practice variation with the help of various tools, including standardized practice guidelines, systematic reviews, and meta-analyses.

Several myths and misconceptions have been propagated about EBM: it is impossible to practice without RCT, EBM disregards clinical proficiency, one needs to be a statistician to practice EBM, there is limited usefulness in the application of EBM to individual patients, finding the evidence and keeping up-to-date is impossible for busy clinicians, EBM is a cost-reduction strategy, and EBM is not evidence-based.[25] These erroneous interpretations resulting from a lack of knowledge are a convenient view of the principles of EBM and contradict the true purpose of EBM, which is to improve patient care.[3] Although the impact of evidence-based practice on patient outcomes remains relatively understudied,[26] EBN provides a stronger scientific foundation for clinical work, to achieve consistency, efficiency, effectiveness, quality, and safety in medical care.[10]

While proponents welcome the stronger scientific foundation of such guidelines, opponents argue that EBM could de-revolutionize care, bringing about stagnation and bland uniformity, derogatorily characterizing it as 'cookbook medicine'.[27] Opponents of EBM disregard it as not having sufficient proven efficacy.[28] They mistakenly suggested that EBM equates 'lack of evidence of efficacy' with the 'evidence for the lack of efficacy'.[3] Questions such as 'Where Is the Evidence for Evidence-Based Medicine?' have been asked.[10] Opponents continue to argue that EBM relies on peer-reviews of literature as their primary source of evidentiary knowledge, which themselves have inherent limitations. Other critics argue that EBM is not a tool for providing optimal patient care but merely a cost-containment tool.[3]

However, the greatest challenge faced by evidence-based neurosurgeons is the overwhelming volume of available evidence of variable quality from a broad range of sources that they must access, analyze, synthesize, and assimilate. This has been remedied by the summarizing of evidence in systematic reviews and evidence-based guidelines.[4]

Furthermore, all evidence has limitations.[4] For example, RCTs, the pinnacle in evidentiary hierarchy, are labour, time, and cost intensive and thus rare diagnoses, and uncommon interventions are unlikely to ever be studied using RCT methodology. 'As a result, there will never be this level of evidence for those diseases or interventions' and, unfortunately, many neurosurgical diseases and interventions fall into this category.

Despite these criticisms, supporters of EBM tend to see it as a panacea for the problems of rising costs, inequity, variability in healthcare delivery, and an attractive philosophy for providing an objective and science-based rationale for healthcare policies.

11.11 Conclusion

The techniques of evidence-based neurosurgery are relevant and essential for effective and safe neurosurgical practice. This requires an understanding of basic concepts about the hierarchy of evidence and critical appraisal methods. Neurosurgeons and neurosurgical trainees should cultivate sound evidence-based practice and strive to improve the available evidence base for neurosurgery.

References

1. Sackett D. L., Rosenberg W. M., Gray J. A., et al. Evidence based medicine: what it is and what it isn't. *Clin. Orthop. Relat. Res.* 2007; **455**: 3–5.

2. Yarascavitch B. A., Chuback J. E., Almenawer S. A., et al. Levels of evidence in the neurosurgical literature: more tribulations than trials. *Neurosurgery* 2012; **71**: 1131–7.

3. Bhandari M., Joensson A. *Clinical Research for Surgeons*. New York, Thieme, 2009.

4. Haines S. Evidence-based practice of neurosurgery: implications for quality and safety. In D. Guillaume, M. Hunt, eds. *Quality and Safety in Neurosurgery*. 1st ed. Minneapolis, Elsevier, 2018: 98–105.

5. Fletcher R. H., Fletcher S. W., Fletcher G. S. *Clinical Epidemiology: The Essentials*. 5th ed. Philadelphia, Lippincott Williams & Wilkins, 2005.

6. Esene I. N., El-Shehaby A. M., Baeesa S. S. Essentials of research methods in neurosurgery and allied sciences for research, appraisal and application of scientific information to patient care (Part I). *Neurosciences (Riyadh)* 2016; **21**: 97–107.

7. Linskey M. E. Evidence-based medicine for neurosurgeons: introduction and methodology. *Prog. Neurol. Surg.* 2006; **19**: 1–53.

8. Esene I. N., Baeesa S. S., Ammar A. Evidence-based neurosurgery. Basic concepts for the appraisal and application of scientific information to patient care (Part II). *Neurosciences (Riyadh)* 2016; **21**: 197–206.

9. Ho P. M., Peterson P. N., Masoudi F. A. Evaluating the evidence: is there a rigid hierarchy? *Circulation* 2008; **118**: 1675–84.

10. Haines S. J. Evidence-based neurosurgery. *Neurosurgery* 2003; **52**: 36–47.

11. Kaiser M. G., Eck J. C., Groff M. W., et al. Guideline update for the performance of fusion procedures for degenerative disease of the lumbar spine. Part 1: introduction and methodology. *J. Neurosurg. Spine* 2014; **21**: 2–6.

12. Carney N. A., B. T. Foundation. Surgeons AAoN, Surgeons CoN, Joint Section on Neurotrauma and Critical Care AANSC. Guidelines for the management of severe traumatic brain injury. Methods. *J. Neurotrauma* 2007; **24 Suppl 1**: S3–6.

13. Robinson P. D., Kalkanis S. N., Linskey M. E., et al. Methodology used to develop the AANS/CNS management of brain metastases evidence-based clinical practice parameter guidelines. *J. Neurooncol.* 2010; **96**: 11–16.

14. Akobeng A. K. Understanding randomised controlled trials. *Arch. Dis. Child* 2005; **90**: 840–4.

15. Carney N., Totten A. M., O'Reilly C., et al. Guidelines for the management of severe traumatic brain injury. *Neurosurgery* 2017; **80**: 6–15.

16. Vandenbroucke J. P. STREGA, STROBE, STARD, SQUIRE, MOOSE, PRISMA, GNOSIS, TREND, ORION, COREQ, QUOROM, REMARK . . . and CONSORT: for whom does the guideline toll? *J. Clin. Epidemiol.* 2009; **62**: 594–6.

17. Mannocci A., Saulle R., Colamesta V., et al. What is the impact of reporting guidelines on Public Health journals in Europe? The case of STROBE, CONSORT and PRISMA. *J. Public Health (Oxf.).* 2015; **37**: 737–40.

18. Kochanek P. M., Carney N., et al. Guidelines for the acute medical management of severe traumatic brain injury in infants, children, and adolescents-second edition. *Pediatr. Crit. Care Med.* 2012; **13 Suppl 1**: S1–82.

19. Eddy D. M. Clinical decision-making: from theory to practice. Designing a practice policy. Standards, guidelines, and options. *JAMA* 1990; **263**: 3077, 81–4.

20. Greenberg S. *Handbook of Neurosurgery*. 8th ed. New York, Thieme, 2016.

21. Anderson P. A., Matz P. G., Groff M. W., et al. Laminectomy and fusion for the treatment of cervical degenerative myelopathy. *J. Neurosurg. Spine* 2009; **11**: 150–6.

22. Rosenberg J., Greenberg M. K. Practice parameters: strategies for survival into the nineties. *Neurology* 1992; **42**: 1110–15.

23. Guyatt G., Oxman A. D., Akl E. A., et al. GRADE guidelines: 1. Introduction-GRADE evidence profiles and summary of findings tables. *J. Clin. Epidemiol.* 2011; **64**: 383–94.

24. Amanda B. *What Is Critical Appraisal?* 2nd ed. Calgary, Hayward Medical Communications, 2012.

25. Poolman R. W., Petrisor B. A., Marti R. K., et al. Misconceptions about practicing evidence-based orthopedic surgery. *Acta. Orthop.* 2007; **78**: 2–11.

26. Grol R., Between evidence-based practice and total quality management: the implementation of cost-effective care. *Int. J. Qual. Health Care* 2000; **12**: 297–304.

27. Timmermans S., Mauck A. The promises and pitfalls of evidence-based medicine. *Health Aff. (Millwood)* 2005; **24**: 18–28.

28. Charlton B. G. Restoring the balance: evidence-based medicine put in its place. *J. Eval. Clin. Pract.* 1997; **3**: 87–98.

Chapter 12

Ethical Challenges of Neurosurgical Care for Brain Tumour Patients

Marike Broekman, Alexander Hulsbergen, Timothy Smith, David Cote, and Jannick Brennum

12.1 Introduction

Brain tumour management is a complex process in which tailoring treatment to disease characteristics and individual patient preferences is key. This process is composed of multiple phases, including diagnosis and preoperative work-up, surgical intervention, post-operative treatment, recurrence, and end-of-life care. Each phase comes with unique challenges, and ethical decision-making can be guided by different combinations of normative frameworks (Table 12.1). These frameworks originate from a variety of domains in medical ethics, including clinical ethics, public health ethics, research ethics, and ethics of innovation. Together, they provide a foundation for the neurosurgeon that can be used to make the best possible decisions in scenarios that are ethically challenging.

12.2 Background Information

Clinical ethics is a practical discipline that provides a structured approach to ethical questions in day-to-day practice. As such, it bears relevance during all phases of care for brain tumour patients. Even though oncology is firmly rooted in evidence-based medicine, many questions that arise during the care for brain tumour patients cannot be answered by simply focussing on medical data, guidelines, or literature. An ethics framework can be a useful adjunct to evidence-based decision-making. Clinical ethics rests on four principles as described by Beauchamp and Childress: non-maleficence, beneficence, autonomy, and justice.[1]

Table 12.1 Phases of brain tumour management and associated ethical frameworks

Management phase	Ethical framework
Preoperative (Diagnosis/screening/surgical workup)	Clinical ethics, public health ethics
Surgery (biopsy, resection)	Clinical ethics, research ethics, ethics of Innovation
Post-operative treatment	Clinical ethics, research ethics, ethics of innovation
Recurrence	Clinical ethics, research ethics, ethics of innovation
End-of-life care	Clinical ethics

Public health ethics deals primarily with the ethical foundations of population health, the various challenges raised by limited resources for promoting health, and the real or perceived tensions between the collective good and individual liberties.[2] Public health ethics are predominantly relevant in the pre-diagnostic phase, for example when considering initiatives such as screening programmes for low-grade, diffuse gliomas.[3] They bear most relevance in large-scale settings as a guide for policymaking. As they are less applicable in individual neurosurgeon's practices, public health ethics will not be covered in detail in this chapter.

Research ethics govern the standards of conduct for scientists and can provide a framework for scientific studies related to the management of brain tumours. Scientific research concerns all stages of brain tumour management; however, neurosurgeons will encounter most trials for malignant brain tumours either at the time of surgery, or, more likely, at the time of recurrence. For example, the majority of glioblastoma trials take place in the recurrent setting. A commonly used framework to assess whether research is ethically sound was proposed by Emanuel, Wendler, and Grady.[4] This framework rests on seven principles: social value, scientific validity, fair subject selection, favourable risk-benefit ratio, independent review, informed consent, and respect for human subjects.

In contrast to clinical and research ethics, ethics of innovation is historically less well-defined, and a precise definition has proven to be challenging in practice.[5] Innovation is characterized by novel, non-validated practices with unknown long-term risks and benefits that aim to contribute to the care of an individual patient, as opposed to research, which has the aim to create generalizable knowledge. Ethics of innovation in neurosurgery is a developing field, and there are at present no generally accepted principles that can aid ethical decision-making. In general, ethics of innovation co-opts principles from both clinical and research ethics.

These normative frameworks (Table 12.2) can help disentangle the complex overlay of issues related to the care for brain tumour patients, and should become an essential part of the neurosurgeon's toolbox. In this chapter, we outline how each framework can be applied in a real-world setting to guide decision-making in different scenarios.

Table 12.2 Definitions of four types of bioethical frameworks relevant to brain tumour management

Framework	Description
Clinical ethics	A practical discipline that provides a structured approach to assist health professionals in identifying, analysing, and solving ethical issues that arise in clinical practice
Public health ethics	A discipline that deals primarily with the moral foundations and justifications for public health, the various ethical challenges raised by limited resources for promoting health, and real or perceived tensions between collective benefits and individual liberty
Research ethics	Govern the standards of conduct for scientific researchers
Ethics of innovation	No clear definition, but involves ethics related to healthcare activities that are non-validated and do not aim to generate generalizable knowledge

12.3 Ethical Issues

12.3.1 Clinical Ethics

Clinical ethics can provide a normative framework that can aid decision-making. For the neurosurgeon, this will be most relevant in the surgical and recurrence phases. As previously mentioned, the four principles of non-maleficence, beneficence, autonomy, and justice are key to this framework.

Non-maleficence is often the first principle invoked. *Primum non nocere* is traditionally translated as 'In the first place, do no harm'. This is often attributed to the Hippocratic oath, although the original phrasing translates into 'abstain from doing harm' rather than 'do no harm', the former phrasing indicating a slightly less absolute rule. If we were to live by the very absolute '*do no harm*' in brain tumour surgery, there would be very little of it at all. Skin incision, craniotomy, durotomy, and corticotomy and all inherently harmful and require a period of healing, even if no tumour is resected or no complications arise. We also have some evidence that brain surgery is harmful in the sense that more patients have post-operative symptoms related to their surgery than most neurosurgeons seem to realize.[6] The term 'post-operative symptoms' is used intentionally rather than complications, as many of these cannot be avoided.

However, this harm or risk is balanced against the benefit of tumour diagnosis and removal. This is true for all types of surgery, and the surgeon's task is to strike a balance between the chances of providing benefit and the risks of harming the patient. In brain tumour surgery, this will often be measured in prolongation of life and possibly the alleviation of symptoms such as epilepsy, increased intracranial pressure, and focal neuro-logic deficits. An additional dimension unique to brain surgery is that this balancing not only influences the decision to operate, but to a great extent the operation itself, as well. Infiltrating tumours, especially those close to eloquent areas, can create intraoperative ethical challenges when determining extent of resection in certain regions. Again, the harms of post-operative deficiencies must be weighed against the survival benefits of tumour resection.

This beneficence versus non-maleficence balance is complemented by the second axis in the clinical ethics framework: autonomy versus justice. Autonomy refers to a patient's free will and ability to make decisions without outside interference or coercion; this should be respected and upheld whenever possible. On the other hand, the justice principle sets guidance for which treatment options are fair on a societal scale. In particular, it concerns how scarce resources can be fairly distributed within a healthcare system. Sometimes, the justice principle prohibits the patient from having access to all innovative treatments despite their autonomous wish, especially if these have no evidence of effect or are extremely expensive.[7] Bringing these two axes of four principles together can be thought of as an ethical intersection, where the surgeon and the patient work together to determine the appropriate treatment pathway.

Besides this traditional framework, two additional factors should be considered, both of which relate to identity. The first is the social and cultural context in which a patient lives and experiences his or her disease. No human being is free from the influences of their environment that have shaped and continue to shape their identity. Most patients are part of a family or other close social network, and the emotions and opinions of these primary relationships influence decision-making. Patients are often faced with extremely important issues involving complex existential decisions, and these close relations are and should be invited to participate in the process. Moreover, the cultural and/or religious background of patients and their families may have profound impact on the way disease courses are experienced and handled.

A second dimension of identity is time itself. Patients change over time as they learn, adjusting preferences, perspectives, and expectations. For example, it is not hard to imagine that a healthy person pondering a glioblastoma diagnosis would make different choices than a patient who has just been confronted with the harsh reality of such a terminal illness and the accompanying dilemma of undergoing something as drastic as brain surgery. Likewise, a patient's wishes for end-of-life may change over the course of disease as their final weeks draw nearer. This temporal self-continuum can result in an altered sense of personhood, and these changing preferences can challenge the concept of patient autonomy. Is the patient capable of expressing his or her preferences at this moment, and will pathology-influenced decisions made now somehow countermand the patient's future self? Again, an additional dimension is relevant in brain tumour patients specifically, as the patients' identity can be influenced both by the disease (e.g., a frontal glioma) or the treatment (e.g., cognitive changes after brain surgery or whole-brain radiotherapy).

It could be argued that this ethical balancing should entirely be up to the patient and that the neurosurgeon's role is therefore simply to provide them with enough information to make a well-informed decision. In other words, 'if the patient wants option A or B, and this seems like a well-considered choice based on available resources, we will go with that'. While the patient should certainly have this autonomy if he or she wants it, this is an oversimplification of decision-making in practice. First of all, providing information is rarely an entirely neutral act, and some inclinations or biases could be communicated to the patient, whether these were intentional or not. Second, patients may view their physicians as authorities not only on medical but also on ethical matters, and may be inclined to go along with the narrative the physician presents. Illustrative Clinical Case 1 provides a good example of some of the ethical challenges

---

Illustrative Clinical Case 1

Mr Adams has just been informed by his primary care doctor that he has a newly diagnosed brain tumour in his left insula, temporal, and frontal regions (Figure 12.1). The most likely diagnosis is low-grade glioma. The only symptom so far has been a seizure. Mr Adams is a 42-year-old architect, married to Louise, a psychologist, and they have two children, Stephanie (age 10 years) and Richard (age 8 years). His primary care doctor recommends a neurosurgical consultation.

Mr Adams first sees the local neurosurgeon, Dr G. T. Resection. This doctor would have explained to him that the MRI demonstrates a slow-growing brain tumour which is the likely epileptic focus, and that surgery aiming for complete resection of the tumour is important in order to increase his survival and reduce lifelong seizure frequency. Of course, there will be some risks, especially language difficulties and some possible cognitive disturbance. However, the risk of long-lasting significant problems related to the surgery is rather small compared to the risk of not having the surgery with respect to the survival prognosis.

Mr Adams is not completely satisfied by this opinion, and therefore seeks another. He consults with another neurosurgeon, Dr Su R. Veillance. She informs Mr Adams that the tumour looks slow-growing and there is no telling how long it has been there or how it is going to behave in the future. What is certain, however, is that surgery in this location will carry significant risks to language and cognition. Such deficits will be likely to have a major influence on his working capacity in the short run and perhaps permanently.

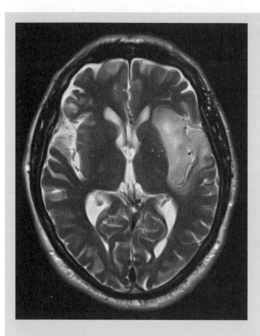

Figure 12.1 Axial T2 weighted MRI demonstrating tumour in the left insular extending into the frontal and temporal regions

Mr Adams is confused by such a disparity between both neurosurgeons and seeks the opinion of a third, Dr Alice Well. She starts out by asking Mr Adams and his wife Louise to tell her a bit about him as a person, what is important to him, and what is important to him looking ahead in life. Only then does she start to explain about the disease and the treatment options and their benefits and risks. She does this based on her knowledge of the patient's disease and functional anatomy, allowing her to predict possible changes in brain function following resection of the tumour, and through realization of her own skills and the relevant success rates and risks of complications in her hands, and not in those of master surgeons published in retrospective personal series.

Dr Well understands that many patients and their relatives in this exact situation tend to dichotomize their options. For most, the right choice will be either to avoid risking harm to their current capabilities or to go for maximum treatment to 'beat' the tumour. She takes her time to discuss to Mr Adams and his wife Louise's expectations for a few years in the future, and in that perspective examine their choices in regard to family including their children, work, and other activities. Dr Well is assessing and sharing information regarding each axis of the ethical balancing board, as well as involving those close to Mr Adams and addressing the continuation of his personhood, given that similar patients who have suffered language impairment and cognitive problems have improved over time with rehabilitation and have adjusted to their new life. In fact, Dr Well finds that she often has to meet with patients such as Mr Adams multiple times before the patient and family are prepared to make a well-considered decision.

It is fascinating to realize simultaneously the multitude of similarities and differences in the importance many patients allocate to these factors. In a small qualitative study with eight low-grade glioma patients, two males both expressed that they left the final decision in the hands of their wives, while others expressed that they really wanted to make the decision themselves and spare their family from the responsibility. Still others expressed that they really would like the neurosurgeon to make the decision for them, as he or she was the expert.[8] Thus the degree of active involvement of the neurosurgeon, the patient, and the patient's friends or family in the decision-making is in itself a factor that depends on the individual patient's preferences.

Ultimately, we know that brain tumour surgery can do both harm and good. We also know that physicians should uphold both a patient's autonomy and societal justice to the best of their abilities. Yet we do not believe these balances can be captured by categorical imperatives. Likewise, rigid flowcharts or treatment algorithms will not be able to provide sufficient guidance in all situations. Rather, neurosurgeons have the ethical obligation to be mindful of these balances. In the context of the provided example, they can ask themselves: Do I sometimes sway too much towards the position of Dr G. T. Resection or Dr Su R. Veillance? Am I involving my patient at every step of the way, prioritizing their needs and wishes, even if they don't necessarily align with my personal convictions? Is my guidance directed towards empowering their autonomy, rather than convincing them of my opinion? In our view, to consider these questions, to answer them in good conscience, and to reflect upon them is to successfully apply clinical ethics to brain tumour management.

12.3.2 Research Ethics

Not all phases of brain tumour treatment have a gold standard of care. For example, the role of surgery in oligometastatic or recurrent brain metastases is controversial. Similarly, recurrent glioblastoma treatment is unstandardized, and surgery or other treatment will often be given in the setting of clinical trials. Illustrative Clinical Case 2 is a good example of this dynamic.

Illustrative Clinical Case 2

Mr Bennett is a 57-year-old man with a left frontal glioblastoma. Twelve months earlier, he underwent craniotomy with gross total resection followed by chemoradiation, the gold standard of care in his situation. His latest scan shows signs of tumour progression in the vicinity of the resection cavity, extending into the left insula. Mr Bennett is discussed at a multidisciplinary tumour meeting and the attending neuro-oncologists notes that he might be a candidate for an ongoing trial that assesses the immunomodulatory effect of a viral vector in recurrent glioblastoma (virotherapy).

In this scenario, two types of bioethics are applicable. First, clinical ethics, as previously described, will be considered. Second, research ethics will play an important role. The seven principles suggested by Emanuel, Wendler, and Grady are the most commonly used principles that can provide structure to ethical reasoning, and many institutional review boards use these principles to assess whether proposed research is ethical (Table 12.3).[4]

In brain tumour patients such as Mr Bennett, the most important role of the treating neurosurgeon revolves around informed consent. Patients with a terminal illness may experience a variety of emotional reactions to their condition such as fear, hope, anger, depression, denial, or a tendency to 'bargain' with their caretakers. Moreover, the very nature of their neurologic disease may influence their capacity to process information or emotions. Both of these factors could hinder a patient's ability to make a rational, well-considered decision. This, in turn, may leave them vulnerable for undergoing procedures for which their consent was not truly informed.[7] Again, by discussing the patient's circumstances, wishes, expectations, hopes, or fears, and by involving friends and family if that is desired, the neurosurgeons can play a crucial role in helping the patient reach a well-considered decision that is in their best interest.

Table 12.3 Principles of research ethics

Principle	Description
Social value	The study should have the potential to provide benefit to society. In the case of virotherapy for recurrent glioblastoma, this benefit would stem from longer survival or better quality of life in these patients.
Scientific validity	This principle aims to ensure that the appropriate preclinical work has been done, that there is reasonable equipoise that precautions have been taken in case of unanticipated side effects of the treatment, that the study is sufficiently powered to find an answer to the research question, and that there is a sound and unbiased statistical approach established a priori.
Fair subject selection	This principle ensures that there is no extra burden to vulnerable patients, nor to patients of a specific background, race, religion, etc.
Favourable risk-benefit ratio	For patients included in the study, the benefits must outweigh the risks. In the case of our example, the anticipated side effects, such as uncontrolled infection, should be balanced against the potential benefits such as longer survival.
Independent review	An independent committee should go over the study and assess it based on the other ethical principles.
Informed consent	Care should be taken that a patient receives information not only about the potential benefits of the study, but also about its risk and about alternative options. Moreover, it should be clear to participants what the primary goal is of any clinical trial: to generate knowledge that can be generalized to future patients with similar conditions. Lastly, needless to say, it should be ensured that the patient receives all this information in a way that is understandable and processable to them and/or their family.
Respect for human subject	It is self-evident that no patient should be treated without respect. However, this does not indicate that a patient can demand participation in any trial or that he or she can demand to be enrolled in a specific treatment arm. Even though neurosurgeons should respect their patients' wishes to the best of their ability, this right to autonomy is not absolute.[7]

12.4 Future Directions

12.4.1 Ethics of Innovation

The broadest definition of neurosurgical innovation would include any practice that is neither the standard of care nor part of a formal clinical trial. This includes a very broad range of surgical care and ranges from minor adjustments to standard techniques to completely novel procedures.[5,9–12] Moreover, off-label or compassionate use of surgical devices would also fall into this category.[10] Surgical adjustments usually do not follow a predefined roadmap, and may only be recognized as innovation in hindsight.

Innovations in neurosurgery can obviously range from extremely unproven and possibly dangerous to merely minor alterations to a well-established treatment. When considering these innovations, neurosurgeons have the obligation to ensure that each innovation meets four key criteria: (1) oversight and regulation, (2) informed consent, (3) efficacy, and (4) no harm to others.[8]

On the one hand, some argue that because of the specific nature of (neuro)surgery and the uniqueness of every case, innovation should not be guided by strict rules, and a surgeon's professionalism will define the ethical way forward. This type of thinking is often referred to as *surgical exceptionalism*. On the other hand, others argue that oversight over innovation is essential and that, for every innovation, research protocols should be in place and assessed by the principles of research ethics. We believe that while oversight that is too strict could stifle innovation, some form of oversight could be beneficial, depending on the potential risks to the patient.[11] For example, use of a new type of drill or dural sealant may fall under surgical exceptionalism. Other innovations might further deviate from the standard of care. An example of this could be laser resection for meningioma or magnetic resonance focused ultrasound for brain metastases.[12] These innovations would require some form of regulation from a person or group of persons other than the neurosurgeon carrying out the innovative treatment. Previous authors have described the formation of a Surgical Innovation Committee (SIC), which could serve in place of an IRB to evaluate necessary protections for different surgical innovations.[7] This group would have the benefit of being independent of the investigation but still specific to surgical innovation. Second, as previously discussed regarding research ethics, one of the key requirements for ethical innovation in neurosurgery is informed consent. Patients undergoing innovative procedures must be fully aware of the risks and benefits of their procedure and should be told exactly how much and what type of testing has been carried out.[7]

Although the efficacy of a proposed innovative treatment is by definition unknown, the treatment should have some scientific basis for benefit based on prior results, animal studies, or analogy to existing treatments. The neurosurgeon should feel that the innovative treatment will be at least as effective or more effective than the current standard of care, to ensure that such a treatment meets the criterion of non-maleficence. Lastly, the innovative treatment should not harm others. While it would be difficult to imagine how even a very dangerous innovative treatment for recurrent GBM could harm someone other than the patient undergoing the innovation, it is important to consider societal costs and other knowledge generation structures. Patients who seek extremely dangerous innovations, and neurosurgeons who provide such treatments, may be harming others both through expending large amounts of healthcare resources, and by subverting ongoing, well-designed trials in the field that need more volunteers.[7]

As ethics of innovation in (neuro)surgery is a developing field, there are to date no absolutely accepted principles available that can drive decision-making. As a pragmatic solution, it is therefore important to estimate the degree of deviation from standard practice along the aforementioned lines, and balance the principles of both clinical and research ethics accordingly.

12.5 Conclusions

Clinical ethics, research ethics, and innovation ethics are frameworks that can guide decision-making during care for brain tumour patients. A thoughtful analysis and integration of these ethical frameworks can augment a treating physician's understanding of a patient's values. Neurosurgeons can also use these tools to assist treatment decision-making, especially for those patients at the end of life.

Funding: National Institutes of Health (NIH) T32 CA009001 (DJC).

References

1. Beauchamp T. L., Childress J. F. *Principles of Biomedical Ethics*, 6th ed. New York, Oxford University Press, 2009.

2. Faden R., Shebaya S. Public Health Ethics, in *The Stanford Encyclopedia of Philosophy*, Winter 2016 Edition, Ed. E. N. Zalta. Available at: https://plato.stanford.edu/arch ives/win2016/entries/publichealth-ethics.

3. Mandonnet E., Taillandier L., Duffau H. Proposal of screening for diffuse low-grade gliomas in the population from 20 to 40 years. *Presse. Med.* 2017; **46**: 911–20.

4. Emanuel E. J., Wendler D., Grady C. What makes clinical research ethical? *JAMA* 2000; **283**: 2701–11.

5. Broekman M. L., Carrière M. E., Bredenoord A. L. Surgical innovation: the ethical agenda. *Medicine (Baltimore)* 2016; **95**: e3790.

6. Brennum J., Engelmann C. M., Thomsen J. A., et al. Glioma surgery with intraoperative mapping-balancing the onco-functional choice. *Acta Neurochir (Wien)* 2018; **160**: 1043–50.

7. Cote D. J., Balak N., Brennum J., et al. Ethical difficulties in the innovative surgical treatment of patients with recurrent glioblastoma multiforme. *J. Neurosurg.* 2017; **126**: 2045–50.

8. Brennum J., Maier C. M., Almdal K., et al. Primo non nocere or maximum survival in grade 2 gliomas? A medical ethical question. *Acta Neurochir (Wien)* 2014; **157**: 155–64.

9. Muskens I. S., Diedersen S. J. H., Senders J. T., et al. Innovation in neurosurgery: less than IDEAL? A systematic review. *Acta Neurochir (Wien)* 2017; **159**: 1957–66.

10. Muskens I. S., Gupta S., Hulsbergen A., et al. Introduction of novel medical devices in surgery: ethical challenges of current oversight and regulation. *J. Am. Coll. Surg.* 2017; **225**: 556–8.

11. Gupta S., Muskens I. S., Fandino L. B., et al. Oversight in surgical innovation: a response to ethical challenges. *World J. Surg.* 2018; **42**: 2773–80.

12. Zaki M. M., Cote D. J., Muskens I. S., et al. Defining innovation in neurosurgery: results from an international survey. *World Neurosurg.* 2018; **114**: e1038–48.

Severe Traumatic Brain Injury

Stephen Honeybul, Kwok Ming Ho, Grant Gillett, and Ignatius Esene

13.1 Introduction

Severe traumatic brain injury (TBI) is a global healthcare problem. It is the main cause of trauma-related death and disability and consumes significant neurosurgical and rehabilitation resources. In some regards the surgical management of patients with severe TBI had changed little over recent years, given the well-recognised need to expediently evacuate significant symptomatic mass lesions such as an acute extradural, subdural, or parenchymal haematoma. However, the medical and certain aspects of the surgical management have evolved considerably over the past few decades.

Better understanding of the complex pathophysiological and haemodynamic responses to neurotrauma, combined with the introduction and refinement of intracranial monitoring, has led to significant modifications in intensive care management. In addition, the results of recent clinical trials have provided important information to guide clinical practice. Finally, advances in our knowledge on prognostic factors and statistical analytic techniques have led to the development of sophisticated and reliable web-based prediction models that can provide consistent and objective information about patients' prognosis when making important surgical decisions.

13.2 Background Information

For many years, the management of severe TBI has been based on information gained from intracranial pressure (ICP) monitoring, which was initially introduced more than 50 years ago and subsequently became widely adopted. The rationale for its use is based on the three Ps of prognosis, perfusion, and pathology of TBI, with the hope that using ICP to guide therapy would prevent secondary brain injury and ultimately improve neurological outcome (Table 13.1).

Current standard management of patients with severe TBI includes endotracheal intubation, sedation (+/- neuromuscular paralysis), head elevation, osmotherapy, and cerebrospinal fluid (CSF) drainage. These therapies are usually introduced in a stepwise fashion, depending on the patient's clinical and ICP response.[1] When these measures fail, more aggressive therapies such as hyperventilation, barbiturate coma, and more recently hypothermia and decompressive craniectomy have been used to manage so-called intractable intracranial hypertension.

The ICP threshold at which these therapies are introduced has been 20 mmHg, and this is based on the strong correlation between outcome and the number of hours the ICP remains above this threshold. However, one of the fundamental challenges in

Table 13.1 The rationale behind intracranial pressure monitoring: the three 'Ps'

The three 'Ps'	Rationale for ICP measurement	Clinical uses
PREDICTION	ICP is an independent predictor of outcome Patients with an ICP < 15 mmHg have a better outcome and less mortality than patients with an ICP > 20 mmHg	Discuss prognosis Monitor treatment response Provide threshold at which therapies are commenced Identify when patients are stable for weaning from sedation
PERFUSION	Cerebral perfusion pressure (CPP) directed therapy Aim for a CPP of 50 – 60 mmHg CPP = mABP – ICP	Optimise cerebral perfusion / avoid hypotension and hypoxia/ prevent secondary insults Avoid hyper perfusion injury in patients with impaired autoregulation
PATHOLOGY	Monitor for changes / development of surgical lesions (e.g., contusion maturation, enlargement of small subdural haematomas)	Early identification of mass lesions such that timely surgical intervention can be performed

Question: Does reducing the absolute value of the ICP result in an improvement in clinical outcome?

mABP – Mean arterial blood pressure

neurotrauma has been the inability to demonstrate that the fall in ICP achieved by these measures is subsequently translated into an improvement in clinical outcome.[2]

For many years, patients with severe TBI were routinely hyperventilated, frequently placed in a barbiturate coma, or more recently rendered hypothermic, because these measures consistently reduce intracranial pressure.[2] However, clinical studies have failed to show that lowering intracranial pressure by these techniques provides clinical benefit, and in some instances they may have caused harm. Although this notion might seem counterintuitive, the negative effects that these interventions have on cerebral blood flow suggest a reason for treatment failure. Notwithstanding the potential neuroprotective role of barbiturates and hypothermia, given their effect on the complex cellular responses to injury, the predominant mechanism by which they reduce intracranial pressure after traumatic brain injury is by cerebral vasoconstriction, and the subsequent reduction in cerebral blood flow has been clearly shown in several studies.[2] In view of the well-known deleterious effect that ischemia has on outcome after traumatic brain injury, it is perhaps not entirely surprising that although these measures reduce intracranial pressure and may reduce mortality, they do not necessarily improve clinical outcome. It is in this regard that the use of decompressive craniectomy was thought to be promising because not only does surgical decompression reduce ICP, but it has also been shown to improve cerebral blood flow.

However, none of these interventions will reverse the effects of the primary brain injury, and it has become increasingly apparent that they are all are associated with significant morbidity.[2] This led to concerns that while they may reduce immediate mortality, they may do so at the cost of an increase in the number of severely disabled survivors or merely change the cause (or time course) of mortality. It was these concerns that prompted researchers to conduct several recent randomised clinical trials.[3-6]

13.3 Current Evidence

13.3.1 ICP Monitoring

ICP monitoring for patients with severe TBI is currently recommended by the Brain Trauma Foundation, and there is some evidence that ICP guided therapy reduces mortality.[1] However, there has only been one prospective randomised controlled trial that was set in South America.

The Benchmark Evidence from South America Trial: Treatment of Intracranial Pressure (BEST: TRIP) trial randomised 324 patients to receive management guided by ICP monitoring or imaging/clinical examination.[3] The trial demonstrated that the monitored group had a slightly better outcome than the non-monitored group (44% versus 39% good outcome, 39% versus 44% deaths, respectively). While this difference was not statistically significant, an additional important finding was that the distribution of serious adverse effects was similar between the groups, suggesting that ICP monitoring was not, as has been suggested, driving overly aggressive interventions that could be harmful.

13.3.2 Hypothermia

Over the past decade, there have been a number of high quality trials that have investigated clinical efficacy of hypothermia; however, none has demonstrated convincing benefit and there has been a tendency to worse outcomes in patients randomised to the hypothermic treatment arm of the trials.[4] The Hutchison paediatric trial showed a higher death rate and incidence of poor neurological outcome in the hypothermia group (23 [21%] of 108 patients in the hypothermia group died versus 14 [12%] in the normothermia group). The NABISH II trial investigated early cooling within two hours of injury, and the outcomes were worse in the hypothermia group, although this was not statistically significant. The 'Cool Kids' trial was stopped on the grounds of futility because hypothermia initiated early, used globally for 48–72 hours, and with a slow rewarming did not improve mortality at three months; there was also a tendency to increased mortality in the hypothermia group. Finally, the most recent 'Eurotherm' trial was halted early because no benefit was seen and there was again a higher mortality in the treatment arm of the trial (34.9% in the hypothermia arm versus 26.6% in the control arm).[4]

13.3.3 Decompressive Craniectomy

There have now been two large multicentre randomised controlled trials comparing surgical decompression with standard medical therapy in patients who have sustained a severe traumatic brain injury. The DECompressive CRAniectomy (DECRA) study investigated the role of early bifrontal decompressive craniectomy in the context of diffuse cerebral swelling.[5] The hypothesis upon which the trial was based was that early decompression would lower the intracranial pressure, optimise cerebral perfusion, and improve clinical outcome by reducing secondary insults. Patients were randomised at the relatively low ICP threshold of greater than 20 mmHg for more than 15 minutes in the hour after first tier medical therapy. The findings of the study were that patients randomised to the surgical arm of the trial had a lower ICP and spent less time in intensive care. However, even though the same proportion survived in both arms of the trial, the neurological outcomes at six months was worse in patients who had been randomised to the surgical arm.

The Randomised Evaluation of Surgery with Elevation of Intracranial Pressure (RESCUEicp) trial randomised patients at a slightly higher ICP threshold of greater than 25 mmHg for 1 to 12 hours despite maximal medical treatment, except barbiturate therapy.[6] Patients were then randomised to ongoing medical therapy with the addition of barbiturates or surgical decompression with the actual technique being at the discretion of the treating surgeon.

The study demonstrated a clear survival benefit in those patients randomised to surgical decompression; however, the reduction in mortality resulted in an increase in the number of survivors in either a vegetative state or with severe disability. At 12 months follow-up there was a small and statistically insignificant increase in the number of patients with a favourable outcome, from 34.6% in the medical arm of the trial to 42% (p = 0.12) in the surgical arm of the trial.

13.4 Ethical Issues

There is no doubt that in the context of severe traumatic TBI raised ICP is prognostically important and can provide useful information to guide therapy. However, it is also apparent the ICP is essentially a measure of end organ injury, and while reducing the absolute value may increase survival, this is not necessarily converted into an improved clinical outcome.[2]

The results of the recent hypothermia trials may have curbed enthusiasm for its routine use; however, this does not necessarily mean that there is no role for its use in the context of severe TBI. It may be that rather like hyperventilation and barbiturate therapy the use of hypothermia needs to be more judicious and applied in circumstances where a patient is thought to be unlikely to survive without some form of intervention. It is also clear that its use must be tempered with the realisation that any reduction in ICP may come at a cost of achieving a greater number of survivors with severe neurological disability. There are similar ethical concerns when considering the ongoing use of decompressive craniectomy.

13.4.1 The DECRA Study

The DECRA trial clearly demonstrated that at an ICP threshold of greater than 20 mmHg for 15 minutes in the hour, there is insufficient ongoing secondary brain injury to justify surgical intervention and any potential benefit obtained from improved cerebral perfusion will be offset by surgical morbidity (from the craniectomy and subsequent cranioplasty) and potential adverse effects on brain parenchyma due to rapid expansion after decompression. Prior to these findings, it was almost assumed that lowering the ICP would be beneficial, and in many ways the results of this study has highlighted the need for a more thorough and considered judgement when making surgical decisions.[7]

The study certainly evoked considerable debate and one of the key criticisms was that the ICP threshold at which patients were randomised was not representative of current clinical practice (which is to intervene at higher ICP thresholds). With the benefit of hindsight this may be a valid observation; however, adopting this position fails to recognise the hypothesis upon which the trial was based. Indeed, if the trial had shown benefit, the patients in the trial would have come to represent the *clinical practice of the future*, and this would have had a significant impact on neurosurgical practice worldwide.[7]

13.4.2 The RESCUEicp Trial

The RESCUEicp trial has provided further evidence to inform the debate and has also raised several ethical issues that require consideration.[7] The first important finding is that there was a clear survival benefit in those patients randomised to the surgical arm of the trial (Deaths at 12 months; 52% in the medical arm, 30.4% in the surgical arm). Nonetheless, this reduction in mortality came as an almost direct result of an increase in the number of survivors in either a vegetative state or with severe disability – a similar finding to that of the hemicraniectomy stroke trials.[7] At 12 months follow-up, there was a small and statistically insignificant increase in the number of patients with a favourable outcome, from 34.6% in the medical arm of the trial to 42% (p = 0.12) in the surgical arm of the trial. This small increase in better outcome after surgery was only seen when patients with upper levels of severe disability were included in the favourable category, in a similar fashion to the hemicraniectomy stroke trials that deemed a modified Rankin Score (mRS) of 4 as favourable. Without this re-categorisation, the number of patients who survived with lower moderate disability or better (traditionally regarded as a genuinely favourable outcome) was very similar (32% favourable in the surgical arm of the trial and 28.5% favourable in the medical arm).[7]

A further, more ethically challenging finding was the increase in the number of survivors in a vegetative state. At six months, the number of vegetative survivors increased from 4 out of 188 patients (2.1%) randomised to the medical arm of the trial, to 17 out of the 201 patients (8.5%) randomised to the surgical arm. This finding is even more ethically problematic when considering outcome findings at 12 months, because 6 of these patients subsequently died – five patients in the surgical arm and one patient in the medical arm. The psychological distress for families involved in these circumstances and the financial cost to society cannot be underestimated.

A final issue that must be taken into consideration is high crossover of patients from the medical arm of the trial to the surgical arm. Among the 196 patients randomised to receive medical therapy, 73 went on to have a decompressive procedure. This seems to indicate that for the patients who crossed over, the attending neurosurgeons were no longer in equipoise regarding efficacy (or benefit) of the procedure, because the patients developed what was considered to be genuinely intractable intracranial hypertension. Indeed, it could be argued that for those patients who were randomised to receive medical therapy, either the ICP was insufficiently intractable to justify surgery, or all those patients with genuine medically intractable ICP had decompressive surgery regardless of allocation.

How that should affect the interpretation of the results is difficult to determine, but as the authors stated, the observed treatment effect may be somewhat diluted. Indeed, it could be argued that there is a strong ethical imperative to assess the outcome in those patients randomised to the medical arm who subsequently underwent surgical decompression. If many of these patients went on to make a good long-term recovery, there would be grounds to argue in favour of the ongoing use of decompressive craniectomy for those patients with failed second-tier therapy resulting in intractable intracranial hypertension. Conversely, if a significant number of survivors in this group of patients had either severe disability or were in a vegetative state (and who were analysed in the medical arm of the trial), support for ongoing use of the procedure would be seriously called into question. However, before this position can be adopted, there are a number of ethical issues regarding survival with severe disability that must be considered.

13.4.3 Survival with Severe Disability and the Disability Paradox

Given the evidence now available, it is clear that surgical decompression can reduce mortality. It is also clear that surgical decompression will not reverse the severity of the primary brain injury and many survivors will be left with severe neurocognitive disability. Traditionally, this outcome has been deemed 'unfavourable', the implication being that patients and their families would perceive or anticipate this outcome to be unacceptable. A further implication of this assumption is that had the patient known their eventual outcome, they would not have provided consent for the surgical intervention.

However, the reality is that patients' perceptions of personal health, well-being, and life satisfaction are often discordant with their objective health status. The disability paradox reflects the observation that many people with serious and persistent disabilities report a good or excellent quality of life when to most observers they would appear to live in a very undesirable state.[8]

Indeed, several outcome studies in the context of survival following decompressive hemicraniectomy for ischaemic stroke and a small study in patients who survived with severe disability following decompressive craniectomy following severe TBI have found that many patients do not regret having had the surgery and would provide retrospective consent for the intervention if they could make that decision again. These responses would seem to confirm the 'disability paradox', and on face value would lend support to the ongoing use of decompressive surgery even if there are an increasing number of survivors with severe neurocognitive disability. However, this does require qualification.

There can be little doubt that obtaining a positive response when asking a patient whether they would agree to an intervention that has enabled them to stay alive, albeit with a considerable alteration in functional status, is certainly a testament to the human will to survive and adapt to adverse and challenging circumstances. It may well be that they have adapted to a level of neurological disability that they might previously have deemed unacceptable, and although it is unknown whether this may have come at the expense of diminished cognitive capacity, this is perhaps of questionable relevance. Just because a person is disabled does not lessen their worth, especially if they feel their quality of life is acceptable. However, it would be injudicious and perhaps misguided to interpret this as a variation of the consenting process and therefore a validation of the surgical intervention, no matter what the eventual outcome.

The illustrative cases further explore the complexity of the ethical issues. All three patients had sustained a severe traumatic brain injury and had developed intractable intracranial hypertension. They had had a secondary bifrontal decompressive craniectomy, survived, and had successful autologous cranioplasties at 2–4 months post-injury (Cases 1–3).

Illustrative Clinical Case 1

Case 1 is a 46-year-old male. At the time of assessment, it was three years since his injury, and he was adjudged to have a good outcome. He had spent eight weeks in rehabilitation following discharge from the acute neurosurgical service and returned to work on a part-time basis in the retail business eight months following his injury. At 12 months he recommenced full-time employment. He reports minor issues with fatigue and occasional memory disturbance but otherwise feels that he has made a full recovery.
Prediction of an unfavourable outcome – 56.6% (44.9–67.5)

Illustrative Clinical Case 2

Case 2 is a 26-year-old male. At the time of assessment, it was six years following his injury, and he was adjudged to have lower severe disability. He was unable to mobilise unaided and required full assistance for all activities such as feeding and attending to his bodily needs. He obeyed single stage commands and appeared to have simple communication with his mother but not easily with healthcare professionals. His mother was his full-time caregiver and she would take him out on frequent day trips and walks. She felt she could communicate with him and felt that he had retained his good sense of humour. While she accepted that he had lost a significant amount of neurocognitive function, she was grateful for the surgical intervention that had saved his life and did not regret providing consent at the time. She felt she would do the same again, even if she had known the final outcome, and felt that her son would have agreed.
Prediction of an unfavourable outcome – 71.6% (58.8–81.7)

Illustrative Clinical Case 3

Case 3 is a 43-year-old male. At the time of assessment, it was five years since he was involved in a motor vehicle accident, and he was adjudged to have lower severe disability. He was unable to mobilise unaided and required full assistance for all activities, such as feeding and attending to his bodily needs. He intermittently followed simple commands but had no coherent communication. He frequently appeared agitated and was occasionally aggressive. Initially following discharge from the neurosurgical facility, he had spent one year at home being cared for by his wife. However, she had found this arrangement to be too difficult to manage and subsequently arranged for him to be cared for in a high-level

care facility with 24-hour support. She visits him frequently; however, she is unsure whether he realises that she is there. He remains reliant on full-time nursing care for all aspects of daily living. His wife is angry that he remains in this condition and is adamant that the husband she knew before the accident would not want to live a life in his current condition.
Prediction of an unfavourable outcome – 91.2 (84.2–95.2)

13.4.4 Survival with Severe Disability – The Futility Debate

These three cases serve in some ways to illustrate the difficulties inherent in dichotomising outcome into favourable or acceptable and indeed the utility or futility of an intervention that converts death into survival with severe disability and dependency. Indeed, the concept of futility has limitations in that it implies a degree of certainty regarding the utility or otherwise of an intervention based on the long-term outcome. It is in this regard that the concepts of 'substantial benefit' and 'risk of unacceptable badness' may of more benefit. Substantial benefit describes an outcome that now or in the future the patient would regard as worthwhile. The 'risk of unacceptable badness' is the probability that a patient will end up living in a state that they would describe as intolerable. These terms were described in order to acknowledge that there may be considerable variability and subjectivity regarding an acceptable outcome for a particular individual, and this can depend on any number of religious, cultural, or social values. More recently, the concepts of 'proportionate' and 'disproportionate' have been introduced to acknowledge that a specific treatment may not necessarily be futile but may have progressively declining benefit and therefore increasing burden in any one particular clinical situation. For a medical treatment to be 'proportionate', the benefits must outweigh the burdens (of the treatment and the likely associated outcome), and this again may vary depending on an individual's aforementioned values and preferences.

Realistically, in the context of an acute TBI, it is difficult to withhold decompressive surgery in a young person who develops intractable intracranial hypertension if it is thought that there was at least some chance of survival with an acceptable level of disability and the possibility of unacceptable dependency is acknowledged and agreed upon by those making the decision. Likewise, certain individuals feel that life is sacrosanct and worth preserving at any cost, or they may want to run the 'risk' of survival with disability in the hope that they might learn to adapt to a level of disability that they might previously have deemed unacceptable. Surgical intervention in any of these circumstances can be considered reasonable and proportionate, even if the eventual outcome turns out unacceptable because there are uncertainties and risks in all fields of clinical medicine, and these must be acknowledged by those involved in the clinical decision-making.

However, the results of the RESCUEicp trial highlight our responsibilities to a patient who has previously expressed a definite view, whether it be voiced or documented, that they would not want to survive with severe disability. In such a case, a surgeon can no longer assume that they would have obtained consent for the operation given the increased chance of survival in either a vegetative state or with severe disability. The difficulty has always been accurately predicting long-term outcome such that these issues can be considered prior to surgical intervention.

13.5 Future Directions

In the context of decompressive craniectomy for severe TBI, there would appear to be a subset of patients who require surgical intervention and go on to make a good long-term recovery. In addition, there are those patients who survive and learn to adapt to a level of disability that they might previously have deemed unacceptable. Given the clear survival benefit demonstrated in the RESCUEicp trial and the difficulties in maintaining randomised allocation, it is unlikely that there will be further trials comparing surgical decompression with standard medical therapy. The question remains as to how to design further studies to investigate clinical efficacy of the procedure, and it is in this regard that sophisticated outcome prediction models and long-term observational cohort studies may be useful.

13.5.1 Predicting Long-Term Outcome Following Decompressive Craniectomy

Traditionally, in the context of severe TBI, prognosis has been based on individual clinical parameters such as age, initial post resuscitation conscious level, pupillary reaction, and extracranial injuries (a surrogate marker for hypoxia and hypotension). Individual radiological features are also known to have prognostic significance. The recently developed CRASH (Corticosteroid Randomization after Significant Head injury) and IMPACT (International Mission for Prognosis and Clinical Trial) prognostic models have incorporated these individual prognostic factors into sophisticated web-based prediction models that provide a percentage prediction of unfavourable outcome at six months.[9,10]

Over recent years, a number of observational cohort studies in Western Australia have used the predicted risk of unfavourable outcome as a surrogate index of injury severity with which to stratify patients according to injury severity.[11] In the two neurotrauma centres that serve a population of approximately 2.2 million, a decompressive craniectomy is performed either as a primary procedure following evacuation of a mass lesion or as a secondary procedure following the development of intractable intracranial hypertension. Given Perth's geographical isolation, it is possible to determine long-term outcome of these patients and confirm the reliability of the relationship between the predicted and observed long-term outcome. This provides an objective assessment of the most likely outcome for patients who are more likely to benefit from surgical intervention (Figures 13.1 and 13.2).

The authors of both models emphasise that the information provided should only be used to support and not replace clinical judgement, and in the emotionally charged circumstances of acute neurotrauma, it would certainly be impractical and potentially inappropriate to discuss statistical data. However, such predictions may act as a prompt to initiate discussions regarding proportionate treatment and the possibility of survival with severe disability, and the acceptability or otherwise of that outcome for the patient concerned.

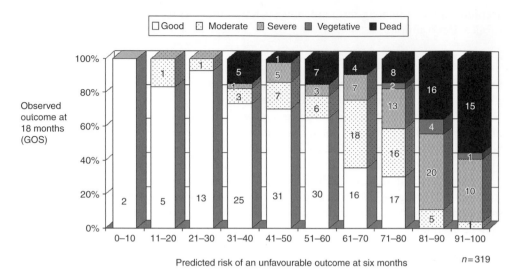

Figure 13.1 The CRASH collaborators prediction model. The prediction of an unfavourable outcome at 6 months (x-axis) and the observed outcome at 18 months among the 319 patients on whom 18-month follow-up was available. Numbers within the bar chart represent absolute patient numbers. *(Reproduced with kind permission by Elsevier.)*

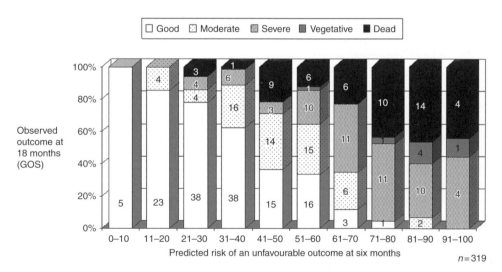

Figure 13.2 The IMPACT investigators model. The prediction of an unfavourable outcome at 6 months (x-axis) and the observed outcome at 18 months among the 319 patients on whom 18-month follow-up was available. Numbers within the bar chart represent absolute patient numbers. *(Reproduced with kind permission by Elsevier.)*

13.5.2 Predicting Long-Term Outcome – Clinical Applications

In the first illustrative clinical case, the prediction of unfavourable outcome was less than 60% (Table 13.2). In these circumstances, surgical intervention may be deemed proportionate, because notwithstanding some uncertainty, the most likely outcome is going to

Table 13.2 Demonstration of the predicted risk of an unfavourable outcome (using the CRASH model) at six months for the illustrative cases based on baseline presentation clinical and radiological findings

Clinical and radiological features required by the model	Illustrative cases		
	Case 1	Case 2	Case3
Basic model			
Country	Australia	Australia	Australia
Age	46	< 40	43
GCS	7	8	7
Pupils react to light	Both	Both	None
Major extracranial injury	No	Yes	Yes
CT model			
Presence of petechial haemorrhages	Yes	Yes	Yes
Obliteration of third ventricle or basal cisterns	No	Yes	Yes
Subarachnoid bleeding	Yes	Yes	Yes
Midline shift	Yes	Yes	Yes
Non-evacuated haematoma	No	No	No
Predicted outcome			
Risk of unfavourable outcome at six months (95% CI)	**56.6%** **(44.9–67.5)**	**71.6%** **(58.8–81.7)**	**91.2** **(84.2–95.2)**

GCS = Glasgow coma score
CRASH = Corticosteroid Randomization after Significant Head Injury

provide the patient with substantive benefit, as indeed was the case. Conversely, for case 3, the prediction of an unfavourable outcome exceeds 80%, and in these circumstances, discussions regarding outcome cannot be dichotomised into life or death because to do so would fail to recognise that the most likely outcome if the patient survives is that of severe disability and dependency. Intervention in these circumstances can be considered disproportionate, especially if a patient had previously expressed a view that they would feel this outcome to be inappropriate or unacceptably bad.

Finally, there is the second case, which in many ways represents the most challenging decision because the prediction is between 60% and 80%. The most likely outcome in these circumstances is indeterminate, and discussions with surrogate decision-makers must reflect the uncertainty. Surgical intervention would seem reasonable if a person's prior wishes are unknown, given the possibility of a good outcome and because they may learn to adapt to a level of disability that they may previously have thought to be unacceptable.

This position is reinforced by the clinical concept of the rule of rescue, which describes the powerful human proclivity to rescue identified endangered lives, regardless of cost or risk. The classic examples of this concept are heroic searches for a sailor lost at sea or daring attempts to rescue someone in a burning building. In such cases, the cost to the community or the risk to those attempting the rescue is extremely high. However, the psychological and moral imperatives are difficult to resist. In the context of medical care, there is always a strong ethical imperative to save an individual already identified life, even when it could be argued from a utilitarian viewpoint that the money and resources might be more efficiently used to prevent deaths in the wider community. People obtain social utility and a feeling of security, knowing that they live in a compassionate society that cares for the needs of each constituent member and where those in most desperate need will not be ignored or abandoned merely on the basis of resource allocation. However, that security is threatened if the rescue system is seen to be a juggernaut that is insensitive to the way people actually value their lives because there will always be circumstances where serious consideration must be given to withholding surgical intervention.

Finally, it must be acknowledged that there are significant limitations when applying population data to individual cases, and there will never be a one-size-fits-all approach to these ethically challenging decisions. However, this type of methodology may provide prognostic assistance and in certain circumstances prompt appropriate discussions regarding the possibility and acceptability of the *most likely* outcome, and perhaps guide clinically and ethically appropriate decisions with the next of kin of individuals who cannot make such difficult decisions themselves.

13.6 Conclusion

The management of patients with severe traumatic brain injury will always be clinically and ethically challenging. While there continues to be advances in the basic science of traumatic brain injury, what is currently lacking are new therapeutic interventions that can have significant clinical impact. Those therapies that are available must be continually evaluated and refined to maximise clinical benefit. Clinical decision-making must also be continually re-evaluated, and although prediction models may provide some assistance when considering surgical intervention, their inherent limitations must be acknowledged. Finally, further work is required to evaluate quality of life for those patients who do survive because unfavourable may not necessarily be unacceptable.

References

1. Bratton S. L., Chestnut R. M., Ghajar J., et al. Brain trauma foundation; American association of neurological surgeons; congress of neurological surgeons; joint section on neurotrauma and critical care, AANS/CNS. Guidelines for the management of severe traumatic brain injury. *J. Neurotrauma.* 2007; **24**, suppl. 1s.

2. Honeybul S., An update on the management of traumatic brain injury. *J. Neurosurg. Sci.* 2011; **55**: 343–55.

3. Chesnut R. M., Temkin N., Carney N., et al. A trial of intracranial-pressure monitoring in traumatic brain injury. *N. Engl. J. Med.* 2012; **367**: 2471–81.

4. Honeybul S. Reconsidering the role of hypothermia in management of severe traumatic brain injury. *J. Clin. Neurosci.* 2016; **28**: 12–15.

5. Cooper D. J., Rosenfeld J. V., Murray L., et al. Decompressive craniectomy in diffuse traumatic brain injury. the DECRA Trial Investigators and the Australian and New Zealand Intensive Care Society Clinical Trials Group. *N. Engl. J. Med.* 2011; **364**: 1493–1502.

6. Hutchinson P. J., Kolias A. G., Timofeev I. S., et al. RESCUEicp trial collaborators. Trial of decompressive craniectomy for traumatic

intracranial hypertension. *N. Engl. J. Med.* 2016; **375**: 1119–30.

7. Honeybul S., Ho K. M., Gillett G. R. Long-term outcome following decompressive craniectomy: an inconvenient truth? *Curr. Opin. Crit. Care* 2018; **24**: 97–104.

8. Honeybul S., Gillett G. R., Ho K. M., et al. Is life worth living? Decompressive craniectomy and the disability paradox. *J. Neurosurg.* 2016; **125**: 775–8.

9. Perel P., Arango M., Clayton T., et al. Predicting outcome after brain injury: Practical prognostic models based on a large cohort of international patients. *BMJ* 2008; **336**: 425–9.

10. Murray G. D., Butcher I., McHugh G. S., et al. Multivariable prognostic analysis in traumatic brain injury: results from the IMPACT study. *J. Neurotrauma* 2007; **24**: 329–37.

11. Honeybul S., Ho K. M. Predicting long-term neurological outcomes after severe traumatic brain injury requiring decompressive craniectomy: A comparison of the CRASH and IMPACT prognostic models. *Injury* 2016; **47**: 1886–92.

'Malignant' Middle Cerebral Artery Infarction

Stephen Honeybul, Volker Puetz, Lars-Peder Pallesen, and Grant Gillett

14.1 Introduction

In the past decade, there have been considerable advances in the management of patients with acute ischaemic stroke. Intravenous thrombolysis with recombinant tissue plasminogen activator (rt-PA) administered within 4.5 hours from symptom onset has been shown to significantly improve outcome.[1] In addition, the clinical efficacy of endovascular thrombectomy for large vessel ischaemic stroke has been clearly demonstrated in a number of recent randomised controlled trials.[2] However, only a minority of patients receive intravenous thrombolysis, and its benefit in large vessel occlusion is limited by a relatively low recanalisation.[3] In addition, notwithstanding the clear-cut evidence for endovascular thrombectomy, there remain major logistical challenges in providing widespread and timely access to this therapy across many healthcare systems.[2]

For those patients who either fail endovascular therapy or who present outside the time-dependent therapeutic window, there is a risk that they will go on to develop life-threatening cerebral oedema, so-called malignant middle cerebral artery infarction (MMCAI; Figures 14.1–14.2). The prognosis for these patients is poor, with a mortality rate in the region of 80% without specific treatment. In these circumstances, consideration may be given to performing a decompressive hemicraniectomy (DH) as a life-saving intervention (Figure 14.3).

14.2 Background Information

Decompressive hemicraniectomy is a technically straightforward surgical procedure that involves the temporary removal of a large segment of the calvarium ipsilateral to the side of the ischaemic stroke. The rationale is that extra space is provided into which the swollen, ischaemic brain can expand, thereby improving cerebral perfusion and preventing death due to transtentorial herniation. The procedure gained popularity in the 1980s and 1990s, and several non-randomised retrospective cohort studies seemed to suggest that mortality could be reduced.

However, unlike the endovascular techniques, surgical decompression will not reverse the effects of what is, by definition, a very extensive infarct, and many patients will be left with significant neurological deficits and a level of disability that they and their families may feel to be unacceptable. In addition, there remained controversy regarding patient selection and surgical timing. It was these concerns that prompted researchers to conduct a number of multicentre prospective randomised controlled trials comparing decompressive hemicraniectomy with standard medical therapy in patients who developed MMCAI.

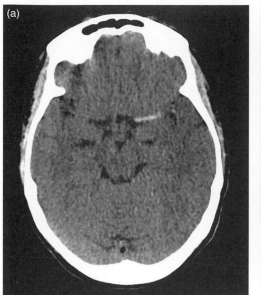
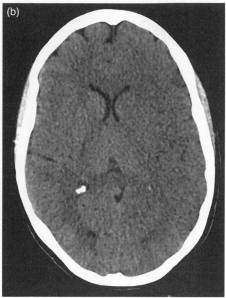

Figure 14.1 (a) 48-year-old female presents at a district hospital three hours following acute onset of right-sided hemiplegia and dysphasia. Axial non-contrast CT brain demonstrating increased density within the left middle cerebral artery to the presence of acute thrombus. (b) There is subtle loss of grey white differentiation and early midline shift.

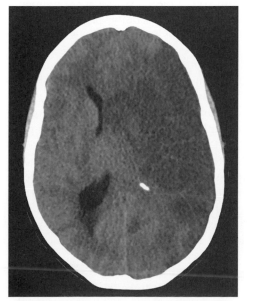

Figure 14.2 The following day she became progressively drowsier and her left pupil became dilated and unreactive. Axial non-contrast CT brain demonstrates an established left middle cerebral artery territory infarct with midline shift.

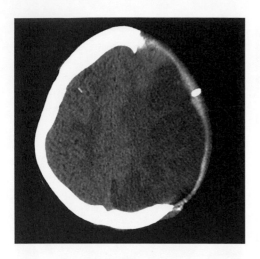

Figure 14.3 Following a left-sided decompressive hemicraniectomy. A subgaleal wound drain has been placed on the left-hand side, and an ICP monitor is seen on the right-hand side

14.3 Current Evidence

14.3.1 The European Stoke Trials

In the early 2000s, three trials were independently conducted in Europe. The DEcompressive Craniectomy In MALignant MCA Infarction (DECIMAL) trial conducted in France randomised patients aged 18 to 55 years who clinically deteriorated within 48 hours.[4] The DEcompressive Surgery for the Treatment of malignant INfarction of the middle cerebral arterY (DESTINY) trial conducted in Germany randomised patients aged 18–60 years who deteriorated within 48 hours.[5] The Hemicraniectomy After Middle cerebral artery infarction with Life-threatening Edema Trial (HAMLET) conducted in the Netherlands randomised patients aged 18–60 who deteriorated up to 96 hours from symptom onset.[6] None of the trials were completed as initially designed.

The DECIMAL and DESTINY trials were interrupted early because of slow recruitment and a significant difference in mortality among the treatment groups favouring surgery. The HAMLET trial was stopped because it was thought unlikely that a statistically significant difference would be seen for the primary neurological outcome measure, which was defined as good (modified Rankin Scale [mRS] score 0–3) or poor (mRS score 4–6).

Although each trial independently demonstrated a significant survival advantage in those patients randomised to receive decompressive surgery, the number of patients included was insufficient to determine whether there was an improvement in favourable outcome. Therefore, the design for a pooled analysis was developed when the studies themselves were still recruiting patients.[7] The outcome measures were defined without knowledge of the results of the individual studies. Patients aged 18 to 60 years were included, and the primary endpoint was defined as a dichotomised mRS score (0–4 versus 5–6) at one year. Only patients with surgery performed within 48 hours after symptom onset were included. This analysis of the 93 patients involved in all three trials confirmed the significant reduction in mortality, and it was concluded that there was an increase in the number of patients with a favourable outcome.

14.3.2 The DESTINY II Trial

The DESTINY II trial investigated use of decompressive hemicraniectomy in patients older than 60 years of age.[8] In a similar design to the previous European trials, patients who deteriorated within 48 hours of presentation following MMCAI were randomised to either surgical decompression or standard medical therapy. The results of this study confirmed that surgical intervention significantly reduced mortality, and the investigators again concluded, that 'hemicraniectomy increased survival without severe disability'.

14.4 Ethical Issues

On initial examination, the findings of the randomised controlled trials would appear to provide compelling evidence for the efficacy of surgical decompression for patients both younger than 60 years of age (as per the pooled analysis of the European trials) and additionally for those patients older than 60 years of age. However, there are a number of issues that require consideration.[9]

14.4.1 Hemicraniectomy for Patients Younger than 60 Years of Age

In the case of the pooled analysis of the three European trials, it was only possible to demonstrate that there was an increase in the number of patients with a favourable outcome if the definition of 'favourable' was changed. Traditionally in the stroke literature, functional outcome of patients with MMCAI has been assessed using the mRS score, and outcome was usually dichotomised into favourable (mRS scores of 0–3) or unfavourable (mRS scores of 4–6) (Table 14.1) – the implication being that the aim of surgery is to achieve an outcome that is felt to be acceptable to the person on whom the procedure is being performed. Notwithstanding some limitations of the mRS score, in that it tends to focus on the physical disability rather than the possibly more important neurocognitive abilities, the fundamental issue that denotes a favourable outcome is that a person has a degree of independence.

In the pooled analysis favourable outcome was reclassified, such that it included patients with an mRS score of 0–4. This would therefore include patients who cannot walk unaided and

Table 14.1 The modified Rankin Scale

Score	Description
6	Dead
5	Severe disability; bedridden, incontinent, and requiring constant nursing care and attention
4	Moderately severe disability; unable to walk without assistance and unable to attend to own bodily needs without assistance
3	Moderate disability; requiring some help, but able to walk without assistance
2	Slight disability; unable to carry out all previous activities, but able to look after own affairs without assistance
1	No significant disability despite symptoms; able to carry out all usual duties and activities
0	No symptoms at all

Table 14.2 The results of the randomised controlled hemicraniectomy trials

mRS	Pooled analysis of the European stroke trials (patients younger than 60 years)	
	Hemicraniectomy n = 51 patients (%)	Conservative n = 42 patients (%)
6	11 pts (22%)	30 pts (71%)
5	2 pts (4%)	2 pts (5%)
4	16 pts (31%)	1 pt (2%)
3	15 pts (29%)	8 pts (19%)
2	7 pts (14%)	1 pt (2%)
mRS	DESTINY II trial (patients older than 60 years)	
	Hemicraniectomy n = 47 patients (%)	Conservative n = 62 patients (%)
6	20 pts (33%)	47 pts (76%)
5	9 pts (19 %)	5 pts (8 %)
4	15 pts (32 %)	7 pts (11%)
3	3 pts (6 %)	3 pts (5 %)
2	0	0

cannot attend to their own bodily needs without assistance – an outcome that has been regarded as unfavourable for many years. The investigators justified the change in outcome categorisation by stating that 'on the basis of increasing experience of long-term outcome in patients with a space occupying infarction, most investigators feel obliged to define a score of 4 on the mRS as favourable'. However, examination of the literature shows little evidence to support this position.[10]

Indeed, closer examination of the data shows that the increase in survival came at the expense of an almost direct increase in the number patients with an mRS score of 4 (i.e., 16/51 patients who underwent hemicraniectomy had this outcome at 12 months). Among the survivors who were randomised to receive standard medical care, 75% (9 of 12) had an mRS score of 3 or less. A similar favourable outcome was achieved in only 55% of the patients treated surgically (22 of 40) (Table 14.2). An alternative interpretation of these results would be that the most likely outcome following medical therapy is either death or a favourable outcome defined as an mRS of 0–3, whereas surgery considerably increases the possibility of survival with dependency. These ethically challenging findings were even more pronounced in the DESTINY II trial.

14.4.2 Decompressive Craniectomy for Patients Older than 60 Years of Age

The DESTINY II trial confirmed the clear survival advantage; however, most of the 27 survivors in the hemicraniectomy group had an mRS score of 4 or 5 at 12 months (Table 14.2). Among

Table 14.3 The Destiny II trial: outcome for hemicraniectomy survivors

Twenty-seven patients survived following decompressive hemicraniectomy

- 2 patients mRS – 3
- 25 patients mRS – 4 or 5

Retrospective consent?

- 16 patients could not answer the question because of severe aphasia or neuropsychological deficits
- Among the 9 that could provide a response:
  - Five said YES
  - Four said NO

this group of survivors, 16 patients had severe aphasia or neuropsychological deficits such that they were unable to provide a response when asked a question regarding retrospective consent (Table 14.3). Given what many commentators would regard as an unacceptable outcome, these findings would appear to lend support to the observation that surgical intervention is associated with a high risk of translating death into survival with severe disability and dependency in this patient cohort.[9]

The two clinical cases serve to illustrate the difficulties when considering a favourable or acceptable outcome based on a patient's social circumstances and healthcare preferences.

Illustrative Clinical Case 1

Case 1 is a 42-year-old female who was married with two children aged 10 and 12. Two years previously, she suffered a right-sided middle cerebral artery infarction at the age of 40. She presented outside the therapeutic window for thrombectomy and became progressively drowsy. She had a right-sided decompressive craniectomy and went on to make a reasonable recovery. Following four months in rehabilitation, she was discharged home. She currently mobilises with the aid of a wheelchair and relies on her husband and her parents for assistance with mobility and many aspects of daily living. However, she can communicate normally and has a good relationship with her husband and children. Overall she is grateful for an intervention that has allowed her to survive so that she can remain part of her children's lives, and when asked a direct question, she was strongly of the opinion that she would have provided consent at the time of her clinical deterioration even if she had known her final outcome.

Illustrative Clinical Case 2

Case 2 is a 68-year-old retired teacher. Twelve months previously, he has suffered a left-sided middle cerebral artery infarct. He had an attempt at stent retrieval of the clot, but this failed for technical reasons. He subsequently deteriorated due to cerebral swelling and had a left-sided decompressive craniectomy. Post-operatively he made a poor recovery. He remained aphasic and fully dependent for all activities of daily living. His family were unable to look after him at home, and he was discharged to a high-care nursing facility. His daughter states that she thinks he is distressed and is certain that the father she knew before the stroke would not want to have ended up with his current outcome.

14.5 Future Directions

Given the life-saving nature of the intervention, it is unlikely that further randomised trials comparing surgical intervention with standard medical therapy will be conducted. It is now clear that surgical intervention is associated with significant long-term morbidity, and while mortality is reduced this comes at expense of an increased number of survivors with dependency. This in itself does not mean that the use of the procedure should be abandoned, but rather that a more patient-centred view should be taken into account when considering surgical intervention that is definitely life-saving but certainly not restorative. Furthermore, given the burden that this outcome may place on the patients and their care givers, factors such as the degree of social support, the biological age, and the preexisting health of the patient must also be taken into account prior to surgical intervention.

This patient-centred approach must incorporate realistic discussions regarding the most likely long-term outcome, and the focus of these discussions must be the acceptability or otherwise of that outcome to the individual patient based on their values and beliefs. The considerations here are not only clinical but also personal and ethical, and require exercise of careful and considered judgement regarding the fundamental issue of informed consent.

14.5.1 Informed Consent

Informed consent forms one of the central tenets of modern clinical medicine, and there are two basic principles that must be fulfilled.[11] In the first instance, the patient must be informed. This requires the individual to have a clear understanding of the facts, implications, and future consequences of an action. Second, the individual concerned must be competent. This requires adequate reasoning faculties in order to fully understand the relevant facts at the time consent is given. In the context of acute ischaemic stroke, both principles are challenged. The patients themselves will be acutely unwell and will often be in no position to participate in any meaningful discussion regarding treatment options or acceptable outcomes. In addition, 'malignant' swelling most commonly occurs in relatively young adults, who are unlikely to have had any prior discussions as to what their wishes would be in such a situation. In these circumstances, family members are often called upon to provide information regarding a patient's known wishes, whether it be in the form of written documentation or previously voiced views, regarding the acceptability or otherwise of the most likely outcome following surgical intervention. If these wishes are unknown, family members are asked to provide substituted judgement based on what they consider to be the person's values and beliefs. Finally, if no surrogate decision-makers are available or if there is conflict among those who are present, a clinician may be required to act in a person's best interests. When considering decompressive surgery for a neurological catastrophe, the decision-making processes can be ethically challenging, and it can place an enormous emotional burden on surrogate decision-makers whose competency to make these decisions may already be compromised due to emotional distress.

14.5.2 Retrospective Consent

The authors of the pooled analysis of the three European trials justified the inclusion of an mRS score of 4 within the favourable outcome category, because they obtained positive responses when they asked survivors whether they regretted having had the surgery, given they had survived but remained disabled. Indeed, it is difficult – if not impossible – to say that it has not been in a person's best interests if they survive a neurological catastrophe but are able to state that they do not regret the intervention, given their eventual quality of life. However, accepting retrospective consent as a variation of the true consenting process, and therefore justifying the surgical procedure is inherently problematic, especially in the light of a commonly invoked ethical concept of 'critical interests' proposed by Dworkin.[12] This concept considers that one's most important values ought to be those made when in full command of one's faculties.

Obtaining a positive response when asking a patient whether they would agree to an intervention that has enabled them to stay alive, albeit with a considerable alteration in functional status, is certainly a testament to the human will to survive and the ability to adapt to adverse and challenging circumstances. However, it would be injudicious and perhaps misguided to interpret this as a variation of the consenting process and therefore a validation of the surgical intervention, no matter what the eventual outcome. When considering the question 'Are you glad to be alive?', one is inclined to answer, 'As distinct from what?', to show up the absurdity of being asked that question. Very few, apart from those who are actually suicidal, are likely to say, 'No, I'd rather be dead.'

Competent individuals have the right to determine their healthcare wishes were they to lose competency, and this is the basis for documentation, such as advance healthcare directives and living wills. Therefore, an alternative approach to seeking retrospective consent is to canvas opinion regarding acceptable outcome among competent healthy individuals. This has been the subject of recent studies in which healthcare workers were specifically asked whether they would provide consent for a decompressive hemicraniectomy if they were unfortunate enough to develop malignant MMCAI.[13,14] They were also asked what level of disability on the mRS they would feel to be acceptable, if they survived. They were then presented with the evidence from the stroke hemicraniectomy studies and were then asked to reconsider their initial responses. The question, which was clearly stated, was whether they themselves would provide consent, based on what they perceived to be the most likely outcome.

Overall the responses reflected that for most of the participants survival with severe disability was unacceptable. It could, of course, be argued that this was a relatively hypothetical situation and not representative of the real-life tension that occurs in the context of acute stroke. However, it could equally be argued that in the real-life acute setting, hasty decisions, which cannot be mitigated, may be made under the pressure of limited time and perhaps limited competency (due to emotional distress) to reflect on the true implications of the decision. Thus the responses of the participants in these studies may be a better reflection of how many people genuinely feel about this outcome for themselves.

14.5.3 The Clinical Decision

There will never be a one-size-fits-all approach when considering the decision to surgically intervene in the context of a catastrophic clinical deterioration. In addition, the timing and manner in which these types of discussion take place may heighten the ethical and emotional tension due to limited time available, situational circumstances, and the experience of the personnel available. Families or surrogate decision-makers often feel under intense pressure to make a decision because the outcome all too often is dichotomised into life or death. However, assuming this position fails to recognise that surgical intervention will not reverse the effects of the stroke, and what clinicians really require is clarification regarding an individual's willingness to survive with that disability. Adopting a more patient-centred position may lessen some of the burden placed on surrogate decision-makers because it may facilitate discussions regarding realistic outcome expectations.

Overall, there would appear to be three broad categories that require consideration. In the first instance, there are those patients whose preferences are unknown; second, there are those patients who have expressed an opinion that survival is paramount, even with severe disability, and finally there are those patients who have expressed a view that survival with disability would be unacceptable.

14.5.3.1   The Patient's Preferences Are Unknown

Realistically, in the emotionally charged atmosphere of an acute stroke, it would be very difficult to withhold therapy in a person younger than 60 years of age if there was at least some chance of survival with an acceptable level of disability and the possibility of unacceptable dependency was acknowledged and accepted by those involved in making the decision. Treatment based on such reasoning can be justified even if the eventual outcome seems unacceptable to the injured party because risks and uncertainties are inevitable in all fields of medicine. It could also be argued that, given the alternative would be not to survive at all, a young person may quite reasonably be given the chance to 'risk' survival with an mRS of 4 in the hope that they will either improve to achieve an mRS score of 3 or even 2, or learn to accept a level of disability that they might previously have deemed unacceptable.

For patients older than 60 years of age, it must be acknowledged that there is only a very small chance that that person may achieve independence, and there is a high chance that they may be left with significant physical, neurocognitive, and neuropsychological deficits. Ideally, the acceptability or otherwise of this outcome for that particular individual must be fully explored prior to surgical intervention.

14.5.3.2   A Patient Wants Survival at Any Cost

There is little doubt that certain individuals may feel that life is sacrosanct and worth preserving under any circumstances, and this may be based on certain religious, cultural, or personal values. These individuals may also be willing to 'run the risk' of survival with severe disability, in the hope that they may achieve a good functional outcome. They might also want the opportunity to adapt and learn to live with a level of disability that they and many others perhaps might previously have thought to be unacceptable. While these views may fall outside what is deemed acceptable to the majority, where possible, these views should be acknowledged and acted upon. For this group of patients, surgical intervention following the development of MMCAI is entirely reasonable.

14.5.3.3   Disability and Dependency Is Unacceptable

The final group will be those patients who have previously expressed a view (either previously voiced or documented) that they would not want to survive with severe disability. In these circumstances, the surgeon cannot reasonably assume that they would be able to obtain consent for the operation and, if they did proceed, would have to justify acting on their own judgement against a properly considered assessment of the wishes of the patient.

It could of course be argued that competent individuals do not necessarily predict what they will later find acceptable or unacceptable as a quality of life, and this may have occurred when investigators have obtained 'retrospective consent' among hemicraniectomy survivors. However, to add determinative weight to this as a variation of the consenting process would undermine one of the fundamental tenets of modern medicine. Notwithstanding the obvious limitations of making somewhat abstract statements such as 'I would rather be dead than live with severe disability', if a person has previously made this assessment, it should be acknowledged and, where possible, acted upon accordingly. Withholding surgical intervention in this situation may further be justified by reviewing the results of the pooled analysis of the three European trials, in which the most likely outcome following standard medical therapy was either death or survival with an mRS score of 3 and thereby some degree of independence.

14.6 Conclusions

The decision to perform a life-saving decompressive hemicraniectomy will always be challenging and requires a number of difficult clinical issues to be considered. There is now clear evidence that surgical intervention can reduce mortality, but this results in an increase in the number of dependent survivors. This is especially important to consider in patients older than 60 years of age, where there is likely to be a significant neurocognitive deficit that may leave a person socially isolated. Before we consign a patient to survival with a severe disability, we have an obligation to establish that this would have been acceptable to them. Informed consent to surgically intervene is not truly informed unless these issues have been openly discussed.

Society as a whole also has to consider the value that is placed on any one particular individual if use of the procedure is to continue and perhaps expand into an ever increasingly aged population.

The considerations here are personal and ethical; however, they are also financial and require considerable judgement to be exercised regarding our actions, responsibilities, and moral values.

References

1. Moussaddy A., Demchuk A. M., Hill M. D. Thrombolytic therapies for ischaemic stroke: triumphs and future challenges. *Neuropharmacology* 2018; **134**(part B): 272–9.

2. Goyal M., Menon B. K., van Zwam W. H., et al. HERMES collaborators. Endovascular thrombectomy after large-vessel ischaemic stroke: a meta-analysis of individual patient data from five randomised trials. *Lancet* 2016; **387**: 1723–31.

3. Bhatia R., Hill M. D., Shobha N., et al. Low rates of acute recanalization with intravenous recombinant tissue plasminogen activator in ischaemic stroke: real-world experience and a call for action. *Stroke* 2010; **41**: 2254–8.

4. Vahedi K., Vicaut E., Mateo J., et al. DECIMAL Investigators. Sequential-design, multicenter, randomized, controlled trial of early decompressive craniectomy in malignant middle cerebral artery infarction (DECIMAL Trial). *Stroke* 2007; **38**: 2506–17.

5. Jüttler E., Schwab S., Schmiedek P., et al. DESTINY study group. Decompressive surgery for the treatment of malignant infarction of the middle cerebral artery (destiny): a randomized, controlled trial. *Stroke* 2007; **38**: 2518–25.

6. Hofmeijer J., Kappelle L. J., Algra A., et al. HAMLET investigators. Surgical decompression for space-occupying cerebral infarction (the Hemicraniectomy After Middle Cerebral Artery infarction with Life-threatening Edema Trial [HAMLET]): a multicentre, open, randomised trial. *Lancet Neurol.* 2009; **8**: 326–33.

7. Vahedi K., Hofmeijer J., Juettler E., et al. DECIMAL, DESTINY, and HAMLET investigators. Early decompressive surgery in malignant infarction of the middle cerebral artery: a pooled analysis of three randomised controlled trials. *Lancet Neurol* 2007; **6**: 215–22.

8. Jüttler E., Unterberg A., Woitzik J., et al. DESTINY II Investigators. Hemicraniectomy in older patients with extensive middle-cerebral-artery stroke. *N. Engl. J. Med.* 2014; **370**: 1091–100.

9. Honeybul S., Ho K. M., Gillett G. Outcome following decompressive hemicraniectomy for malignant cerebral infarction: ethical considerations. *Stroke* 2015; **46**: 2695–8.

10. Honeybul S., Ho K. M., Gillett G. R. Long-term outcome following decompressive craniectomy: An inconvenient truth? *Curr. Opin. Crit. Care* 2018; **24**: 97–104.

11. Beauchamp T. L., Childress J. F. The meaning and justification of informed consent. In *Principles of Biomedical Ethics*, 5th ed. New York, Oxford University Press, 2001, 69–98.

12. Dworkin R. Life past reason. In *Life's Dominion: An Argument about Abortion, Euthanasia, and Individual Freedom.* New York, Alfred A. Knopf, 1993, 218–37.

13. Honeybul S., Ho K. M., Blacker B. W., ORACLE stroke study: opinion regarding acceptable outcome following decompressive hemicraniectomy for ischaemic stroke. *Neurosurgery* 2016; **79**: 231–6.

14. Olivecrona M., Honeybul S. A study of the opinions of Swedish healthcare personnel regarding acceptable outcome following decompressive hemicraniectomy for ischaemic stroke. *Acta Neurochir (Wien)* 2018; **160**: 95–101.

Chapter 15

Aneurysmal Subarachnoid Haemorrhage

Stephen Honeybul and Albert Chiu

15.1 Introduction

Acute aneurysmal subarachnoid haemorrhage (aSAH) is associated with significant morbidity and mortality. The worldwide incidence is approximately 9 per 100,000 per year; however, there are regional differences. Approximately 10–15% of patients die before getting to hospital, and of those patients that actually get to hospital, 25% die within the first 24 hours. Overall, 40–50% of patients die within 30 days of the ictus. For those patients that do survive, up to 20% can be left with significant neurocognitive deficits such that they are dependent. In addition, many survivors have significant neuropsychological problems, such as depression and anxiety, and this can present problems with issues such as difficulty returning to the workplace and reintegration into family and social networks.

Accurate, timely diagnosis and treatment is imperative to avoid aneurysmal re-rupture, which has a mortality in the region of 80%. For patients that survive the initial aSAH, the re-rupture rate is approximately 5% in the first 24 hours and, thereafter, approximately 1% per day. Patient outcome may be further compromised by complications such as seizures, cerebral vasospasm, cerebral infarction, electrolyte disturbances, and hydrocephalus.

Management of patients admitted with acute aSAH is based on early exclusion of the aneurysm from the circulation in order to prevent rebleeding, and for many years, the treatment of choice was an open craniotomy and surgical clipping of the aneurysm.

15.2 Background Information

The first clipping of a brain aneurysm was in 1937. At the time, Dandy observed that 'an aneurysm at the circle of Willis is not entirely hopeless', and thereafter surgical techniques were developed such that clipping of aneurysms became widely adopted as the treatment of choice. However, the invasive nature of surgical intervention with the inherent need for a craniotomy, brain retraction, and arachnoid dissection led scientists to seek alternative, less traumatic approaches.

Initial attempts in the 1940s focused on various methods of thermocoagulation, and early techniques involved puncturing the aneurysm via a burr hole craniotomy and heating the puncture needle to promote thrombosis. Initial results were mixed and certainly not as good as the developing field of microsurgery and surgical clipping. The same desire for minimal invasiveness, however, lead to the development of endovascular treatments in the 1970s, and initial techniques involved occluding the aneurysms with detachable balloons. The results were again mixed, given the relative inability to control balloon morphology relative to the aneurysmal lumen, manifesting as a high aneurysmal rupture and mortality rate. However, the concept of an endovascular approach to intracranial aneurysms gained momentum.

Two particular bridging technologies deserve special mention leading up to the modern basis for endovascular treatment of intracranial aneurysms. For a time, short pushable coils were utilized for the treatment of intracranial aneurysms endovascularly via a catheter. This technique, however, was limited in its ability to control deployment of the coil, in that the coil could not be repositioned, rendering a high risk of incomplete occlusion and/or deposition of the coil in the parent artery. The other is that of attempted intra-aneurysmal thermocoagulation to aid thrombosis. A particular endovascular attempt to promote targeted intra-aneurysmal occlusion involved the introduction of a micro-magnet at the end of a stainless steel wire into an aneurysm, with the aim of attracting injected iron microspheres to form a mass. Unfortunately, as enlargement was insufficient to completely occlude the aneurysm, a small current was applied to the stainless-steel wire in an attempt to promote thermocoagulation on top of microsphere formation. However, because of the differing resistance between the stainless-steel wire and the magnet, application of the current led to erosion at the point where they joined. So rather than enlargement of the microsphere mass, separation occurred and a serendipitous mechanism of reliable intra-vascular catheter-delivered device detachment was discovered. The rest is history. Further developments led to the ubiquitous detachable platinum coils that were named after their developer Guido Guglielmi.[1]

The subsequent years saw many technical refinements that avoided early issues of coil migration and compaction, and these were paralleled by improvements in the surgical management of aneurysms with the introduction of the operating microscope and the refinement of microsurgical techniques for open clipping.

These developments led to considerable debate regarding clinical efficacy and appropriate choice of treatment modality. On the one hand surgeons, who may have seen their subspecialty (and possibly their livelihoods) threatened, argued that complete aneurysm occlusion was not always possible, and the long-term stability of the coils was unknown. On the other hand, endovascular radiologists claimed that the reduction in brain manipulation resulted in better patient outcomes.

These clinical and ethical issues prompted researchers to conduct several large multi-centre randomized controlled trials.

15.3 Current Evidence

15.3.1 The Kuopio Trial

The first randomized controlled trial comparing GDC coil embolization with surgical clipping was carried out at the Kuopio University Hospital in Finland.[2] The trial was conducted between 1995 and 1997, and all patients admitted with an acute subarachnoid haemorrhage were considered. There were a number of exclusion criteria, such as age over 75, late presentation (more than three days post ictus), or the presence of hematoma requiring evacuation. There were also aneurysm-related factors, such as a wide neck, fusiform morphology, or a size less than 2 mm. The rationale was that patients were randomized if it was felt that the aneurysm could be treated either surgically or endovascularly.

A total of 192 patients were randomized (52 endovascular, 57 surgical), and at 1 year after treatment, more patients who had undergone surgery had a poor outcome (33% in the surgical group versus 23% in the endovascular group). While this difference was not statistically significant, it represented the first attempt at a direct comparison of the two techniques, and it suggested a trend towards a better functional outcome with endovascular therapy. There were slightly better angiographic results in the surgical group (for anterior circulation but not posterior circulation), but this was probably a reflection of the early experiences of a technology in its relative infancy.

15.3.2 The International Subarachnoid Aneurysm Trial (ISAT)

The ISAT was conducted at multiple centres, mostly in the United Kingdom and Europe, and patients with an acute aSAH were randomized to either surgical clipping or endovascular coiling.[3] Between the years 1994 and 2002, 2,143 patients were randomized out of 9,559 that were screened. Most patients were of good grade on presentation and had small (< 10 mm) anterior circulation aneurysms. The trial was halted early because an interim analysis found that there was a statistical difference in outcome between the two groups. The primary outcome measure (death or dependency rate) was better with the coiling group (23.5%) compared with the surgical clipping group (30.9%) ($p = 0.0019$). Subgroup analyses also suggested that the incidence of seizures, and ischaemic complications from vasospasm were lower in patients undergoing endovascular treatment.

The results of the ISAT led to a major change in the management of aSAH in many (but not all) centres around the world; however, there remained concerns regarding the long-term durability of occlusion in a coiled aneurysm. The study demonstrated that there was a higher incidence of incomplete angiographic obliteration among the endovascular group (although not all surgical patients had a post-operative angiogram), and the question arose as to whether the initial outcome advantage of endovascular therapy diminished over subsequent years due to either rebleeding or retreatment related morbidity. In order to address these issues, the ISAT investigators reviewed the original cohort at 10 and 18 years and found that the functional outcome advantage was maintained. There was a slightly higher risk of rebleeding in the endovascular group, but this was very small (0.0216 in the endovascular versus 0.0064 in the surgical group) and did not translate into a significantly worse clinical outcome when compared with that of the surgically treated group. Indeed, one of the key findings from these follow-up studies was that long-term outcome of these patients did not relate to treatment failure but rather to a high incidence of cardiovascular disease and cancer.

Notwithstanding the impact that the results of the ISAT had on the global management of aSAH, there were some limitations of the study. One of the main criticisms was the potential for lack of generalization of the results, given the relatively small number of patients that were actually enrolled versus those that were screened (2,143 enrolled from 9,559 screened). There were also concerns regarding the level of surgical expertise. The experience parameter of 30 coiling procedures was set for participating physicians performing the coiling procedure; however, no such standard was set for the surgeons performing the surgical clipping.

In order to address these issues, a trial was performed at the Barrow Neurological Institute in Phoenix, Arizona.

15.3.3 The Barrow Ruptured Aneurysm Trial (BRAT)

This institution based the study on the premise that the skill level of surgeons performing aneurysm surgery in the ISAT was not specified, and this may in part have resulted in the poorer outcomes in the surgical arm of the trial.[4] The clinicians at the Barrow Institute had a high degree of sub-specialization and expertise in both surgical clipping and endovascular procedures, which was an indication of modern-day aSAH management, in high volume, highly subspecialized units.

The trial design was such that the investigators enrolled every patient that presented with an acute subarachnoid haemorrhage into the study irrespective of neurological grade, location, or geometry of the aneurysm. This methodology allowed a large number of patients to be enrolled in a relatively short time frame; however, it did result in a high rate of crossover between modalities, especially from those randomized to endovascular therapy to surgical clipping (38% [75 of 199] of patients assigned to coiling crossed over to clipping). The outcomes were initially analyzed according to intention to treat; however, there was improved clinical outcome for endovascular coiling at the end of 1 year, regardless of how the results were analyzed (intention to treat or as treated). Indeed, the results of the study were strikingly similar to the ISAT and the Kuopio trials. A subsequent analysis at the end of three and six years found the difference between the two methods lessens with time in anterior circulation aneurysms, but the coiling group had a better outcome for aneurysms located at the posterior circulation both at short term and long term. A further important finding was the absence of recurrent haemorrhages in the patients randomized to coiling, which may be a reflection of technological advances or improvements in technique since the ISAT (during the first year of ISAT, there were 20 [4.2%] recurrent haemorrhages).

15.4 Ethical Issues

The publication of the aforementioned trials has led to significant debate in the literature regarding the best treatment modality for patients with acute aSAH, and the arguments have centred on two key issues. In the first instance, there has been debate regarding the applicability or otherwise of the evidence gained from the randomized controlled trials. Second, concerns have been voiced on whether results have been biased by the potential conflicts of interest among those voicing their opinion.

15.4.1 Randomized Controlled Trials

For many years, a well-designed randomized controlled trial published in a reputable medical journal was seen to be the only way to advance clinical practice because this method can produce valid results by limiting bias and confounding using techniques such as randomization and blinding.

There can be no doubt that within the field of neurosurgery there are notable examples, such as the Clifton studies investigating the role of hypothermia in traumatic brain injury (TBI)[5,6] and the MRC CRASH study that investigated the role of steroids also in the field of TBI.[7] However, it has become increasingly apparent that randomized controlled trials can have some limitations. They can be expensive to conduct, take many years to complete (during which time therapeutic options may change), and often have very strict inclusion/ exclusion criteria, which can limit the degree to which the results can be applied to the general population. Some of these limitations were highlighted in the subarachnoid trials.

The ISAT trial randomized 2,143 patients that were mainly good grade, small (< 10 mm), anterior circulation aneurysms, out of 9,559 patients that were screened. Because of these relatively narrow selection criteria, questions remained regarding the role of coiling for larger aneurysms and for aneurysms in the posterior circulation. In addition, the slightly higher incomplete obliteration rate among those patients randomized to coiling led the ISAT investigators to conclude that surgical clipping might be superior to coiling in young patients (< 40 years). At the time, these would appear to be valid observations; however, adopting this position failed to recognize the rapid advances in endovascular technology that have subsequently occurred. Improvements in basic coil technology have significantly decreased the incidence of coil compaction and aneurysm regrowth that were common in the early days of endovascular therapy. In addition, there have been huge technological advances that have seen the introduction, refinement, and adoption into practice of adjunctive techniques such as balloon and stent-assisted coiling, as well as completely new technologies such as flow diversion and the more recent intrasaccular flow disruptor devices. None of these devices has been the subject of a randomized controlled trial, and this would seem unlikely; however, they have allowed neuro-interventional practitioners to expand their practice to include wide-necked, complex aneurysms in both the anterior and posterior circulation, leaving a rapidly decreasing number of aneurysms that are surgically treated.

Notwithstanding these advances, there remains considerable debate as to the role of surgical clipping. While there may be appropriate theoretical concerns regarding the long-term durability of some endovascular techniques given their underlying method of causing aneurysmal occlusion relative to aneurysm clipping, ongoing discussions must acknowledge that there is considerable potential for conflict of interest.

15.4.2 Conflict of Interest

Conflicts of interest occur in many political, business, and medical circumstances. In general, they can be divided into conflicts that provide a personal benefit for an individual or their families, or bias such that financial or other considerations may compromise (or appear to compromise) a person's judgement.

In the field of medicine, there are many instances where a conflict of interest may arise, whether it be a doctor prescribing a drug that is produced by a company in which they have shares or receiving gifts from a company that manufactures a device that a surgeon implants in patients. Over recent years, these conflicts and the influence that they may have on clinical practice have been increasingly recognized, and in most jurisdictions, there are stringent guidelines that seek to limit conflict and, where conflict exists, for it to be openly declared.

When considering the management of aSAH, there is clear potential for conflict of interest, given that surgeons were having the use of a procedure that may have been a substantial part of their clinical practice (at least in the early days) challenged. If endovascular treatment proved superior to surgical clipping, then this would have major implications for their surgical practice, both financially and in terms of career reputation. Indeed, given the relatively noninvasive nature with minimal need for brain manipulation, combined with the current durability of modern endovascular techniques, it could be argued that it is only necessary to prove that endovascular therapy is equal to surgical intervention in terms of safely excluding the aneurysm from the circulation.

The hypothesis on which the BRAT was instigated was that surgical outcomes in the ISAT were not as good as coiling because the level of surgical expertise was less than in the highly subspecialized units such as the Barrow Neurological Institute. The obvious implication was that there already existed a significant conflict of interest among the investigators who seemed to have designed the trial to protect surgical interests. Notwithstanding the limitations of how the BRAT was designed in terms of enrolment and randomization (leaving unsuitable aneurysms in the endovascular arm, consequently causing crossover), what the trial unequivocally determined was that for aneurysms deemed appropriate for coiling, outcome at one year was significantly better than for those patients treated surgically.

There will continue to be debate on an intellectual and scientific level regarding the relative merits of open surgery versus endovascular therapy for aSAH. However, given the evidence currently available, there is a strong ethical imperative for discussions with patients and relatives surrounding consent for aneurysm treatment to reflect the available evidence and to acknowledge that the clinician obtaining consent may have a potential conflict of interest based on their clinical background, expertise, and currency of practice.

The question now remains as to the future direction on clinical research for aSAH, how the management may evolve in future years given the decline in surgical clipping, and the implications that this will have for surgical training.

15.5 Future Directions

15.5.1 The ISAT II Trial

The ISAT II is a randomized, multicentre, pragmatic trial comparing clinical outcomes for patients with ruptured intracranial aneurysms treated with endovascular treatment or with surgical clipping. The hypothesis on which the trial is based is that certain aneurysms were unrepresented in the initial ISAT trial, and for many clinicians there is still clinical equipoise. The study will be multicentre and will involve centres performing both surgical clipping and endovascular coiling of aneurysms. The trial will aim to enrol 1,896 patients over a 10-year period, and recruitment commenced in November 2012. There is no doubt that this is an ambitious, well-constructed clinical trial, with hopes to address whether the expanding armamentarium of endovascular therapy available, such as balloon- and stent-assisted coiling and flow diversion, improves outcome. However, it may face similar problems to previous trials, especially considering the rapidly evolving nature of endovascular techniques and technology. There may also be difficulties recruiting patients, given the ethical requirement to counsel patients regarding the results of previous trials. Clinicians will also have to be confident that they are in genuine equipoise regarding treatment options, and as previously mentioned, there will be a strong ethical imperative among clinicians randomizing patients to acknowledge any conflict of interests based on their clinical expertise and counsel patients accordingly. In a final reflection of the relevance of trials in a rapidly developing field, one interesting exclusion criterion is that of basilar tip aneurysms, which are now treated almost exclusively by endovascular therapies.

15.5.2 Implications for Future Training

There is little doubt that in the future most patients with an aSAH should be treated in high volume, specialized units in which clinicians are highly trained in microvascular neurosurgery and endovascular techniques. Currently this would seem to be a good potential working model because many of these neurosurgeons will have been trained in an era where there was a significant, albeit declining, number of aneurysms treated with open surgery, and they have also been exposed to a significant amount of microsurgery for other intracranial pathologies, which at least share some similar techniques.

The difficulty will be sustaining this training model. Currently in many centres most relatively straightforward, narrow-necked aneurysms are treated endovascularly, and this would appear reasonable in the light of the evidence currently available. However, adopting this policy will result in a gradual decline in the number of aneurysms treated surgically and the cases that are operated on will be the most technically challenging. Maintaining specific microvascular surgical expertise in this environment will be problematic, especially if the dual-trained vascular neurosurgeon takes on the rapidly enlarging workload of clot retrieval for ischaemic stroke. While this might superficially appear extraneous, a robust argument can be mounted for how it would be unethical for such time-critical and experience-dependent work to be left to other practitioners who have not had the recency of elective endovascular practice in the neurovasculature, which in today's neurointervention practice predominantly comes from aneurysm treatment. Similar parallels have long been drawn in the interventional cardiology guidelines for coronary stenting.

This fact may have significant implications in the organization of neurointerventional services and the necessity of availability of an endovascular neurosurgeon for clot retrieval, limiting his or her ability to participate in other elective surgery. If the only time that the surgeon goes to theatre is to clip a highly complex and challenging aneurysm, it is easy to see that over time, enthusiasm for surgical intervention may diminish as endovascular techniques continue to evolve. While this will not affect his or her endovascular technical expertise, arguably a different skill set to microsurgery, it can impact on the theoretical ability for a dual-trained neurosurgeon to provide a balanced view between open and endovascular treatment over time, which can already be a challenge from the outset, as all individuals inherently carry biases based on training and experience.

It has been suggested that neurosurgeons should continue to clip aneurysms in order to maintain their surgical skills; however, this is ethically problematic, given the evidence currently available. In addition, in the era of the Internet, patients and their families are increasingly well informed and can easily gain access to information from a multitude of websites. If a surgeon is genuinely of the opinion that the most appropriate treatment option is surgical clipping or if they are in equipoise (allowing that they are reasonably up to date with the possible mechanisms of endovascular treatment), then it is entirely reasonable to offer a patient operative intervention. However, if they do not work in an environment where they are exposed to the possibilities of treatment via endovascular technique, their impression of equipoise may be inappropriate, and given the overall positive trend of the published evidence towards endovascular therapy, then offering surgery without a proper consideration of potential endovascular approaches is problematic and can be interpreted as an attempt to protect their surgical interests.

These considerations will of course work both ways, because there are a significant number of clinicians not trained in surgical therapy, including not only interventional neuroradiologists but also neurologists. Some of these providers may not necessarily work at high volume neurosurgical centres where comprehensive treatment modalities are available and will understandably favour treatment by the only means at their disposal. Finally, the same argument may also potentially apply to dual-trained neurosurgeons; should they not be able to keep abreast of the entire repertoire of neurointerventional therapy (including clot retrieval), they are at risk of becoming a 'jack of all trades but master of none'. The fact that stroke requiring clot retrieval can be a significant complication of endovascular aneurysm treatment reinforces this position.

15.5.3 Implications for Service Developments

There has been no uniform approach to the transition of management of aSAH from initially completely neurosurgically managed through joint care between neurosurgeons and interventional neuroradiologists to what may become the sole care of endovascular clinicians from a variety of backgrounds, with the formation of a new neurointervention specialty, similar to the development of intensive care and practicing neurointervention full-time. However, notwithstanding the results of the trials, there will, at least for the foreseeable future, be a small but significant number of aneurysms for which surgery should at least be considered.

The management of aSAH is highly variable throughout the world based on clinical practices, geography, and local resources. However central to any health provision is a clinician's responsibility to act and offer treatment that they feel to be in a patient's best interests, especially in situations where that patient or their family's decision-making capacity may be compromised due to either a neurological deterioration or emotional distress due to a loved one having had an aSAH. The considerations here are not only ethical but also financial, and in an increasingly litigious environment, they may also eventually become medico-legal and will require the exercise of well-considered judgement.

15.6 Conclusion

Medical care is in perpetual evolution and is constantly being evaluated and re-evaluated in the light of evidence gained from randomized controlled trials. The modern-day management of aSAH provides a good example of how the treatment of a medical condition can be affected by evidence but is also affected by the availability of local expertise, practice patterns, and service demands. It can be seen how despite aneurysmal treatment traditionally forming a significant component of the workload for the neurosurgeon, this work is now shared through the better outcomes delivered by endovascular therapy, which requires training in an entirely different skill set and environment to deliver results that reflect the evidence. Furthermore, with the introduction of newer workloads on the neurointerventional practitioner (whether they be from a neurosurgical or other background), with the most recent and significant being clot retrieval for ischaemic stroke, there will need to be significant ethical considerations as to the maintenance of skills and recency of practice in all their arenas of work. The demands for specific skill sets may not necessarily obey the boundaries of traditional specialty delineation, and these boundaries are inadequate in an ethical debate. This may in turn have implications whether it is possible to provide a balanced view as a dual-trained neurosurgeon, or whether separate but collegiate neurointerventionists working with a smaller number of microsurgical vascular neurosurgeons (on whom the appropriate cases can be concentrated) is more appropriate.

References

1. Guglielmi G. History of the genesis of detachable coils. *J. Neurosurg.* 2009; 111: 1–8.

2. Koivisto T., Vanninen R., Hurskainen H., et al. Outcomes of early endovascular versus surgical treatment of ruptured cerebral aneurysms. A prospective randomized study. *Stroke* 2000; 31: 2369–77.

3. Molyneux A., Kerr R., Stratton I., et al. International Subarachnoid Aneurysm Trial (ISAT) Collaborative Group. International Subarachnoid Aneurysm Trial (ISAT) of neurosurgical clipping versus endovascular

coiling in 2143 patients with ruptured intracranial aneurysms: a randomised trial. *Lancet* 2002; **360**: 1267–74.

4. McDougall C. G., Spetzler R. F., Zabramski J. M., et al. The Barrow Ruptured Aneurysm Trial. *J. Neurosurg.* 2012; 116: 135–44.

5. Clifton G. L., Miller E. R., Choi S. C., et al. Lack of effect of induction of hypothermia after acute brain injury. *N. Engl. J. Med.* 2001; **344**: 556–63.

6. Clifton G. L., Valadka A., Zygun D., et al. Very early hypothermia induction in patients with severe brain injury (the National Acute Brain Injury Study: Hypothermia II): a randomised trial. *Lancet Neurol.* 2011; **10**: 131–9.

7. Roberts I., Yates D., Sandercock P., et al. CRASH trial collaborators. Effect of intravenous corticosteroids on death within 14 days in 10008 adults with clinically significant head injury (MRC CRASH trial): randomised placebo-controlled trial. *Lancet* 2004; **364**: 1321–8.

8. Darsaut T. E., Jack A. S., Kerr R. S., et al. International Subarachnoid Aneurysm Trial – ISAT part II: study protocol for a randomized controlled trial. *Trials* 2013; 14: 156.

Chapter 16

Paediatric Neurosurgery

Naci Balak, Ulrika Sandvik, and Stephen Honeybul

16.1 Introduction

A thorough understanding of clinical ethics is essential in all areas of medicine but no more so than in the complex and evolving field of paediatric neurosurgery.[1,2] Many of the issues encountered are similar to those seen in adult patients; however, there are inherent differences because the circumstances are constantly evolving as the child develops both physically and intellectually.

Advances in antenatal care have also led to a number of ethical issues that are unique in that they need to consider not only the health of the foetus but also maternal welfare. Thereafter, as the child develops through infancy, early school age, and onto early adolescence, discussions regarding ethical problems will need to evolve to reflect the child's intellectual maturation. In the early years of development, parents will have to be the sole decision-makers and will be called upon to make decisions that are in the best interests of the child. However, as children approach adulthood and begin to develop an opinion regarding their self-interests, discussions must become more patient centred, and the child must have a more significant role regarding clinical decisions that may affect their developing values and quality of life.

16.2 Background Information

As with adults, the field of bioethics in the paediatric population has emerged relatively recently and has needed to evolve in parallel with surgical advances. This has affected many aspects of paediatric neurosurgery, and a good example of the issues that require consideration comes with the evolving management of neural tube defects.[3]

In 1954 Ingraham and Matson published a book entitled *Neurosurgery of Infancy and Childhood*.[4] At the time, there were very limited treatments available for these patients, and many children either died early due to infection or survived with extensive disabilities requiring constant medical and surgical care. The prospects for anything approaching a normal life were poor, and the authors expressed the widely accepted view at the time that withholding treatment from these infants was ethically justified. Over subsequent years as surgical expertise improved, it became increasingly apparent that some patients could benefit from surgical closure of the defect and make a good recovery, despite having some degree of disability. In 1974 Lorber published an article on 'Selective Treatment of Myelomeningocele', in which certain adverse clinical criteria – such as high-level myelomeningocele (MMC), deformation of the spine, severe hydrocephalus, and associated anomalies – deemed cases to be inoperable.[5] However, as surgical treatments continued to advance, the use of these criteria became increasingly infrequent. In addition, social attitudes to disability were changing such that it was becoming increasingly apparent that there were significant ethical problems when intervention was withheld, based on a somewhat paternalistic notion of unacceptable disability and poor quality of life. These changes in attitude were reflected in government legislation at around the same time.

In 1973 the US federal government had passed the Rehabilitation Act, prohibiting discrimination against handicapped individuals, and public attention was drawn to several high-profile paediatric cases. The Baby Doe was one such case that provoked considerable debate. On April 9, 1982, he was born with Down's syndrome and a tracheoesophageal fistula. At the time, it was felt that the defect was correctable and the child would eat normally after surgery. The prognosis was felt to be good, and a nearby hospital was available to perform the procedure. However, Baby Doe's obstetrician advised the parents that instead of surgery they could simply do nothing, which would result in death due to dehydration or starvation after a few days. The doctor's advice was based on the belief that he thought survival with Down's syndrome was unacceptable. The parents agreed, and the baby died six days after birth. The hospital had brought the case before a judge, who ruled that the parents had the right to decide between treatment options, including the option that provided no actual treatment. An appeal to the Indiana Supreme Court resulted in a 3–1 vote to let Baby Doe die. At the centre of the ethical debate was whether the life of a child with Down's syndrome should be valued any less than that of other people. This is an instance where contemporary opinion would fall in favour of survival. The publicity surrounding this case was shortly followed by another case of nontreatment of a spina bifida patient with multiple myelomeningocele, microcephaly, and hydrocephalus. The parents did not consent to surgery and the case went to court, where it was decided that the Rehabilitation Act was not violated by their refusal.

At the time, these cases caused such legal and ethical debate that President Ronald Reagan ordered the Department of Health and Human Services to refuse federal funding to hospitals that withheld medical care in order to allow disabled infants to die. In 1984 this regulation was modified by the provision of several exceptions for the nontreatment of neonates, including irreversibly comatose infants and cases where intervention merely prolongs dying. These regulations regarding life-prolonging treatment continue to be a source of considerable clinical and ethical debate.

16.3 Current Evidence

Paediatric neurosurgery, like other branches of medicine, is gradually shifting towards being a more stringent, evidence-based discipline. However, randomised controlled trials of paediatric neurosurgical procedures have been infrequent. As a result, most paediatric neurosurgical practice is not supported by class I evidence.

This may in part be due to the fact that clinical research using children requires more rigorous standards than research using competent adults. In addition, children are in a potentially vulnerable position. Several trials of neurosurgical techniques that are frequently performed on children have either excluded children from participation or include an insufficient number of children to draw strong conclusions. Finally, those trials that have been conducted have had methodological problems due to difficulty with recruitment, such that they are insufficiently powered to provide substantive conclusions.

16.3.1 Randomised Trials in Paediatric Neurosurgery

Taylor et al. studied the role of decompressive craniectomy and randomised children with elevated intracranial pressure following head trauma to either early decompressive craniectomy or medical management alone.[6] The study demonstrated that the intracranial pressure (ICP) was consistently (but not significantly) lower in patients randomised to surgery, and it was also concluded that functional outcomes were better in children randomised to surgery. However, the number of patients in the trial was very small, and the results of subsequent studies in adults (discussed elsewhere in this book) have confirmed that surgical intervention reduces mortality at the expense of an almost direct increase in the number of survivors with dependency. This in many ways highlights the difficulties in obtaining conclusive findings in paediatric studies; however, this is not always the case, as was demonstrated in the Management of Myelomeningocele Study (MOMS).[7]

Human prenatal myelomeningocele repair by hysterotomy was first performed in 1997, and initial analysis of the results suggested a significant improvement in Chiari malformation and a reduction in post term hydrocephalus. However, there also appeared to be an increased risk of maternal compromise in terms of preterm labour and uterine dehiscence, as well as increased risk of foetal or neonatal death and preterm birth. In order to address these issues, the MOMS study randomised 183 patients (of a planned 200) to either prenatal surgery before 26 weeks of gestation or standard postnatal repair, at three institutions in the United States. The findings of the study were that there was indeed an improvement in outcome in terms of reduction in shunt insertion and improvement in mental development and motor function; however, these benefits came at the cost of increased maternal and foetal risks, as previously mentioned. Currently the field of in-utero surgery continues to evolve, with some centres continuing to offer prenatal open repair, some centres offering endoscopic surgery, and some developed countries such as Australia where until recently no centres were offering this service.

These trials demonstrate that randomised controlled trials are possible in the paediatric population; however, they do serve to highlight the difficulties and limitations facing paediatric researchers. Both the aforementioned trials were well designed and executed; however, given the relatively small numbers involved and advances in surgical management that have subsequently occurred, the influence that they have had on clinical practice is debateable.

Currently most paediatric neurosurgical practices, including surgery for epilepsy, spasticity, and CNS tumours, are not supported by class I evidence. However, this does not mean that there has been no research in these areas. There are an ever increasing number of shunt registries and clinical outcome databases for a variety of conditions that gather a significant amount of clinically useful information. While evidence from this type of data may not conform to the 'gold standard' of a randomised controlled trial, the information obtained can form the basis of comparative effectiveness research (CER), aiming to directly compare existing healthcare interventions to determine what works best for which patients and what provides the greatest benefit and possible harm. The data can also be used to generate hypotheses on which to base future studies. This field has been developed because it has become increasingly recognised that not all types of neurosurgical interventions are best examined by randomised controlled trials.

16.4 Ethical Issues

There are many ethical issues in all aspects paediatric neurosurgery; however, the major problems have been encountered within: prenatal diagnosis, palliative care for children with intractable serious disease, and medical neglect.

16.4.1 Prenatal Diagnosis

In general, the same ethical principles for children and adults should be applied to the foetus for new and innovative management strategies. When a central nervous system malformation has been diagnosed in utero, the decision regarding management can vary depending on both the foetal and maternal conditions. Although it is becoming increasingly apparent that in selected cases intrauterine treatment can be effective, it is mandatory that the mother's welfare be considered. Accurate morphological diagnosis and prediction of the long-term outcome of some central nervous system malformations are still challenging. If the malformations of the foetus can be improved by treatment, the time and the method of the delivery should be discussed with the family, and broad support for the parents should be provided. If there are multiple untreatable anomalies, consideration may be given to either termination of pregnancy or withholding or withdrawing treatment after the birth of the child, should this confirm the severity of the prenatal diagnosis. Whatever the course of action, it is important to provide support to the parents throughout this period in order to alleviate the distress experienced due to the commonly experienced feelings of loss or guilt.

16.4.2 Palliative Care

Depending on the condition of the newborn, there are several management options available for children born with severe developmental anomalies. These can be broadly categorized into active treatment, restrictive treatment, relief treatment, and terminal care. In active treatment, all available treatments are administered. In restrictive treatment, certain interventions such as cardiac surgery and haemodialysis are either withdrawn or withheld. Relief treatment means that already established maintenance and nonmedical care are administered without escalating treatment any further in the event of a clinical deterioration. In terminal care, all treatments are suspended.

This sounds like a very reasonable and measured approach; however, in what can be a very emotionally charged atmosphere, clear and concise clinical reasoning with parents can be problematic. One of the fundamental issues has always been making an objective assessment as to whether a quality-of-life threshold exists, beyond which life can be considered not worth living and further intervention deemed futile. In an attempt to address this issue and make decisions regarding end of life more transparent, physicians in the Netherlands have developed a somewhat controversial management strategy.

16.4.3 Groningen Protocol for Euthanasia in Newborns

Management of newborns with serious medical conditions and the initiation or withdrawal of life-sustaining treatments is one of the most difficult aspects of paediatric neurosurgical practice. In ancient Greece, there were detailed methods for dealing with handicapped newborns, which included killing weak and deformed infants. Modern-day management of these infants remains challenging. From an ethical viewpoint, there is deemed to be no difference between initiating treatment and withdrawing that treatment, and in most countries, the majority of neonatologists feel that intensive care treatment is not a goal in itself. However, in most jurisdictions, active termination of an infant's life is illegal, no matter how severe the illness or deformity, and it is in this regard that the Groningen Protocol has attracted significant debate.

In 2005 a group of paediatricians at the University Medical Centre in Groningen, The Netherlands, published the Groningen Protocol for Euthanasia, which was produced mainly to apply to children born with nonterminal, severe congenital anomalies.[8] The case that triggered the protocol was that of a baby girl with severe epidermolysis bullosa. The parents had requested euthanasia; however, the doctors refused because of the concern regarding possible legal action. This prompted clinicians to develop a protocol that legislated for an effective and transparent regulation of end-of-life practice.

The protocol grouped patients into three categories (Table 16.1), and there was an exhaustive list of requirements that needed to be fulfilled in order to consider euthanasia (Table 16.2).

The critical response to the protocol in many ways reflects the difficulties when making moral judgements regarding societal values in different jurisdictions (Table 16.2). Most commentators accepted that the originators of the protocol truly believed that they were acting in the infant's best interest. Indeed, the aim of the protocol was to protect physicians who were already carrying out some form of euthanasia by putting in place clear guidelines, to ensure accurate reporting to legislative authorities. A publication in the *New England Journal of Medicine* outlining the protocol was intended to combat the 'blood-chilling accounts and misunderstanding concerning the protocol'. However, in spite of these attempts, certain commentators still doubted the ethical position adopted and continued to use unhelpfully emotive descriptions of the protocol, such as 'a blood-chilling crime against a helpless population'.

While some of the criticisms of the protocol stem from genuine moral (and reasonable) ethical disagreements, some originate from misinterpretation. Indeed, one of the major misunderstandings regarding the protocol is that it is aimed at infants with spina bifida. The authors of the protocol are partially to blame for this, as they presented 22 cases of infant

Table 16.1 Infants and newborns for whom end-of-life decisions might be considered

Category	Disease severity	Examples
No chance of survival	Infants who will die soon after birth despite optimal care	Very severe underlying disease such as lung or kidney hypoplasia
Very poor prognosis	Patients will be dependent on intensive care. They may survive after a period of intensive treatment, but expectation regarding future development is bleak	Severe brain abnormalities Extensive organ damage due to hypoxia
Hopeless prognosis	Infants experience what parents and doctors deem to be unbearable suffering	Infants not dependent on intensive care treatment but for whom a very poor quality of life, associated with sustained suffering, is predicted

Table 16.2 The Groningen Protocol for Euthanasia in Newborns

The protocol	Criticisms of the protocol
Requirements that must be fulfilled	
1. The diagnosis and prognosis must be certain.	The protocol fails to distinguish with clinical precision between babies whose prognosis of death is certain and those who could continue to live.
2. Hopeless and unbearable suffering must be present.	Determining suffering in a newborn is almost impossible, as is assessment of quality of life. Physicians tend to overestimate the importance of quality of life and the acceptance or otherwise of survival with severe disability – the so-called disability paradox.
3. The diagnosis, prognosis, and unbearable suffering must be confirmed by at least one independent doctor.	It lets doctors decide what is unbearable suffering and what is an unacceptable quality of life. Neonates cannot suffer because they lack the ability to realise intentions, desires, and hopes for the future.
4. Both parents must give informed consent.	Questions relate to the quality of the consent, violation of the infant's autonomy, the parent's reliance on experts to predict the future, and bias introduced by emotional distress to the parents and a physician's personal ethical perspective. There is also potential bias from the state whose role should be to protect those most weak and vulnerable, rather than remove them and thereby abrogate the financial and moral responsibilities that come with survivors with severe disability and dependency. The protocol potentially allows parents to commit infanticide as a means of escaping an unwanted burden of care.
5. The procedure must be performed in accordance with the accepted medical standard.	A detailed protocol, with internal and external checks and balances, minimises the impact of a morally unacceptable act. The protocol provides a purely procedural response to the problem of measuring subjective suffering.
Information needed to support and clarify the decision about euthanasia (abridged)	
1. Diagnosis and prognosis Details regarding test results, opinions, assessments, and treatments	
2. Euthanasia decision	

Table 16.2 (cont.)

The protocol	Criticisms of the protocol
Personnel involved, parental involvement, and all opinions expressed	Doctors alone are, in essence, determining the morality of their actions. There is lack of input from nurses, social workers, clergy, and ethicists. There is a history of doctors and scientists who distorted morality for what they felt to be the benefit of the individual or society.
3. Consultation	
Second opinions obtained	
4. Implementation	
Procedure method	
5. Steps after death	
Coroner findings, reports to authorities, parental support, case follow-up	Legalising the taking of a life is morally indefensible and crosses a major boundary line.

euthanasia, all of whom had spina bifida. However, nowhere in the protocol is spina bifida represented as a condition associated with an unacceptable outcome, and as critics have pointed out, many people with surgically managed spina bifida report a good quality of life. While the variable spectrum of disabling conditions associated with this condition may cause a burden on parents and society at large, society has an obligation to shoulder that burden, and the social utility gained from protecting and caring for the most vulnerable individuals in the community must be openly acknowledged.

Many critics of the protocol feared that the protocol would lead to a slippery slope of rising infant euthanasia. However, paradoxically there has been a fall in the number of reported cases. In the Netherland's this may have been as a result of an increase in the use of maternal ultrasound at 20 weeks gestation, leading to an increase in terminations of pregnancy for foetuses with severe neural tube defects.

Notwithstanding these findings, the overall effect of the protocol has been to highlight some of the difficult issues faces by clinicians in these circumstances, such that they can enter the wider ethical debate. No other country has introduced such legislation, and the ethical and moral debate regarding these issues will no doubt continue.

Notwithstanding the broader debate societal debate, the position of the parents in these circumstances must always be carefully considered and supported. Setting aside the legal and moral discussion, for any decision to be considered ethical, must be one that can be included in the narratives of those involved with integrity, so that for the child whose life may end and for those who are left grieving, there is closure and a sense of having done what is right in a tragic situation.

16.4.4 Medical Neglect

Medical neglect is broadly defined as a parent's failure to provide adequate medical care for their child, especially when it is needed to treat a serious physical injury or illness. Some jurisdictions may also hold other parties liable for medical neglect, such as custodians or guardians who have a legal duty to care for the child.

It is generally considered to be a form of child neglect that is usually listed under a state's child abuse laws, and there are two broad categories. Parents or caregivers either do not seek medical treatment when a child is clearly ill or they do not follow medical advice once it has been sought. This can take various forms (Table 16.3).

When it comes to religious exemptions, legislation varies. Many jurisdictions do allow parents to refuse both preventative care and treatment for children. Generally, the exemption must be based on sincere religious beliefs and the parents' membership in a recognised faith or religious tradition. For example, the Followers of Christ Church is an established sect, known for distancing themselves from modern medicine and placing its belief in faith healing. Notwithstanding these beliefs, there have been a number of cases of criminal charges and imprisonment of parents from this sect who have been found guilty of neglect. In addition, some jurisdictions do not allow parents to refuse medical treatment for their children based on religious beliefs.

In the case of neurosurgery, there are several important specialty-specific considerations. First, parents may have genuine anxieties and not fully understand the rationale and potential benefits of surgical intervention. They may also have genuine fears regarding the potential for complications and impact on functional development. In these circumstances, every effort must be made to communicate effectively and, where necessary, obtain a second opinion. It must always be kept in mind that their fears may be well founded, and the surgeons themselves may sometimes need to reconsider their opinion. This is especially the case for surgery that may have limited long-term benefit, as may occur in certain aggressive intracranial tumours.

Table 16.3 Types of medical neglect

Neglect	Comments
Refusing or denying the child access to medical care in an emergency	In these cases, signs of older untreated or unreported injuries must alert the clinician to the possibility of abuse.
Refusing to support the child's medical expenses or attendance for treatment of an illness without good reason	It must also be shown that the treatment recommended would substantially benefit the child, that there is access to healthcare, and that the caretaker understands the situation (i.e., is mentally competent).
Ignoring medical recommendations by a physician with regards to a treatable condition	Where this stems from religious reasons, laws vary between jurisdictions. Where this stems from genuine concerns regarding treatment (which may be valid in the case of neurosurgical intervention), these concerns must be explored hopefully without recourse to legal intervention. Again, it must also be shown that the treatment recommended would substantially benefit the child.
Failing to administer medicine to the child as prescribed by a doctor	

Where conflict remains, it may be possible to involve extended family members and community resources, and work with the family to develop a surgical plan that everyone understands. Ultimately, if it is felt that the parents are obstructing an intervention that is in the child's best interests, it may be necessary to refer the matter to child services. This may lead to a suspension of parental rights, and selection of a substitute consent provider may be necessary. A substitute consent provider can also be an ethical review board or another legal institution.

16.4.5 Jehovah's Witness

The management of children whose parents are Jehovah's Witnesses can present difficult clinical and ethical issues. Jehovah's Witnesses believe that the Bible prohibits ingesting blood and that Christians should not accept blood transfusions or donate or store their own blood for transfusion.[1] The belief is based on an interpretation of scripture that differs from that of other Christian denominations, espousing that the refusal of transfusions of whole blood or its four primary components – red cells, white cells, platelets, and plasma – is a nonnegotiable religious stand.

It must be acknowledged that a mentally competent adult individual has an absolute moral and legal right to refuse consent, and many Jehovah's Witnesses carry an advance directive or have executed a detailed healthcare advance directive (living will). Copies are usually lodged with their general practitioner, family, and friends, and case law is now very clear that such an advance directive is legally binding. For children, the ethical and legal issues require careful navigation. Depending on the age at which a child is deemed a minor (e.g., 16 in the United Kingdom, 18 in the United States), parents have the right to give consent by proxy to medical intervention, based on the belief that they are safeguarding the best interests of the child.

However, it is important to recognise that a doctor's final legal and ethical obligation rests with the child and not the wishes of the parents. Courts throughout the world generally recognise parental rights, but also recognise that these rights are not absolute and exist only to promote the welfare of children.

If parents refuse consent to give blood for an elective procedure, a full and candid discussion among anaesthetists, surgeons, parents, and the child (if old enough to understand) is essential. It is important to emphasise that every attempt will be made to minimise blood loss but also be clear that the surgeon would not allow a child to die for lack of a blood transfusion. In most jurisdictions, there are strong recommendations to obtain assent from the child rather than ask the child to provide consent. This is particularly important where the child is in doubt such that they may feel that providing formal consent would place them in conflict with their parents and threaten their rights as a patient.

It must also be acknowledged that there are instances where a child younger than 16 may have matured sufficiently such that they can form their own opinions and provide consent. In the UK, the test of 'Gillick Competence' states that parental right to determine whether or not their child below the age of sixteen will have medical treatment terminates if and when the child achieves sufficient understanding and intelligence to fully understand what is proposed.

There will always be situations where all avenues of discussion have been exhausted and consent for transfusion from either the parents or a competent child is refused. In these circumstances, if it was thought to be unreasonable to go ahead with surgery without the freedom to transfuse, a request to the appropriate courts for 'specific issue order' can be made, which allows transfusion without removing all parental authority. Where time does not permit application to the courts, blood should be given. Failure to give life-saving treatment to a child could render the doctor vulnerable to criminal prosecution.

16.4.6 Brain Death and Organ Transplantation

Unlike tests for brain death in adults, bedside tests for brain death in children may be difficult to thoroughly validate.[5] Age-specific neurological examination findings should be carefully done and interpreted by two physicians, and at least one of them should be a child neurologist or paediatric neurosurgeon.

In newborns, diagnosing brain death is more complicated because of the small number of brain-dead neonates reported in the literature and uncertainty about intrinsic biological differences in neonatal brain metabolism, blood flow, and response to injury.[9] Open fontanel and sutures may allow for higher intracranial pressure and create incompatible findings between cerebral angiography studies and brain death. There are also limitations of the clinical examination and ancillary studies in this age group. It is therefore imperative to carefully and repeatedly examine term newborns, paying particular attention to brainstem reflexes and apnoea testing.

In children, particularly term newborns, assessment of neurologic function may be unreliable immediately following an acute catastrophic neurologic injury or cardiopulmonary arrest. In these circumstances, a 24-hour period is recommended before evaluating for brain death. Preterm infants younger than 37 weeks gestational age are not included in guidelines for the determination of brain death, because some brainstem reflexes are not developed until late in gestation.[9]

The main indication of formal brain-death determination is for the infant to serve as a potential organ donor.[5] There have been reports of using living anencephalic infants as multiorgan donors because they are usually stillborn, and even if they survive birth, only 5% remain alive at one week. However, they can cry, suck, swallow, breathe, cough, and have sleep-wake cycles mediated by the brainstem.[5] Therefore, an anencephalic infant is not technically brain dead and cannot be treated as a nonperson. Indeed, to do so would violate the ethical principle of organ transplantation.

16.4.7 Informed Consent in Children

It is a legal and ethical duty for paediatric healthcare providers to provide a standard of care that meets the child's needs and not necessarily what the parents desire or request. Parental decision-making does not imply a right for parents to make their own autonomous choices; instead, it should primarily be understood that the parents' responsibility is to support the best interests of their child. As a rule, medical decision-making in children is centred on the best-interest standard, not on the interests of the caregiver. The parents or surrogate should be advised to maximise benefits and minimise harms to the minor and prevent neglect of the child.[10] Collaborative communication and the exchange of information between the medical team and the family, which leads to a shared family-centred decision-making, are an increasingly preferred approach to paediatric medical decision-making. In addition, developmental maturation of the child allows for increasing longitudinal inclusion of the child's opinion in medical decision-making in clinical and research practice.[10] It is noteworthy that medical decision-making in paediatrics is informed by the cultural, social, and religious diversity of physicians, patients, and families.[10] Regardless of parents' religious beliefs, children deserve the best medical treatment when such treatment is not excessively burdensome and is likely to prevent substantial harm, serious disability, or death.[10] At the same time, it is the duty of surgeons to respect the parents' culture, religion, and autonomy.

16.5 Future Directions

The field of paediatric neurosurgical bioethics will continue to evolve as new surgical techniques are introduced, developed, and refined. With each new advance will come new ethical issues that require consideration, and surgical boundaries will continue to expand, as occurs in all aspects of surgery. One of the issues that are unique to paediatrics is the need to involve parents in difficult decisions, given that they are often placed in a highly vulnerable and emotionally compromised position. The decision to proceed with treatment can be relatively straightforward; however, withholding treatment can present difficulties as demonstrated by the following two illustrative clinical cases.

Illustrative Clinical Case 1

A male was born with a large thoracic myelomeningocele, severe hydrocephalus, spinal kyphosis, and a Chiari II malformation. He is the fourth child in his family. The attending paediatric neurosurgeon proposed surgical treatment to close the defect and treat the hydrocephalus. Initially the parents were reluctant to give consent for the surgery to proceed. They realised that the child would survive but would be left with significant neurological disability, and they did not think that this would constitute a good quality of life. They were also concerned regarding the possible burden he may place on the family.

Eventually, after several discussions with the parents, the surgeon persuaded the parents to provide consent for surgical intervention. This was successfully completed, and after a lengthy stay in hospital, the child was discharged home. As time goes by, the child develops into a healthy young man. He has significant cognitive defects and is dependent on a wheelchair for mobility. He attends a special school; however, he interacts positively with his siblings, who seem not to notice his disability and interact with him as part of the family.

16.5.1 Discussion of Illustrative Clinical Case 1

In previous years, withholding intervention for Case 1 would have been deemed acceptable. However, clinical experience of such cases has demonstrated that patients with severe hydrocephalus, paraplegia, spinal kyphosis, or Chiari malformation can still maintain an acceptable quality of life.[11] This young man and his family have never known him to be anything other than the person who he is, and if you asked him if he was happy to be alive, the most likely answer would be 'As opposed to what?' Unless one is actually suicidal, judging quality of life based on abilities is inherently problematic and is reflected in the ethical concept of the 'disability paradox'.

While it must be acknowledged that a good quality is difficult to define, it is often associated with good health, subjective well-being and freedom from disability. The reality is that patients' perceptions of personal health, well-being, and life satisfaction are often discordant with their objective health status. The disability paradox reflects the observation that many people with serious and persistent disabilities report a good or excellent quality of life when to most observers they would appear to live in a very undesirable state.

This does not mean that every child with a case of myelomeningocele should be treated. When there are potentially fatal congenital malformations or chromosomal abnormalities, a decision to withhold treatment may be considered reasonable. It is best to treat each case on an individual basis after a frank and realistic discussion with the parents about the most likely outcome, with an emphasis on realistic outcome expectations and an acknowledgement that most survivors find their outcome acceptable. Despite their disabilities, the majority of these children, when successfully treated, become independent adults, and although only about one-third of them become remuneratively employed, it is a societal duty to support these individuals where facilities are available for appropriate management.

Illustrative Clinical Case 2

An 11-year-old female child presented with a one month history of headache and vomiting. She was admitted to the hospital following a collapse, and a CT scan revealed a 7 by 4 cm parieto-occipital mass and hydrocephalus. Emergency surgery was performed, the mass lesion was debulked, and an external ventricular drainage was inserted. Histopathological diagnosis confirmed a high-grade glioma. She was commenced on chemotherapy and radiotherapy; however, one month later she clinically deteriorated, and serial imaging confirmed rapid regrowth of the tumour and severe cerebral oedema. She had a second procedure but failed to wake following surgery and remained ventilator dependent. She was continued on chemotherapy, but four weeks later repeat imaging showed that the tumour had regrown almost to its original size. The treating neurosurgeon and physician colleagues thought that any further treatment would not improve the condition of the patient and would therefore be deemed futile. The family requested active treatment to be continued in the hospital and requested a third operation.

16.5.2 Discussion of Illustrative Clinical Case 2

In the second case, there may be several alternatives for the ongoing management of this patient, but serious consideration must be given to withholding further treatment. The parents certainly have the right to request ongoing treatment because they are surrogate decision-makers and they may feel that surgery may be in the child's best interests. However, while they have a right to make decisions on behalf of the child, they cannot be abandoned to make what may be an inappropriate decision.

Likewise, the neurosurgeon must be cautious when making decisions based on so-called *futility* because the term itself is difficult to define and implies a degree of certainty. More recently, the concepts of 'proportionate' and 'disproportionate' have been introduced in order to acknowledge that a specific treatment may not necessarily be futile and therefore regarded as useless, but may have progressively declining benefit and therefore represent an increasing burden in any one particular clinical situation. For a medical treatment to be 'proportionate', the benefits must outweigh the burdens, and this may vary depending on an individual's values and preferences and the cost to the healthcare system.

There is little doubt that the treatment up to now has been proportionate and appropriate to the needs of this patient. It could, of course, be argued that the decision to operate a second time could be questioned, indeed considered futile, given that the tumour was known to be aggressive and had recurred quickly despite surgery, chemotherapy, and radiotherapy.

It could also be argued that further surgery with the attendant need for intensive care has placed an unacceptable burden on the patient's health and general well-being for management of an aggressive disease that will always recur, and this brings to the discussion the utilitarian theories of value and justice. These acknowledge that resources are scarce and must be allocated optimally to ensure that the overall performance of a healthcare system is maximised. An egalitarian assumption adds a further constraint of fairness to try and ensure universal access to adequate healthcare. From this standpoint, it is difficult to justify the doubtless life-saving nature of the second operation, when the *most likely* outcome is eventual tumour recurrence and death of the patient. However, adopting this position fails to recognise the considerable social value in caring for those most vulnerable in society, especially if this is undiluted by considerations of cost. While attempts to preserve life at any cost may prove incompatible with a utilitarian resource allocation, conveying the message that life is precious and worth a great deal of effort to preserve can be a source of social utility. People obtain benefit from the belief that they are living in a caring and humane society, and heroic attempts to save a young child's life serve to reinforce this belief. This can provide a feeling of security, knowing that one lives in a compassionate society that cares for the needs of each constituent member and where those in most desperate need will not be ignored merely on the basis of resource allocation, and this is embodied in the ethical concept of the 'rule of rescue'. The considerations prior to the second operation would favour surgical intervention, and the actions of the neurosurgeon would seem to be proportionate.

The difficulty comes in this case when it is no longer clear that providing a third operation is in the best interests of the child and further surgery may be deemed disproportionate and inappropriate, despite the parents' request at a further attempt at rescue. This puts intense ethical pressure on the point at which the utilitarian value of demonstrating compassion fails to justify the utilitarian value of arguably poorly allocated resources. Even at this stage, any strategy aimed at rationalising healthcare resources must take into account what is acceptable to society. There is an inescapable fact about human nature that will always challenge the utilitarian rationality that is implicit in cost-benefit analysis.

The difficulty lies in how to determine whether in fact a disease is incurable or not, as improvements in medicine always occur. At present, because high-grade gliomas always recur despite aggressive treatment, innovative surgical treatment can be considered. Therefore, patients with recurrent high-grade gliomas should have a right to innovative surgical treatments, due to the ethical principle of patient autonomy. However, innovative treatments must have adequate evidence before implementation, and there should not be a risk of harm to the child.[12] Additionally, an endless fight for life can result in unnecessary physical suffering for a seriously ill child. This can also result in distress for the family. In this particular case, the child could have been discharged home to spend the remainder of her life with her family. However, it was agreed with the parents that the treatment should be continued in the hospital using established symptom relief treatment without further aggressive treatment.

16.6 Conclusions

Children deserve the best medical treatment when such treatment is not excessively burdensome and is likely to prevent substantial harm, serious disability, or death. Collaborative communication and the exchange of information between the medical team and the family, which leads to shared family-centred decision-making, are an increasingly preferred approach to paediatric medical decision-making. However, parents cannot be abandoned to make what may be deemed disproportionate decisions. Ultimately, medical decision-making in children is centred on the best-interest standard, not on the interests of the caregiver. Surgical intervention based on this standard must always be considered proportionate and reasonable, with the aim of providing clear benefits to the child in question.

References

1. Yamasaki M. Life and medical ethics in pediatric neurosurgery. *Neurol. Med. Chir. (Tokyo)* 2017; **57**: 101–5.

2. McDonald P., Gupta N., Peacock W. Ethical issues in pediatric neurosurgery. In *Principles and Practice of Pediatric Neurosurgery*, 2nd ed., A. L. Albright, P. D. Adelson, I. F. Pollack, eds. New York: Thieme; 2008.

3. McLone D. G. The diagnosis, prognosis, and outcome for the handicapped newborn: a neonatal view. *Issues Law Med.* 1986; **2**: 15–24.

4. Ingraham F. D., Matson D. D. *Neurosurgery of Infancy and Childhood*. Springfield, IL, Charles C. Thomas, 1954.

5. Lorber J. Selective treatment of myelomeningocele: To treat or not to treat? *Pediatrics* 1974; **53**: 307–8.

6. Taylor A., Butt W., Rosenfeld J., et al. A randomised trial of very early decompressive craniectomy in children with traumatic brain injury and sustained intracranial hypertension. *Childs Nerv. Syst.* 2001; **17**: 154–62.

7. Adzick N. S., Thom E. A., Spong C. Y., et al. MOMS Investigators. A randomised trial of prenatal versus postnatal repair of myelomeningocele. *N. Engl. J. Med.* 2011; **364**: 993–1004.

8. Verhagen E., Sauer P. J. The Groningen protocol: euthanasia in severely ill newborns. *N. Engl. J. Med.* 2005; **352**: 959–62.

9. Nakagawa T. A., Ashwal S., Mathur M., et al. Committee for Determination of Brain Death in Infants' guidelines for the determination of brain death in infants and children: an update of the 1987 task force recommendations – executive summary. *Ann. Neurol.* 2012; **71**: 573–85.

10. Katz A. L., Webb S. A. Committee on bioethics. Informed consent in decision-making in pediatric practice. *Pediatrics* 2016; **138**(2).

11. Barry S. Quality of life and myelomeningocele: an ethical and evidence-based analysis of the Groningen Protocol. *Pediatr. Neurosurg.* 2010; **46**: 409–14.

12. Cote D. J., Balak N., Brennum J., et al. Ethical difficulties in the innovative surgical treatment of patients with recurrent glioblastoma multiforme. *J. Neurosurg.* 2017; **126**: 2045–50.

Spinal Neurosurgery

Cara Sedney

17.1 Introduction

Spinal surgery is unique to other neurosurgical subspecialties such as trauma, tumour, and vascular neurosurgery in that it is generally for preservation of quality of life rather than preservation of life. This, along with the nature of degenerative disease as well as the unique relationship with and influence of industry, has created unique ethical issues within the spine surgery field.

17.2 Background

Spinal neurosurgery as a field is exploding at an exponential rate, with spinal procedure volumes increasing yearly. However, patient outcomes may not necessarily be improving in line with the increase in surgical procedures. This suggests a number of ethical issues in the field that require exploration and resolution. Spine surgery is unique in the nature of degenerative processes, which are both universal and inexorable, but not always symptomatic. Furthermore, the heavy influence of industry in research that moves the field forward presents additional ethical dilemmas to the individual practicing neurosurgeon as well as the field of spinal neurosurgery as a whole. In discussing these issues, it will be assumed that the ethical implications of spinal surgery decisions are governed by their effect, rather than the intention of the surgeon, and therefore resolutions to such ethical issues are strongly data driven.

17.3 Ethical Issues

17.3.1 Informed Consent

Spinal surgery is generally not life-saving and is rather geared towards improving quality of life. This differentiation changes the risk-benefit assessment and places a higher responsibility upon the surgeon with regard to surgical decision-making, technique, and outcomes. It is furthermore imperative that the patient understands the likely post-operative course and outcome of surgery, and that the surgeon and patient agree on the goals of surgery, which should be both symptom-based and activity-based.

The idea of informed consent in turn reflects the importance of a patient's autonomy, or agency, in medical decision-making. It is important to note that many aspects of the informed consent process have been influenced by previous case law.[1] Park and colleagues suggest a number of best practices for the informed consent process, such as the following: a discussion that includes both the patient and their family; utilization of both direct verbal communication and supplementary educational materials; outlining alternatives, including the option of no treatment; a full description of pre-, intra-, and post-operative expectations; encouraging the patient to ask questions; and appropriate time between consent and procedure for the patient to consider their options.[1]

Given spine surgery's unique goal of improving quality of life rather than as a life-saving enterprise, the accurate assessment of risk is key. Kelly and colleagues have reported that retrospective reviews, extremely common in the neurosurgical field in general and spine surgery in particular, often underestimate the risks involved with various types of surgical procedures.[2] Having an accurate and up-to-date knowledge of both benchmark complication rates, as well as a sense of personal complication rates, may assist the surgeon in providing an accurate assessment of risk during the informed consent process.

Patient goals of surgery should be known to the surgeon during the decision-making process, and may include both symptom-based goals (fixing back pain versus fixing radiculopathy pain or posture), as well as activity-based goals (for example, being able to play with grandchildren). A number of instruments have been utilized in the spinal surgery clinic on an experimental basis to assess patient-reported goals, such as the Patient Generated Index.[3]

17.3.2 New Technology

Spine surgery abounds with new technology, including techniques, biologics, and devices. The ethical dilemma here (aside from conflict of interest, which is discussed later) is whether such new technologies would be considered 'experimental' by the surgeon or, more importantly, the patient. According to Roger's Diffusion of Innovation theory, such techniques are often developed by innovators in an experimental setting, and then adopted in an either early or late fashion.[4] In daily spinal surgery practice, these techniques are often learned in an informal setting that might consist of industry-provided literature and training, or other surgeons who may represent innovators or early adopters. The potential benefit of being an early adopter of new technology lies in its opportunity to solve issues unresolved by more traditional techniques, while the downside may lie in incomplete knowledge of complications or subtleties in indications.

In achieving a balance between these conflicting values, an intentional approach may assist both the surgeon and patient, with an underpinning in patient autonomy as well as avoidance of harm. Is the surgeon (or patient) a traditionalist, or do they want the newest technology? In deciding whether to be an early or late adopter of a new technology, a number of questions might be considered by the surgeon with regard to safety and efficacy. Specifically, are meaningful complication rates known and reported? Are long-term outcomes known, and if so, what is the duration of follow-up? Is a new approach or technique very similar to previous approaches with which the surgeon is familiar (such as disc arthroplasty for a surgeon familiar with anterior cervical discectomy and fusion) or significantly different (for example, an oblique lateral fusion for a surgeon who has not done direct lateral approaches in the past). In certain circumstances, it may be preferable that some degree of supervision is provided when new procedures are introduced.

17.3.3 Conflict of Interest in Practice and Literature

Spine surgery is perhaps the subspecialty of neurosurgery with the strongest ties between industry and literature. The most famous example is that of Medtronic's involvement in the reporting of data regarding its product InFuse. According to a US Senate Finance

Committee investigation, Medtronic officials significantly altered the written publications of physician consultants responsible for clinical studies, including removing the mention of adverse events and including statements favouring the use of InFuse over other products.[5] Furthermore, it was determined that Medtronic paid those consultants approximately $210 million dollars for leading such research endeavours.[5] This remains a cautionary tale regarding the influence of industry on scientific literature, and the significant negative publicity surrounding the InFuse debate has possibly tempered acceptance of industry-supported studies. However, industry support is largely inescapable when industry-driven innovations are often the subject of such studies. Recent examples of research that remains heavily industry-driven includes that relating to disc arthroplasty and interlaminar spacer devices.

The conflict-of-interest debate still remains murky with regard to its effect on the scientific literature, but without doubt conflict of interest between researchers and industry remains common. A review of abstracts from an international spine research meeting revealed that in 79% of abstracts evaluating a device, biologic, or proprietary procedure, authors reported a conflict of interest of which the cumulative amount minimum among authors of the abstract was US$219,634.[6] Bartels and colleagues have reported that authors who declare a financial relationship are less likely to publish negative or neutral studies than those without.[7] Furthermore, Janssen and colleagues have noted that 29% of journal editorial board members declare an industry conflict of interest, of which 42% of those reported a financial relationship of more than US$10,000 during the prior year.[8] In the words of the former editors of *The Spine Journal* regarding the InFuse incident:

> [T]he entire research system, at least for commercial products, has broken down in a fundamental way and needs to be redesigned. After more than a decade of high-profile research, 'no one seems to have known' what the full body of data on rhBMP-2 actually said: not the FDA, not the sponsored researchers, not the incoming CEO of Medtronic, not the research and development team of Medtronic, and certainly not the authors of the TSJ review.[9]

17.3.4 Prevalence of Degenerative Spine Disease in a Normal Population

Degenerative spinal disorders are universal, inexorable, and not always symptomatic. This is both unique and significant in neurosurgery, because degenerative disease of the spine is therefore very unlike an aneurysm, brain tumour, or subdural haematoma. The 'lesion = surgery' or 'symptoms = surgery' treatment paradigm in other areas of neurosurgery does not translate well in spinal neurosurgery, again leading to inaccurate assessments of success or risk for planned interventions. Having a clear sense of surgical indications is paramount.

17.3.5 Lack of Standardization of Care

The issue of surgical indication and informed consent is compounded by lack of consensus in the field regarding the need for surgery for even basic spinal conditions. It remains exceedingly difficult to accurately counsel a patient when there is little consensus on the best course of action for multiple spinal diagnoses. Lenza and colleagues found a 'large discordance' between first and second opinions regarding the need for spinal surgery.[10] This phenomenon is further illustrated by the variation in spinal fusion rates based upon myriad surgeon demographic factors.[11] This may reflect both uncertainty regarding valid scientific data as well as disciplinary siloing, wherein 'if one has a hammer, everything is a nail'. A number of strategies may be utilized to minimize the effect of the current knowledge gap. Yanamadala and colleagues have noted that spinal fusion utilization decreases if patients are evaluated by a multidisciplinary team who are involved in multi-modality spine care.[12] Ultimately, high-quality meta-analyses, large prospective database studies, and pragmatic clinical studies are needed to help clarify these issues.

Illustrative Clinical Case 1

A 55-year-old male presented to the neurosurgical clinic after 15 spinal surgeries. A careful history revealed that his first surgery, an L5-S1 fusion, was done for pure back pain without radiculopathy. He did well from that operation for five years, then required an additional operation extending his fusion up to L4. This, in turn, resolved his back pain satisfactorily for about 1 year. His subsequent procedure was to extend his fusion up to L1. He suffered a compression fracture at T12 with recurrent pain which was resistant to vertebroplasty, and so he had an additional surgery extending his fusion up to T10. This failed to resolve his back pain, and he suffered recurrent loss of fixation at the end-to-end rod connectors that had been placed even after multiple revisions, so he underwent an additional four-rod construct and anterior support, which helped his pain for about a year when the back pain resurfaced. He had a spinal-cord stimulator placed, which helped for six months with again recurrence of the back pain. Finally, he presented to a referral centre neurosurgical clinic and was diagnosed with iatrogenic flat back syndrome, eventually undergoing pedicle subtraction osteotomy (Figure 17.1).

It is worth noting that this patient had 17 spinal surgeries (including staged PSO), all for back pain, which is typically not considered a surgical symptom. This case illustrates the ethical conflicts in operating for pure axial back pain, as well as the consequences of starting down a surgical pathway with questionable operative indications – essentially a risk-benefit

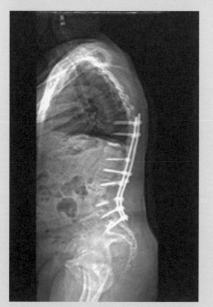

Figure 17.1 Final x-rays after 17 spinal surgeries for axial back pain.

tension, as well as communitarian or utilitarian concerns over healthcare expenditure. Individual surgeons, as well as the field as a whole, must be vigilant regarding operative indications when devising a risk-benefit analysis for their patients. Even considering the 'five good years' experienced by the patient after his first operation, the ethical acceptability and clinical value of these procedures is subject to debate. The healthcare expenditure is further-more questionable and might be considered to be contributing to an unsustainable health-care model.

Illustrative Clinical Case 2

A 32-year-old female is seen in the neurosurgical clinic for a second opinion. She previously had a cervical MRI done for axial neck pain and was found to have cervical stenosis (Figure 17.2). She denies any symptoms of myelopathy or radiculopathy, and neurological exam is unremarkable. She was originally seen by a neurosurgeon who told her she would 'likely become paralyzed' and needed 'urgent spinal surgery to decompress the spinal cord'. She was pressured to make her decision within 24 hours. She stated that she felt uneasy with the urgency of the situation and wished to see another surgeon. Ultimately, she elected to continue with watchful waiting and serial exams for myelopathy.

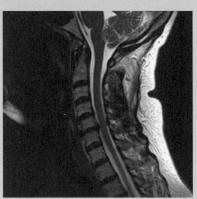

Figure 17.2 Sagittal T2 weighted magnetic resonance imaging of a patient with asymptomatic cervical stenosis who had been told she needed surgery or would be paralyzed.

Similar to the previous case, the ethics of this issue surround the surgical indication and risk-benefit of surgery, which in turn affects informed consent and patient agency in the decision for surgery. In this case, understanding the natural history of asymptomatic cervical stenosis is helpful.

17.4 Future Directions

17.4.1 Future Directions for the Spine Surgery Field

The field of spinal neurosurgery has dealt with many of ethical issues at an organiza-tional and disciplinary level, particularly with regard to the involvement of industry, for many years. Schofferman and colleagues note that conflict of interest among professional medical associations may have even more far-reaching consequences than conflicts of interest among individual surgeons,[13] so such vigilance is imperative within the surgical societies. Currently much more stringent conflict-of-interest report-ing is required of many organizations and publications, but the risk of conscious or unconscious bias remains real. It has previously been suggested that to improve transparency of industry sponsored research, separate journals specifically for company-sponsored trials should be developed.[9]

Improving the quality of reported data aside from conscious or unconscious conflict of interest bias is also of significant interest in improving the ethical strength of the field, particularly given the quality-of-life goals of spine surgery. Bartels in 2013 called for more accurate reporting in the scientific literature regarding clinically relevant outcomes, and eschewing 'obscuring expressions' such as 'reached nearly statistical significance' or 'seems to' in the conclusions of scientific papers.[14] Prospective studies and the utilization of large prospectively collected data sets may improve the quality of clinical data upon which risk/benefit analyses may be conducted. Additionally, an editorial requirement of full access to data would avoid issues with data fidelity.

Overall, these organizational directives may be useful in ensuring progressive growth and avoidance of pitfalls of the past.

17.4.2 Strategies for the Practicing Neurosurgeon

Strategies for avoiding questionable ethical practices in spine surgery are somewhat different for individual practicing neurosurgeons. Given the known and unknown biases of industry-sponsored data which may be difficult to discern, individual surgeons may wish to avoid obtaining their scientific literature from industry representatives and remain sceptical of all literature with industry support. Remaining active in continuing medical education and national organizations may allow one to continuously compare one's current practice with that of others and avoid drift in surgical indications. Furthermore, consideration should be given regarding whether it is better to be an 'early adopter' or a 'late adopter' of new surgical techniques and devices, depending upon whether a full assessment of sequela and complications is known. A number of surgeon-level or practice-level interventions have been shown to decrease unneeded spinal surgeries, including utilizing second opinions, multidisciplinary evaluation prior to surgical decision-making, and payment models that are not purely productivity based.

References

1. Park J., Park H. Surgical informed consent process in neurosurgery. *J. Korean Neurosurg. Soc.* 2017; **60**(4): 385–90.

2. Kelly M. P., Lenke L. G., Godzik J., et al. Retrospective analysis underestimates neurological deficits in complex spinal deformity surgery; a Scoli-RISK-1 Study. *J. Neurosurg. Spine* 2017; **27**: 68–73.

3. Scheer J. K., Keefe M., Lafage V., et al. Importance of patient-reported individualized goals when assessing outcomes for adult spinal deformity (ASD): initial experience with a Patient Generated Index. *Spine J.* 2017; **17**(10): 1397–1405.

4. Rogers E. M. *Diffusion of Innovations.* New York, Free Press, 2003.

5. United States Senate Finance Committee. Staff report on Medtronic's influence on INFUSE clinical studies. *Int. J. Occup. Environ. Health* 2013; **19**(2): 67–76.

6. Walcott B. P., Sheth S. A., Nahed B. V., et al. Conflict of interest in spine research reporting. *PLoS One* 2012; 7(8): e44327.

7. Bartels R. H., Delye H., Boogaarts J. Financial disclosures of authors involved in spine research: an underestimated source of bias. *Eur. Spine J.* 2012; **21**: 1229–33.

8. Janssen S. J., Bredenoord A. L., Dhert W., et al. Potential conflicts of interest of

editorial board members from five leading spine journals. *PLoS One* 2015; **10**(6): e0127362.

9. Weiner, B. K., Hurwitz E. L., Schoene M. L., et al. Moving forward after YODA. *Spine J.* 2013; **13**: 995–7.

10. Lenza M., Buchbinder R., Staples M. P., et al. Second opinion for degenerative spinal conditions: an option or a necessity? A prospective observational study. *BMC Musculoskeletal Disord.* 2017; **18**: 354.

11. Schallmo M. S., Cook R. W., Weiner J. A., et al. Do demographic factors of spine surgeons affect the rate at which spinal fusion is performed on patients? *Spine* 2017; **42**(16): 1261–6.

12. Yanamadala V., Kim Y., Buchlak Q. D., et al. Multidisciplinary evaluation ideas to the decreased utilization of lumbar spine fusion: an observational cohort pilot study. *Spine* 2017; **42**(17): E1016–23.

13. Schofferman J. A., Eskay-Auerback M. L., Sawyer L. S., et al. Conflict of interest and professional medical associations: the North American Spine Society experience. *Spine J.* 2013; **13**: 974–9.

14. Bartels R. H. Influence of industry on scientific reports. *Eur. Spine. J.* 2013; **22**: 1690–1.

Ethical Challenges in Psychosurgery: A New Start or More of the Same?

Paul A. Komesaroff and Jeffrey V. Rosenfeld

18.1 Introduction

Psychosurgery, which was discredited following public condemnation of practices that were widely applied in the mid-twentieth century, has in the last decade experienced a resurgence of interest. This has resulted from the introduction of deep-brain stimulation for the treatment of movement disorders such as Parkinson's disease, essential tremor, and dystonia in the early 1990s, which was followed by a range of additional applications. The scientific and medical literature is now replete with reports of new insights and achievements in psychosurgery. Refined imaging techniques and the availability of less-invasive operative techniques, we are told, have opened up novel possibilities for the treatment of an increasing range of conditions. Awareness of the risks and public sensitivities has led to more careful approaches to patient selection and communication. Regulatory processes provide independent scrutiny of both research proposals and treatment programmes. Overall, optimism is high that the misadventures of more than half a century ago can be put behind us and we can move forward to a new era of safe and effective therapies.

As encouraging as this picture may be, the confident claims in support of psychosurgery have to be viewed with caution. With only a few exceptions, the procedures are still experimental. Data collection under rigorous controls remains difficult. Long-term safety and efficacy continue to be uncertain. Public sensitivities remain high. The troubled historical background cannot be dismissed without careful scrutiny of what went wrong and clear recognition of the lessons that must be learnt from it.

This chapter examines the current prospects for psychosurgery and the ethical challenges confronting it. After a brief overview of current practices and indications, it summarises some aspects of the earlier history. A number of specific ethical issues are then discussed, followed by questions about the broader social implications of a greatly expanded neurosurgical practice. The article ends with a discussion of the requirements of a regulatory framework that might be able to support the continued growth of the discipline while maintaining the support and confidence of the medical, neuroscience, and general community.

18.2 The Context and Promise of the New Psychosurgery

Driven forward by advances in neuroscience, including enhanced imaging techniques, knowledge about function, and refined surgical techniques, now approaches are being applied to the treatment of a variety of psychiatric disorders.[1-6]

An impressive array of neurological targets has been developed, some of which have undergone testing. These include the anterior capsule, cingulate gyrus (particularly Brodmann area 25), nucleus accumbens, limbic system, lateral hypothalamus, and so forth. The surgical techniques include deep brain stimulation (DBS), which is now favoured because it is significantly less invasive than earlier lesioning techniques. DBS is also reversible because it can be turned off, and in some cases the device can be explanted. Stereotactic lesioning, however, is still in use and includes anterior capsulotomy, cingulotomy, stereotactic subcaudate tractotomy, and limbic leucotomy.

These techniques have been, or are proposed to be, applied to the treatment of a wide and ever increasing range of conditions. A partial list of these is as follows: Parkinson's disease, epilepsy, Tourette's syndrome, major depression, obsessive compulsive disorder (OCD), eating disorders such as anorexia nervosa and bulimia, body dysmorphic disorder, schizophrenia, trichotillomania, morbid obesity, alcohol abuse, facial pain, migraine, anxiety, and essential tremor. Beyond this list, multiple additional proposals have been advanced: for example, it has been suggested that conditions also treated by psychosurgery might include traumatic brain injury, substance abuse, dementia, memory deficits, disorders of consciousness, and antisocial and criminal behaviour, including uncontrolled aggression.[7,8]

In spite of the enthusiasm generated and the impressive volume of work that has already been accomplished, it is accepted that, with only a few exceptions, little conclusive evidence is yet available regarding the efficacy or long-term safety of these procedures. The main exceptions are Parkinson's disease, benign essential tremor, dystonia, and epilepsy, for which neurosurgery and the use of DBS has become an accepted practice. While the data from these two areas of practice are extremely valuable, it can be observed that both conditions may be regarded as exceptional, in the sense that they are not strictly psychological and the ability to localise their respective neurological targets has for many years been far in advance of all the other conditions mentioned.

A DBS system for the treatment for OCD is currently approved by the US Federal Food and Drug Administration (FDA) on a Humanitarian Device Exemption. The first prospective multicentre sham-controlled trial of DBS for chronic unremitting depression (the BROADEN Study) was terminated by the trial sponsor (St. Jude Medical) because of the ineffectiveness of the treatment at six months.[9] A number of patients in the latter trial have since had the device removed, and reports of adverse effects have appeared.[10] Researchers continue to refine the selection of patients and the optimal targets for DBS in depression. DBS treatment for severe depression or bipolar disorder is not currently approved by the FDA.

Less-invasive treatments of psychiatric illness are also emerging. Transcranial magnetic stimulation is non-invasive and reversible. A vagal nerve stimulation device has been approved by the FDA for use in depression. This remains a somewhat controversial treatment because of the weak evidence for its success. Radiosurgery (stereotactic focused radiotherapy) employing the Gamma Knife is being used to treat OCD. This is a non-invasive method of making small lesions deep in the brain.[11] It probably will not be too long before it is applied to the treatment of other psychiatric disorders. Focused stereotactic delivery of ultrasound is being used to create brain lesions to treat tremor, and the deep brain lesions could also move to 'psychiatric' targets. The less-invasive treatments using a Gamma Knife or ultrasound raise concerns about possible proliferation of 'uncontrolled' psychosurgery because of the ease of application compared with the placement of deep brain electrodes.

18.3 Skeletons in the Closet: The Recent History of Psychosurgery

Before proceeding to consider some key ethical issues confronting psychosurgery, in the present context it is important to review the history that has for so long obstructed progress in this area. This is because the history enables us both to understand the main concerns that continue to preoccupy the community, the profession, and the regulators, and to ensure that the lessons of the past have been learnt.

It is well known that the modern history of psychosurgery goes back to Gottleib Burckhardt (1836–1907) of Switzerland, who in 1891 published a series of six cases of institutionalised patients experiencing chronic psychiatric illness associated with aggressive behaviour. Burckhardt performed bilateral cortical resections in areas identified on the basis of contemporary neuroanatomic models and claimed that, despite the persistence of psychosis, the patients had become more placid. Burckhardt's reports were not well received by his contemporaries, and he did not pursue his initial investigations further.[12]

The major turning point occurred nearly half a century later when the Portuguese neurologist and politician Egas Moniz (1874–1955) developed the concept of frontal leucotomy, involving the introduction of a frontal cortical brain lesion, which he showed produced behavioural and affective changes. Moniz went on to postulate that anxiety and other psychiatric states could be treated surgically. In 1936 he developed an instrument – the 'leucotome' – designed specifically to achieve this.

Moniz's work was quickly taken up in the United States by Walter Freemen (1885–1972), who popularised and extended the treatment across the country. Freeman developed streamlined techniques, including the 'transorbital prefrontal lobotomy', that allowed rapid treatments to be administered to a wide range of psychiatric patients. It is estimated that Freeman himself performed or supervised 4,000 lobotomies and that up to 20,000 in total were performed in the United States and the United Kingdom over the next 20 years.[12]

Freeman's work was widely accepted by the medical profession and highly celebrated in the popular media. Approval was so great that Moniz was awarded the Nobel Prize for Medicine 'for his discovery of the therapeutic value of prefrontal leucotomies in certain psychoses' in 1940. At the time, it was argued that the new treatment would provide an effective response to the overwhelming need for psychiatric treatments among former soldiers from World War I and their families, as well as the large number of psychiatric inpatients for whom no treatments existed. Indeed, lobotomy became a recommended practice of the Veterans Administration for the treatment of psychologically disabled soldiers returning from World War II, with more than 2,000 of them subjected to the procedure in the late 1940s and 1950s.[13]

Although there were critics from the very beginning, it is important to understand the manner in which psychosurgery was discussed in the scientific literature and the high level of support it received in the wider community. It was argued that despite incomplete evidence, psychosurgery was justified by the great social need it purportedly addressed. It was claimed to be based on up-to-date scientific knowledge and to employ novel, precise, 'modern' imaging techniques.

In addition to Moniz's Nobel Prize, Freeman had accolades heaped upon him, and the popular press was full of supportive stories about psychosurgery. In 1968 *Life* magazine ran a cover story on the 'Psychobiology of Violence', which promoted the work of psychiatrists and neurosurgeons who claimed that psychosurgery could be used to treat individuals considered to be likely to commit violence. The article carried the subheading 'A young science offers insight and a potential of remedy for a worried society' and concluded that 'violence is a public health problem' and psychosurgery could help deliver 'a better and safer world for all of us'.[14] The doctors whose work was so highly praised in this article went on to receive significant amounts of US federal and state government funding to support their continuing research.

Opposition to psychosurgery mounted during the 1960s, with a number of clinical and philosophical works that criticised the practices of psychiatry and psychosurgery, but these were widely discounted as representing marginal viewpoints. Books such as *The Myth of Mental Illness* by Thomas Szasz, published in 1961,[15] and anti-psychiatry texts stimulated by the work of R. D. Laing and others,[16–18] which were to become profoundly influential in years to come, had little impact at the time, especially among the medical profession. During the early 1970s, strongly critical reviews were published in the *Congressional Record* and *Medical Opinion*.[19]

Even in spite of mounting criticism, however, the vigorous support continued well into the 1970s. An editorial in the *Lancet* on 8 July 1972 argued that 'such was the enormous pool of psychotic patients vegetating as chronic sick in the closed wards of mental hospitals, without effective drug control and without hope, that, when it became possible to help them in any way, this new method was taken up with more enthusiasm than caution'.[20] The main indication of the 'modern operations of lower-quadrant frontal lobotomy was said to be not schizophrenia but 'intractable psychotic depression, especially in a previously obsessional personality. The editorial went on:

> No-one who has suffered (and who has not suffered, however briefly?) the agonising experience of acute depression can either doubt or forget the genuine anguish that this represents. It is in some ways more devastating than physical pain. If no more effective medical means become available to treat this condition, it can be taken without further argument that some form of lobotomy is here to stay. The results are excellent, usually permanent, and on occasion almost miraculous.

The editorial concludes with the rather breathless exhortation: 'Already individual results are so strikingly good that this time there can be no turning back.'

An expert review under the chairmanship of Harvard physician J. Kenneth Ryan conducted in 1974 by the US National Commission for Protection of Human Subjects of Biomedical and Behavioural Research concluded that 'some very sick people had been helped by it and . . . it did not destroy their intelligence or rob them of their feelings. Their marriages were intact. They were able to work. The operation should not be banned.'[21]

Perhaps most worrying of all was the wide promotion and acceptance of psychosurgery as a tool to be used for overtly political purposes. As Peter Breggin pointed out at the time:

> [S]everal of the nation's leading psychosurgeons have persistently linked their work to the control of urban violence, ghetto disorders and political dissent. These men rode the wave of hysteria generated by the urban uprisings of the late 1960s and parlayed the nation's fear into federal and state grants for themselves. . . . Each of the psychosurgeons targeted potential patients according to well-recognized political categories. They began with a political issue of grave national concern, the inner-city uprisings of 1967 and 1968, and then attempted to redefine it as a medical disease or syndrome to justify their own interventions. This is analogous to the Russian practice of redefining political dissent into psychiatric categories in order to subject the dissenters to psychiatric authority and treatment.[22]

Psychosurgery fell out of favour from the mid-1970s – well after the advent of neuroleptic drugs, which have often been credited with its demise. When the evidence was finally fully examined, it had become apparent that the effectiveness of the treatments was very limited and that in many cases the adverse effects were overwhelming. It was recognised that tens of thousands of vulnerable individuals had been subjected, without proper discussion, consent, or oversight, to what was now seen as a cruel and barbaric treatment.

Today, looking back, it is important for us to recognise what this episode entailed. The advent of psychosurgery in the 1930s was not an aberration manufactured by criminals or charlatans. It was a mainstream medical practice that arose from within the normal operation of the profession subject to the usual scrutiny to which medical innovations and discoveries were subjected. It was undoubtedly driven by a powerful and genuine social need. It was widely observed and discussed by the profession, government, and popular media. It was supported by imprecise claims about 'new scientific knowledge', refined imaging and targeting techniques, and significant social benefits. While the lack of evidence was acknowledged, the science was described as 'emerging' and the results 'promising'. It was supported by multiple grants from public sources following standard processes of review, on the basis that the work promised to deliver significant cost savings in relation to public funds by saving on healthcare and social support.

It is notable that very similar arguments are advanced today to support contemporary versions of psychosurgery. The latter additionally provide assurances that the brutal excesses of the past cannot be repeated. However, it is not obvious that we are less vulnerable today: at the least, this is a refutable proposition. As with other outrages of the twentieth century, the ability of the medical profession to adopt practices later judged to be ethically unconscionable remains troubling and the reasons for it elusive. These sobering facts inevitably colour any review of psychosurgery today, which carries the responsibility to prove – to the profession and the wider society – that the ethical standards and safeguards that exist today can provide us with sufficient confidence that history will not be repeated.

18.4 Selected Ethical Issues in Contemporary Psychosurgery

In addition to coming to terms with its own history, psychosurgery today faces a number of ethical challenges. While in many cases the issues themselves are not unfamiliar or surprising – for example, issues related to consent, the assessment of benefits and harms, and management of conflicts of interest – the details which they encounter may be highly specific to psychosurgery. In addition, there are some novel issues that are largely peculiar to this area of practice, such as its potential social or political implications, challenges to the concepts of medicine and illness, and, more deeply, philosophical issues concerning the relationship between body and mind and the ethical implications of treatments designed to alter mental states or personality traits.[23–30]

The review of the current understanding of ethics in this field highlights the inadequacy of some of the conventional bioethical formulations and the need for a more radical theoretical critique, as well as for an appropriately critical approach to existing concepts. It also highlights the potential value of vigorous cross-disciplinary dialogues involving medicine, philosophy, social theory, psychology, and politics.

In what follows, we do not seek to present a comprehensive account of all ethical issues raised by psychosurgery. Rather, we draw attention to a few key, fundamental questions to enable a return to the primary question of whether current understanding and regulatory structures are sufficient to guarantee protection against a repeat of the failures of the past.

18.4.1 The Question of Evidence and Research

A first and fundamental issue concerns the nature of the evidence that is available about psychosurgery and the difficulties in adding to it. It is widely agreed that there is no strictly psychological or psychiatric indication for which existing data are sufficiently robust to justify adopting a surgical approach as standard practice. Accordingly, in all cases, psychosurgical treatments must still be regarded as experimental. This means that any procedures must be limited to a research context and therefore subject to the usual regulatory requirements and restrictions of clinical trials.

While this is now recognised, however, both the design and conduct of clinical trials in psychosurgery present significant obstacles. The diagnoses in general lack the usual precision demanded for clinical research, being based largely on phenomenological criteria rather than rigorously testable physiological markers. The interventions themselves are often unstandardised or difficult to standardise. The outcomes may contain qualitative and subjective elements or be otherwise difficult to assess with precision. The duration within which long-term effects might be expected to appear is unknown, and these may be very subtle, including disruptions in relationships, mood, or personality that may be difficult for a research project to discern. Numbers may be limited, meaning that studies are often unlikely to achieve adequate statistical power. As discussed below, consent issues may be very complex. Placebo studies are largely impossible, and other controls are elusive.

Recruitment for phase one studies may present a particular challenge. The difficulty of introducing novel techniques into humans is increased by the absence or unreliability of animal models in relation to psychiatric phenomena. Where studies are conducted across institutions, countries, and cultures, the heterogeneity of diagnosis, techniques, and outcomes may limit the utility of data.

In these circumstances, the design of clinical trials is difficult and the task of ethics committees is complex. In the absence of reliable data, and the possibility of resolving fundamental uncertainties, further discussion about the implications and applications of psychosurgery becomes very difficult. This means that many of the decisions that must be made in relation to this practice – including its safety and efficacy, indications, and outcomes, together with the ethically relevant issues – must often be undertaken in settings where the data are incomplete or unreliable. This uncertainty itself is of ethical significance.

18.4.2 Assessment of Outcomes and the Balance of Benefit and Harm

If the data are insufficient or unreliable, it is difficult to assess with full confidence the nature of the purported outcomes. This adds to the risk that is often cited in relation to novel therapies of producing more harm than good.

In this context, the reliability of the literature itself is uncertain, even in relation to elementary issues relating to the procedures and their outcomes. It is also possible, as has often been pointed out, that where the number and quality of clinical trials are limited, publication bias favouring anecdotal reports of a positive nature becomes a problem. The nature of the procedure itself may be presented in an excessively favourable light: for example, DBS is often described as a 'reversible' treatment, despite the obvious invasive nature of the procedure that it entails and the lack of long-term data about the local effects it may produce.

From the point of view of defining the safety of the neurosurgical procedures, it is obviously of great importance to document the full range of side effects and complications and their incidence. It is common in the literature for a rather limited range of negative side effects to be referred to in comparison with an extended list of potential benefits. Typically, discussion of adverse effects relates to the low risk of common or familiar surgical complications such as infection or haemorrhage. However, a careful analysis of the literature raises concerns about less easily identifiable outcomes, some of which may only become apparent over an extended period of follow-up.

For example, in a review by Clausen[31] it was shown that although the variability may be high, significant rates of adverse events remain possible. In this study, the risk of speech disturbances was 10.8–33%, memory impairment up to 20%, dementia up to 24.5%, depression up to 25%, patient's 'self-perception' 66%, and family problems up to 71%.

Another study[32] commented that a substantial proportion of DBS patients treated for movement disorders showed 'severe and lasting behaviour disturbances, which were credibly not present in the ultimate preoperative phase'.[4] These behavioural disturbances were said to include 'reckless driving or other forms of risk-seeking behaviour and even aggressive and contemptuous behaviour toward relatives and spouses'.[32] According to this author, the psychiatric effects could only be managed by markedly reducing or switching off the stimulation.

Various other reports describe adverse effects such as hypomania, suicidal ideation, and actual suicide.[33–37] According to Drapier et al.,[38] hypomania 'may be systematically underestimated in its frequency' and 'depression and apathy may stay for years'. It has been claimed that measurements are rarely taken to exclude less-obvious changes in behaviour and personality,[39] but that relatives may often report reckless and risk-seeking behaviour that lasts well beyond the post-operative phase. Examples of such behaviours may result in car accidents and marital conflicts.[40] Although these patients were receiving DBS for Parkinson's disease, similar side effects have been described after DBS for depression.[10,41]

While not contesting their likely existence, some authors[42] have dismissed concerns about changes in cognitive and affective aspects of personality on the basis that this is exactly an aim of treatment, so that any such outcome would be regarded as representing success, although it is unclear whether such changes were presented among the intended goals during the consent process.

Frederick Gilbert[43] draws on the concept of 'burden of normality' (BoN), first characterised by Wilson and Bladin et al.,[44] in relation to epilepsy treatment, which describes the adjustment response process that occurs following efficacious psychosurgery in which patients experience a transformation from being 'chronically ill' to being 'well'. In seeking to apply the concept to patients with Parkinson's disease who have undergone a DBS intervention, Gilbert argues that a reduction in debilitating symptoms might not necessarily be experienced as enhancing well-being, but rather as negative outcomes, such as a threat to a patient's identity, 'highlighting challenges with respect to ethical obligations (such as providing access to information, preoperative psychometric self-image measurements, postoperative follow-up, etc.)'. Gilbert summarises case reports of such outcomes in patients with epilepsy and Parkinson's disease. The latter lists a variety of outcomes under the headings of 'psychological', 'behavioural', 'affective' and 'social' changes, 'change in self-image', 'apathy and difficulties in initiating action', and 'change in couple and work dynamics'.

These reports highlight the fact that the outcomes of DBS may go far beyond conventional physical complications of surgical procedures and extend to subtle changes in mood, behaviour, personality, and relationships that are difficult to conceptualise let alone measure. In addition, any attempt at assessing them may need to include the effects on marital or other family or social relationships over an undetermined period of time.

Because of the deep significance of the possible outcomes and the high levels of uncertainty about short- and long-term outcomes, detailed and reliable assessments of the balance between benefits and harms may be very difficult to undertake, even in apparently straightforward clinical cases. This makes a fundamental determination of the value of a procedure difficult and greatly complicates the process of consent, as will now be discussed.

18.4.3 Consent

As with other areas of medicine in which work is being undertaken to test and introduce innovative treatments, consent is a major issue for psychosurgery. Furthermore, many of the complexities that present themselves here are similar to those that arise in the other settings. Key problems that arise relate to the assessment of decision-making capacity, the uncertainty of the balance between risks and benefits, the possibility that dependent relationships might distort the consent process, the social context of stigmatisation of mental illness, and ambivalence about psychosurgery itself.

As previously discussed, in the research setting the complexities of trial design, the difficulties associated with establishing adequate control processes, and the absence of reliable animal models or other preclinical data complicate decision-making. In clinical contexts, the innovative nature of treatments and the absence of long-term data limit informed choice.

These issues are well recognised in the psychosurgical literature, where responses are often sought in familiar and conventional terms, perhaps without full recognition of the limitations they may encounter in the unique setting of this discipline. For example, it is often assumed that the difficulty in determining a patient's capacity to decide can be overcome by a reliance on formal psychometric instruments, such as the MacArthur Scale or other psychosocial measurement tools. However, putting aside well-discussed concerns about cultural and other biases within these tests, in most cases such instruments have not been validated for the particular context, including the unique conceptual issues and the array of philosophical complexities raised by psychosurgery.

The problem here is not unique to psychosurgery but exposes a deeper flaw in the bioethical concept of consent as it is often presented. While it is true that consent entails the agreement of a patient or research volunteer to participate in a programme of treatment or investigation, the granting of such agreement is not a purely formal or mechanical process.[45] Further, it cannot be reduced to a series of abstract steps such as receipt and processing of information, followed by validation or approbation by a patient of a course of action proposed by a practitioner. As has been recognised in more modern theories of consent, such formal mechanisms may largely miss the point about what is most important, which is that a particular kind of conversation has taken place involving relevant stakeholders, who certainly include the patient himself or herself and the key medical practitioners, but may also include family members and other participants in the healthcare team.[46]

Both the form and content of the consent conversation are important, and both must be appropriate to the clinical context. The participants in the conversation may be determined by the cultural background of the patient and the nature of his or her medical condition. The content may need to address complex and difficult philosophical issues such as the possibility of personality changes or disruptions to marital and other relationships. It may be necessary to explore difficult personal, social, physical, and emotional issues that evoke intense anxiety in a patient, who is likely already to be experiencing significant stress. In the setting of unproven therapies or unknown risks, the conduct of such a conversation may be especially difficult.

It is often correctly pointed out that the fact of mental illness itself does not necessarily exclude or invalidate the integrity of a consent process. Nonetheless, because mental illnesses frequently involve disturbances of volition and insight and may be associated with self-harming behaviour each, case must be considered on its own merits in relation to its particular details.

Independent of the effect of the underlying condition on a patient's ability to decide, all consent conversations may be vulnerable to the influence of treatment resistance, outcome expectations, the therapeutic misconception, and external pressure to participate.[47]

In cases where a patient is not able to participate adequately in a consent conversation, and therefore is considered to lack the capacity to consent, other alternatives, such as substitute decision-making, are often proposed.[48] Such cases include those where the patient is a child. The subject of substitute decision-making is a difficult one, especially in the setting of research projects with uncertain, and possibly seriously adverse, outcomes. Indeed, many people consider that in such circumstances it is impossible to speak of 'consent' at all. Furthermore, legally based procedures do not solve the ethical problem. In these settings, it therefore may be difficult or impossible to proceed with recruitment into the research project.

There is an inherent potential power imbalance between medical specialists and their patients, which is especially evident in cases involving mental illness. The influence of the doctor may be accentuated further in cultural settings where the views of authority figures tend to be accepted without question, where medical research expertise is weak, or where ethics and hospital credentialing committees are not yet well established. This would result in weaker constraints on the conduct of psychosurgery.

The establishment of independent, government-administered processes involving psychiatrists, neurosurgeons, lawyers, and lay persons may provide additional checks and balances in relation to the processes of consent, particularly where psychosurgery procedures are being contemplated outside of clinical trial settings.

18.4.4 Conflicts of Interest

As with consent, familiar and well-established issues concerning conflicts of interest may apply to psychosurgical procedures as they do to other areas of medical practice. However, here too it is important to be aware of the special features of the psychosurgical context, as well as the limitations of conventional theory.

As in some other areas of surgery, psychosurgery may involve the implantation of devices developed and manufactured by commercial enterprises. The largely experimental nature of psychosurgical practice, and increasing requirements that research data be made publicly available, highlight the likely commercial value of information that may be obtained. Both of these factors inherently raise the possibility of a material interest that may affect decision-making processes in clinical or research practice. In some cases, practitioners may stand to personally gain from their association with the device manufacturer. In all cases, research projects need to be funded and, in particular, need to be able to obtain supplies of the equipment or devices that are being tested.

Regardless of the specific circumstances of a particular research project, it is well-recognised that clinical practitioners are often engaged in mutually supportive relationships with pharmaceutical companies and device manufacturers. Often, industry assists with training and provides equipment and support, along with funds for conferences and educational and research activities. It may also play a role in the publication process, marketing, advertising, and other media activities.[49] The closeness of these relationships leads to the risk that they may influence judgements in the clinical or research context.

As with consent, the modern theory of interests requires a somewhat broader approach that may have implications for the psychosurgical context. From this perspective, the identification of a 'conflict of interest' requires a precise description of the interests that are in play in a particular setting. Here, an 'interest' is defined as a 'goal, commitment, obligation or duty that arises in relation to a social relationship or practice' – that is, as a value within a practical context that may direct or otherwise influence decision-making. Where two interests give rise to contradictory or incompatible obligations, it is natural to speak of the existence of a 'conflict of interest'.[50]

From this formulation, it is clear that conflicts of interest may occur in the normal course of everyday practice, simply as a result of the fact that individuals occupy multiple roles and in doing so serve a range of different interests. In these settings, there is nothing untoward or ignominious about a conflict; it is a normal event that must be dealt with systematically. In addition, interests are not limited to financial matters, but can also include personal, non-pecuniary interests; indeed, at least in medicine, it is such non-financial interests that are in general the most powerful drivers of behaviour.

In the case of psychosurgery, both these considerations apply. To the extent that surgeons occupy multiple roles – as clinicians, researchers, educators, advisors to industry, and so forth – they are likely at times to encounter conflicting interests. In addition, their values and beliefs, commercial interests, personal goals, aspirations, commitments, and obligations also constitute interests, the significance and influence of which must be considered in every clinical and research setting.

The processes for identifying and managing interests and conflicts of interest are well described in the literature and will not be repeated here, apart from drawing attention to the need for the establishment of independent decision-making bodies to consider individual cases, as has also been mentioned above in relation to informed consent. Where conflicts of interest are found to arise, these committees can assist in separating the contending roles to ensure that no more than one set of interests is operating in any particular decision-making context.

Various sets of guidelines exist to provide assistance with the management of conflicts of interest. In the psychosurgical context, much of the focus is on disclosure of financial interests, ties with industry, sources of funding for research, and the influence of any other relevant interests that may affect decision-making.[51] Where commercial information is involved, this should be provided as widely as possible to avoid the possibility of doubt about the considerations that are being taken into account.

18.4.5 Special Considerations Relating to Particular Populations

The patients who may be considered for psychosurgical research studies or, where appropriate, clinical treatments often belong to groups with special needs or concerns that may require particular consideration. Such patients may come from cultural backgrounds in which mental illness carries particular connotations, or surgical interventions (especially into the brain) may be understood in particular ways. From their earlier experiences, whether because of their illnesses or for other reasons, they may have particular fears or anxieties. Individuals who have been institutionalised for long periods may harbour suspicions about people in authority. The dependent nature of their relationships may complicate decision-making contexts in relation both to health professionals and to family.

Levels of education, income, and social status may also affect the nature of participation in clinical and research programmes. Understanding of the complex concepts and uncertainties associated with a field of such complexity as psychosurgery may be diminished in patients unable to speak English or where past experiences erode the ability to engage with authority (as with refugees or patients with past traumatic experiences).

Patients with particular diagnoses may have limited ability to resist medical recommendations. These include highly institutionalised patients, owing to their illnesses or underlying personality factors, patients in urgent or desperate need of an effective treatment (including patients with unrelieved depression or psychosis), or (possibly) patients who have previously undergone psychosurgery. A special case of such dependency is that of children and young people.

Some of the issues raised in relation to such groups have been addressed in the discussion of consent, but it is important to recognise that consent is not the only question that is at stake here. Cultural sensitivity may require acknowledgment of the belief systems and vulnerabilities of whole communities. Engagement of a patient in a research project requires more than simple acquiescence to participate. Anxiety about relationships with authority in itself can skew the assessment of outcomes or even the outcomes themselves.

In ethical discourse, particular groups such as the ones mentioned have in the past often been considered under the heading of 'vulnerable populations'. However, the concept has recently come under critical scrutiny on the basis that it ignores the inherent vulnerability of all patients and suggests that vulnerability can be measured, proven, or discounted, or minimised through specific intervention. The approach currently favoured considers the particular issues or concerns relevant to each individual in his or her personal, social, or cultural context and responds as appropriate in all applicable dimensions. In addition to the question of consent, the latter may include communication strategies, approaches to recruitment, study design, choice of outcome measures, conduct of study or clinical procedures, and formulation and dissemination of results.

The case of children may be particularly difficult. Established guidelines about the participation of children in research usually recommend against the inclusion of minors in invasive programmes or where the chance of individual benefit is limited. In most cases, children will therefore be excluded from psychosurgery altogether. It is possible that there will be rare exceptions to this, but these would need to be considered on a case by case basis, and compliance with local regulatory requirements – legal and ethical – would need to be assured.

18.4.6 The Social and Cultural Context of Psychosurgery and Its Possible Applications

As discussed above, the early proponents of psychosurgery saw it not just as a therapy for medical conditions affecting individuals but also as a social tool to oppose dissent and violence in the political arena. Their proposals received widespread support in the profession and the popular media, as well as US government grant funding. They also attracted significant opposition; indeed, much of the popular resistance to psychosurgery that developed in the 1960s and 1970s focused on its potential and actual applications for controlling behaviour.

To contemporary sensibilities, the use of brain surgery as a technique to enforce social control appears to be unequivocally objectionable. However, the general principle that medicine may play an important role in stabilising social systems and supporting existing regimes of power is by no means out of the ordinary. On the contrary, extensive sociological theory and research over more than half a century has identified this as one of medicine's key social functions.[52,53] What is more, much work in the social sciences on the nature of mental illness and the history of psychiatry has focused on the role of mental asylums in establishing and maintaining socially current concepts of reason and rationality. Less subtle applications of medicine to control behaviour and enforce conformity to contemporary norms are also familiar, such as treatments in the recent past to reverse homosexuality.[54,55]

If, on the one hand, it is part of the normal functioning of medicine to support or enforce accepted behaviours and, on the other, the direct application of brain surgery to stifle dissent evokes widespread revulsion, then a key problem for psychosurgery will include the clear delineation of the boundary between acceptable and unacceptable interventions according to existing standards. The process of establishing such a boundary will require a detailed account of the full range of possible – or, at least, conceivable – psychosurgical interventions and a process according to which these interventions can be assessed and regulated. It is possible that in the course of this analysis a case can be made by some in support of surgical intervention to alter the minds of criminals, to limit dissent, or to abolish impulses considered to be antisocial. However, even to attempt this, fundamental ethical and philosophical questions will need to be addressed, such as the nature of mind and its relationship with the brain; the meaning of embodiment; the concepts of self and person-hood; the nature of free will, agency, and moral judgement; and the role and status of brain function in social and moral decision-making.

Obviously, these fundamental questions cannot be discussed in detail here. However, their contemporary relevance has been accentuated by the rapid advance of neuroscience – which itself is based on contestable philosophical assumptions about the relationship between mind and brain – and the knowledge it has generated about the role of certain neural pathways in cognition and affective states. At least in principle, this knowledge raises the possibility of applications of psychosurgery for purposes that have hitherto been limited to science fiction, such as the deliberate creation of emotional states or the enforcement of compliance with or opposition to authority. While the realisation of such practices may lie outside present capabilities, it is by no means unthinkable that research in this area might be attempted. Further, it is even within the bounds of possibility that individuals might 'freely' consent to participate in such studies. Prisoners of the state in jail would be particularly vulnerable, especially if they were rewarded with reduced sentences or freedom. The intense concerns research of this sort might provoke, along with its potential far-reaching consequences, suggest that formal mechanisms for regulating future directions in psychosurgical may need to be explored.

18.4.7 Potentially Controversial Uses of Psychosurgery

The list of possible and imaginable developments and applications of psychosurgery is long and complex. Many of its elements would undoubtedly evoke controversy, and many would stimulate demands for outright rejection. If it were possible – as some people have claimed – to identify neural pathways subserving particular attitudes, beliefs, or emotional states, surgical interventions could be applied to interfere with or direct these. Racist attitudes and criminal dispositions could be identified and corrected. Specified emotional states could be created or abrogated. Highly traumatic memories of the past could be eliminated. Cognitive abilities could be stimulated, enhanced, or reduced. Particular needs could be implanted. Personality traits could be created or eliminated. Dispositions favouring participation in certain professions or social roles could be supported or inhibited.[31,42,56,57]

While these examples may seem fanciful, at least some of them have been the subject of serious discussion in the scientific literature. It is likely that over time they will need to be considered comprehensively and in full detail, and whether they exceed the legitimate ethical purposes of medicine will need to be determined.

18.5 Some Principles for the Ethical Regulation of Psychosurgical Research and Practice

The novel, potentially powerful techniques of neuroscience combined with psychosurgery raise the possibility not only of beneficial but also of harmful and ethically troubling applications.

Whatever opinion or views might exist about the ethical and philosophical issues listed above, it is clear that there is a strong basis for concern about their potential impact on society. The seriousness of the questions asked and the risk of harm is sufficient to justify the establishment of a formal process of review and regulation.

While most contemporary practitioners of psychosurgery undoubtedly reject the excesses of the past, much of their language and the ways in which their ideas are formulated remain largely unchanged: the techniques applied are recognised to address major, urgent social needs; they are said to be based on 'modern' scientific knowledge and to utilise refined imagining techniques; although actual data are limited, the techniques are referred to as 'promising' and 'emerging'; and little reflection is undertaken on the underlying values or assumptions that provide the contexts within which both clinical practice and research occur. Apart from assurances about commitments to respecting the 'autonomy' and 'dignity' of patients – which were already well established half a century ago – there is little to indicate that the current ethical climate is significantly different to that previously or that the professional and social judgements that were so favourable in the past would not be favourable again.

A number of key ethical issues require attention, such as the design of studies, assessment of evidence, consent, management of conflicts of interest, and issues relating to specific populations. Many of these can be addressed on the basis of contemporary approaches in research ethics, with attention to the special questions raised by psychosurgery.

However, there also needs to be a broader social discussion about the wider social, ethical, and philosophical context in which the field is developing and its potential malign (or at least ethically questionable) applications. The ease with which such applications were introduced and supported in the past suggests a need for great caution.

Proposed ethical criteria for the conduct of clinical research in psychosurgery are useful but may not go far enough (Table 18.1).[58]

Table 18.1 Ethical criteria for clinical trials in neurosurgery

Criteria
Transparent discussion of patient selection
Evidence-based rationale for disease and target selection
Demonstration of disease burden and clinical need
Rigorous attention to consent process
Multi-disciplinary review and assessment
Independent oversight of all aspects of research
Systemic process of evaluation and review

The recommendations developed by the consensus conference in 2009 (see below) are also helpful but require wider debate and the establishment of formal processes to enable their implementation.

It is unlikely that a formal legal process will provide sufficient flexibility, openness, or responsiveness to local needs. A better model may be a devolved system of community-based deliberative forums, as with the networks of ethics committees that regulate research.

Independent registries containing data on all individuals undergoing DBS and their outcomes should also be developed using common standards so that experience can be tracked and scrutinised.

A consensus conference held in 2009[59] has generated a number of recommendations for the regulation of psychosurgery that addresses the main questions of an ethical nature. Drawing on our discussion, and on these and other recommendations,[60-63] we propose the following principles as the basis for any regulatory framework that may be considered in the future:

1. Psychosurgery for disorders of mood, behaviour, and thought is presently at an early proof-of-principle stage and must be considered investigational.
2. Research in DBS, and other techniques in psychosurgery such as stereotactic radiosurgery and focused ultrasound, for such disorders is justified.
3. Studies should include comparisons of the efficacy and safety of DBS with those of other treatments, including ablative surgery.
4. Studies should take the form of carefully designed trials conducted at expert centres.
5. DBS should only be undertaken by multidisciplinary teams in duly constituted research settings subject to independent oversight and review.
6. Inclusion criteria for trials should be disease specific and may change over time. At present, such trials should be limited to adults.
7. Trial outcomes should include both symptoms and outcomes in domains such as activities of daily living, cognition, quality of life, and global improvement.
8. Research centres should collaborate to develop an agreed upon, common framework for assessing potential subjects' capacity to consent. Assessment of capacity should be carried out for each potential subject.
9. The consent process should include detailed discussion of the current knowledge about DBS, including potential consequences and the limitations of such knowledge.

10. Studies to determine long-term safety are essential, with follow-up data at 1, 2, 5, 10, and 15 years.
11. Independent registries should be established to store data on all individuals who undergo DBS for disorders of mood, behaviour, and thought.
12. Patients must be free to withdraw from studies at any time.
13. Patients should not incur financial costs, either by participating in or withdrawing from a study.
14. No recommendation can be made at the present time about patient control of stimulation.
15. The various specialist practitioners involved in psychosurgery should undertake appropriate training and be subject to a rigorous credentialing process.

18.6 Conclusion

This chapter has presented an overview of some of the key ethical issues that arise in relation to psychosurgery. The egregious history of the mid-twentieth century misuses of psychosurgery has undoubtedly generated lasting suspicion and hostility among many medical practitioners, ethicists, community members, and regulators that will need to be overcome before psychosurgery can be accepted as a routine practice at any time in the future.

Many specific questions will need to be addressed, including those related to the assessment of the balance of good and harm – especially given the difficulties in obtaining reliable evidence, along with the questions of consent, conflicts of interest, the needs and vulnerabilities of specific populations or cultural groups, and the possibility of a malign misuse of psychosurgical procedures for social or political purposes. Some principles to guide the regulation of the field have been proposed.

References

1. Burchiel K. J. Deep brain stimulation and depression. *J. Neurosurg.* 2012; **116**: 313–14.
2. Delaloye S., Holtzheimer P. E. Deep brain stimulation in the treatment of depression. *Dialogues Clin. Neurosci.* 2014; **16**: 83–91.
3. Kuhn J., Gründler T. O., Lenartz J., et al. Deep brain stimulation for psychiatric disorders. *Dtsch. Arztebl. Int.* 2010; **107**: 105–13.
4. Moro E. Impulse control disorders and subthalamic nucleus stimulation in Parkinson's disease: are we jumping the gun? *Eur. J. Neurol.* 2009; **16**: 440–1.
5. Schlaepfer T. E., Bewernick B., Kayser S., et al. Modulating affect, cognition, and behavior – prospects of deep-brain stimulation for treatment – resistant psychiatric disorders. *Front. Integr. Neurosci.* 2011; **5**: 29.
6. Sen A. N., Campbell P. J., Yadla S., et al. Deep brain stimulation in the management of disorders of consciousness: a review of physiology, previous reports, and ethical considerations. *Neurosurg. Focus* 2010; **29**: E14.
7. Clausen J. Ethical brain stimulation – neuroethics of deep brain stimulation in research and clinical practice. *Eur. J. Neurosci.* 2010; **32**: 1152–62.
8. Heller A. C., Amiar A. P., Liu C. Y., et al. Surgery of the mind and mood: a mosaic of issues in time and evolution. *Neurosurgery* 2006; **59**: 720–39.
9. Holtzheimer P. E., Husain M. M., Lisanby S. H. et al. Subcallosal cingulate deep brain stimulation for treatment-resistant depression: a multisite, randomised, sham-controlled trial. *The Lancet Psychiatry* 2017, 4(11): 839–48.
10. Egan D. Adverse effects: The perils of deep brain stimulation for depression. Available

at: https://www.madinamerica.com/2015/09/adverse-effects-perils-deep-brain-stimulation.

11. Gupta A., Shepard M. J., Xu Z. et al. An international radiosurgery research foundation multicentre retrospective study of gamma ventral capsulotomy for obsessive compulsive disorder. *Neurosurgery* 2018; **85**(6): 808–16. doi:10.1093/neuros/nyy536.

12. Heller A. C., Amar A. P., Liu C. Y. et al. Surgery of the mind and mood: a mosaic of issues in time and evolution. *Neurosurgery* 2006; **59**: 720–39.

13. Fins J. From psychosurgery to neuromodulation and palliation: History's lessons for the ethical conduct and regulation of neuropsychiatric research. *Neurosurg. Clin. N. Am.* 2003; **14**: 303–19.

14. Hunt G. P. The two accused: the psycho-biology of violence. *Life*, 21 June 1968. Available at: www.amazon.com/Life-Magazine-Accuese-Psycho-Biology-Violence/dp/B0013SHPPG.

15. Szasz T. S. *The Myth of Mental Illness: Foundations of a Theory of Personal Conduct*. New York, Harper & Row, 1974.

16. Laing R. D., Esterton A. *Sanity, Madness and the Family*. London, Tavistock, 1964.

17. Laing R. D. *The Self and Others*. Harmondsworth, Penguin, 1969.

18. Cooper D. *Psychiatry and Anti-Psychiatry*. London, Tavistock, 1967.

19. Breggin P. R. Psychosurgery as brain-disabling therapy. In *Divergent Views in Psychiatry*, eds. M. Dongier and E. Wittkower. Hagerstown, MD, Harper and Row, 1981, 302–26. Available at: http://breggin.com/wp-content/uploads/2008/01/psychosurgeryas.pbreggin.1981.pdf.

20. Editorial. 'Psychosurgery.' *Lancet*, July 8, 1972, pp. 69–70.

21. Ryan J. K. US National Commission for Protection of Human Subjects of Biomedical and Behavioural Research. *US Statut. Large.* 1974; **88**: 342–54.

22. Breggin P. R. Psychosurgery for political purposes. *Duquesne Law Review* 1975; **13**: 841–62.

23. Fisher C. E., Dunn L. B., Christopher P. P., et al. The ethics of research on deep brain stimulation for depression: decisional capacity and therapeutic misconception. *Ann. NY Acad. Sci.* 2012; **1265**: 69–79.

24. Fuchsa T., Schlimme J. E. Embodiment and psychopathology: a phenomenological Perspective. *Curr. Opin. Psychiatry* 2009; **22**: 570–5.

25. Hansson S. O. Implant ethics. *J. Med. Ethics* 2005; **31**: 519–25.

26. Kringelbach M. L., Aziz T. Z. Neuroethical principles of deep-brain stimulation. *World Neurosurg.* 2011; **76**: 518–19.

27. Lipsman N., Giacobbe P., Bernstein M., et al. Informed consent for clinical trials of deep brain stimulation in psychiatric disease: challenges and implications for trial design. *J. Med. Ethics* 2012; **38**: 107–11.

28. Lipsman N., Glannon W., Brain, mind and machine: what are the implications of deep brain stimulation for perceptions of personal identity, agency and free will? *Bioethics* 2013; **27**: 465–70.

29. Rabins P., Brian S., Appleby J. B., et al. Scientific and ethical issues related to deep brain stimulation for disorders of mood, behavior and thought. *Arch. Gen. Psychiatry* 2009; **66**: 931–7.

30. Schmitz-Luhn B., Katzenmeier C., Woopen C. Law and ethics of deep brain stimulation. *Int. J. Law and Psychiatry* 2012; **35**: 130–6.

31. Clausen J. Ethical brain stimulation – neuroethics of deep brain stimulation in research and clinical practice. *Eur. J. Neurosci.* 2010; **32**: 1152–62.

32. Cyron D. Mental side effects of deep brain stimulation (DBS) for movement disorders: the futility of denial. *Front Integr. Neurosci.* 2016; **10**: 17.

33. Herzog J., Reiff J., Krack P., et al. Manic episode with psychotic symptoms induced by subthalamic nucleus stimulation in a patient with Parkinson's disease. *Mov. Disord.* 2003; **18**: 1382–4.

34. Morgan J. C., DiDonato C. J., Iyer S. S., et al. Self-stimulatory behavior associated

with deep brain stimulation in Parkinson's disease. *Mov. Disord.* 2006; **21**: 283–5.

35. Schupbach M., Gargiulo M., Welter M. L., et al. Neurosurgery in Parkinson disease: a distressed mind in a repaired body? *Neurology* 2006; **66**: 1811–16.

36. Witt K., Daniels C., Reiff J. et al. Neuropsychological and psychiatric changes after deep brain stimulation for Parkinson's disease: a randomised, multicentre study. *Lancet Neurol.* 2008; 7: 605–14.

37. Voon V., Krack P., Lang A. E. et al. A multicentre study on suicide outcomes following subthalamic stimulation for Parkinson's disease. *Brain* 2008; **131**: 2720–8.

38. Drapier D., Drapier S., Sauleau P. et al. Does subthalamic nucleus stimulation induce apathy in Parkinson's disease? *J. Neurol.* 2006; **253**: 1083–91.

39. Florin E., Muller D., Pfeifer J., et al. Subthalamic stimulation modulates self-estimation of patients with Parkinson's disease and induces risk-seeking behaviour. *Brain* 2013; **136**: 3271–81.

40. Schupbach M., Gargiulo M., Welter M. L., et al. Neurosurgery in Parkinson disease: a distressed mind in a repaired body? *Neurology* 2006; **66**: 1811–16.

41. Hobbs D. What went wrong in the first-ever clinical trial of deep brain stimulation for depression? Available at: http://dig.com/2018/deep-brain-stimulation-depression-trial.

42. Pacholczyk A. DBS makes you feel good! – why some of the ethical objections to the use of DBS for neuropsychiatric disorders and enhancement are not convincing. *Front Integr. Neurosci.* 2011; 5: 14

43. Gilbert F. The burden of normality: from 'chronically ill' to 'symptom free'. New ethical challenges for deep brain stimulation postoperative treatment. *J. Med. Ethics* 2012; **38**: 408–12.

44. Wilson S., Bladin P., Saling M. The 'burden of normality': concepts of adjustment after surgery for seizures. *J. Neurol. Neurosurg. Psychiatry* 2001; **70**: 649–56.

45. Komesaroff P. A. *Experiments in Love and Death.* Seattle, University of Washington Press, 2008.

46. Manson N. C., O'Neill O. *Rethinking Informed Consent in Bioethics.* Cambridge, University of Cambridge Press, 2007.

47. Lipsman N., Bernstein M., Lozano M. Criteria for the ethical conduct of psychiatric neurosurgery clinical trials. *Neurosurg. Focus* 2010; **29**: E9.

48. Morse S. J. New therapies, old problems, or, a plea for neuromodesty. *AJOB Neuroscience* 2012; **3**: 60–4.

49. Laura Y., Cabrera H. M. K., Boyce R. M., et al. Conflicts of interest and industry professional relationships in psychiatric neurosurgery: a comparative literature review. *Neurosurg. Focus* 2108; **45**: E20.

50. Komesaroff P. A., Lipworth W., Kerridge I. Conflicts of interest: new thinking, new processes. *Int. Med. J.* 2109; **49**(5): 574–7.

51. Fins J. J., Schlaepfer T. E., Nuttin B., et al. Ethical guidance for the management of conflicts of interest for researchers, engineers and clinicians engaged in the development of therapeutic deep brain stimulation. *J. Neural. Eng.* 2011; **8**: 033001.

52. Parsons T. *The Social System.* Glencoe, IL, Free Press, 1951.

53. Illich I. *Medical Nemesis.* London, Random House, 1976.

54. Foucault M. *Madness and Civilization: A History of Insanity in the Age of Reason.* London, Random House, 1988.

55. Szasz T. S. The myth of mental illness. *American Psychologist* 1960; **15**: 113–18.

56. Lipsman N., Zener R., Bernstein M. Personal identity, enhancement and neurosurgery: a qualitative study in applied neuroethics. *Bioethics* 2009; **23**: 375–83.

57. Synofzik M., Schlaepfer T. E. Stimulating personality: ethical criteria for deep brain stimulation in psychiatric patients and for enhancement purposes. *Biotechnol. J.* 2008; 3: 1511–20.

58. Lipsman N., Bernstein M., Lozano M. Criteria for the ethical conduct of

psychiatric neurosurgery clinical trials. *Neurosurg. Focus* 2010; **29**: E9.

59. Rabins P., Brian S., Appleby J. B., et al. Scientific and ethical issues related to deep brain stimulation for disorders of mood, behavior and thought. *Arch. Gen. Psychiatry* 2009; **66**: 931–7.

60. Lipsman N., Bernstein M., Lozano M. Criteria for the ethical conduct of psychiatric neurosurgery clinical trials. *Neurosurg. Focus* 2010; **29**: E9.

61. Fins J. From psychosurgery to neuromodulation and palliation: history's lessons for the ethical conduct

and regulation of neuropsychiatric research. *Neurosurg. Clin. N. Am.* 2003; **14**: 303–19.

62. Bell E., Racine E. Ethics guidance for neurological and psychiatric deep brain stimulation. *Handbook of Clinical Neurology: Brain Stimulation*, Vol. 116, 3rd series, ed. A. M. Lozano, M. Hallett. London, Elsevier, 2013, 313–25.

63. Synofzika M., Schlaepferb T. E. Electrodes in the brain: ethical criteria for research and treatment with deep brain stimulation for neuropsychiatric disorders. *Brain Stimul.* 2011; **4**: 7–16.

Chapter 19

Brain Death and Organ Donation

George Skowronski and Ian Kerridge

19.1 Introduction

Transplantation using organs obtained around the time of death began in 1962 and has become a large and very successful enterprise. In Australia, around 500 organ donors currently provide about 1,500 organs for transplantation per year. Success rates of the order of 90% are now achievable, but currently the demand for organs for transplantation greatly exceeds supply.

Around three quarters of all donated organs are acquired around the time of the donor's death, and the majority of these donors have a neurosurgical pathology as the cause of death. The process by which organs are obtained is constrained by the so-called dead donor rule (DDR), which requires that the donor be declared dead before organs are removed. Most commonly, this is achieved by the development of the syndrome of 'brain death'. However, 'donation after circulatory death' (DCD) is now responsible for a growing proportion of organs obtained around the time of death. Ethical and religious controversies surround both brain death and DCD, and there have been legal challenges to their validity.

The legalisation of physician-assisted suicide and euthanasia in many jurisdictions has raised new ethical questions regarding the place of organ donation in these forms of death.

Consent for organ donation is controversial, with arguments for opt-in, opt-out, mandatory request, and mandatory choice all supported by various advocates. The provision of financial incentives has also been widely debated.

In potential DCD donors, it has become commonplace to undertake a number of interventions before death has been declared, including anticoagulation, blood transfusion, placement of large-bore intravenous catheters, and even coronary angiography. These raise ethical questions around their justification in the best interests of the donors.

Peri-mortem organ donation also raises potential conflicts of interest, particularly in ICUs where actual and potential transplant recipients may be cared for alongside each other. Another potential conflict arises when transplant doctors to attempt to influence the process of donor identification and recruitment.

19.2 Background – The Diagnosis of Death

The ancient Egyptians and Greeks regarded the absence of a heartbeat as the primary criterion for death. Their understanding of cardiac physiology was that the heart created the vital spirits, so that without cardiac pulsation, life was impossible. Traditional Jewish sources, by contrast, focus on respiration as the primary criterion for life. The Old Testament contains several references to this idea, beginning in Genesis where God 'breathes life' into Adam via his nostrils. The Talmud also emphasises the absence of breathing as the primary sign of death and contains few references to the role of the heart.

Despite the elucidation by William Harvey in 1628 that the heart is nothing more than a biological pump, none of this was especially controversial until around 1960, when two medical developments made matters much more complicated. The first was the development of modern intensive care, which grew primarily out of the European polio epidemics of the 1950s. The second was the invention of cardiac defibrillation and cardiopulmonary resuscitation, both around 1960. These developments meant that life could be maintained, potentially indefinitely, in the absence of spontaneous breathing, while the absence of a heartbeat became a medical emergency rather than a sure sign of death. Further advances in extra-corporeal techniques now allow life to continue in the complete absence of cardiac activity.

The first reference to the brain as a primary source of life also comes from a Jewish scholar, Maimonides (1135–1204). He argued that the twitching movements seen after decapitation should not be taken as signs of life, as they were not under central control. This is relevant, as some modern scholars, both Jewish and secular, have argued that brain death with absent cerebral blood flow is equivalent to decapitation.

In 1959 two French neurologists described an extreme state of unconsciousness, which they termed *coma dépassé* (beyond coma), in patients maintained using these new intensive care 'life support' technologies. By 1968 the problem of withdrawing life support had become sufficiently concerning that a special committee was set up by the Harvard Medical School with the aim of defining *brain death*.[1] They proposed that *irreversible coma*, described as a state virtually identical to *coma dépassé*, might be defined as a new kind of death for medical and legal purposes, and that this definition could be used to justify the withdrawal of life support. A further statement from the combined Royal Colleges of the UK in 1976[2] further endorsed the position that the criteria proposed for the diagnosis of brain death should be accepted as amounting to the death of the individual.

While these concepts are now very widely accepted, Japan, Romania, and Pakistan still do not recognise brain death as a valid criterion for the death of the individual. When Japan's first heart transplant was performed by Juro Wada in 1968, using a brain-dead donor, Wada was charged with murder, though he was eventually acquitted after years of litigation. Japanese legislation now recognises brain death for the purposes of organ donation, but death of the individual is still deemed not to have occurred until after removal of donated organs is completed.

19.3 Death and Organ Transplantation

In 1968 the Judicial Council of the American Medical Association declared, 'When a vital, single organ is to be transplanted, the death of the donor shall have been determined by at least one physician other than the recipient's physician.'[3] This was later popularised as the 'dead donor rule' and, in combination with the definition of brain death, has been widely accepted as one of the main ethical foundations for organ donation at the end of life.

In more recent years, a new basis for organ donation has emerged in many parts of the world and is responsible for most of the increase in previously low organ donation rates in Australia in the last few years. In what has been called 'non-beating heart' organ donation, or 'donation after cardiac (or circulatory) death (DCD)', a patient with profound brain pathology, whose prognosis is agreed to be hopeless, but who is not brain dead, has life support withdrawn, either in the intensive care unit (ICU) or in the operating room. After heartbeat and respirations cease (provided this happens within a reasonably short time interval), a further period of a few minutes (two to eight minutes, depending on local guidelines) is allowed to pass without intervention, in order that the DDR can be deemed fulfilled by traditional cardio-respiratory criteria, before organ removal can begin. DCD limits both the quality and number of organs, which can be used for transplantation, but the results are nevertheless quite acceptable.

19.4 Ethical Issues

19.4.1 Is Brain Death Really a Form of Death?

There is no doubt that family members confronted with the prospect of brain death find it difficult to accept that their loved ones should be regarded as dead, even though they appear warm and pink, their hearts are beating, and their chest rises and falls with respiration.

In fact, while the early statements from the Harvard group and the UK colleges comfortably justified 'brain death' as a valid criterion for the removal of life support, which was their primary aim, both were more vague about whether this state truly constituted a form of biological death. Current legislation defining death in the United States, Australia, and many other countries requires either the irreversible cessation of all functions of the entire brain or the irreversible cessation of circulatory function. There are two main problems with this legal definition.

19.4.2 Is Brain Death Really Irreversible?

Fifty years of experience with the concept of brain death have taught us that it probably is irreversible in the sense (contrary to urban myths that arise from time to time) that there is no properly documented case of a patient having regained consciousness or returned to a life off life support after meeting brain death criteria, when rigorously and expertly determined. But, setting aside the extent to which this fact might represent a self-fulfilling prophesy, it can equally be argued that these patients are more correctly described as being in a state of permanent, profound coma that renders them ventilator-dependent, with no basis for equating such a state with death, any more than other cases where consciousness is profoundly impaired, such as permanent vegetative states (now called 'post-coma unresponsiveness' in Australia[4]).

For some years after brain death was recognised, it was believed that 'bodily death' would inevitably follow brain death within a few days, even if maximal life support was provided, and this argument was sometimes used to support the idea that brain death really did represent a form of death. Unfortunately, this is no longer the case. Abhorrent as the idea is to most of us, it is now possible to maintain brain dead patients for prolonged periods, if not indefinitely.

As for the cardiac/respiratory component, when does an absent heartbeat become irreversible? In exceptional circumstances (such as extreme cold), people have been restored to normal after 20–30 minutes of cardio-respiratory arrest. Many of the people meeting current DCD criteria could readily be resuscitated after their mandatory 2 minutes (the current Australian standard) of pulselessness, but it has been argued that after this length of time 'auto-resuscitation' (i.e., the spontaneous recommencement of cardiac and respiratory activity) is extremely unlikely if not impossible. Since a decision has been made not to resuscitate on the grounds of futility, the donor can now be deemed to be dead.

Whether this somewhat convoluted rationale really meets the requirement of irreversibility is doubtful; the situation is only irreversible because we *choose* not to reverse it.

19.4.3 The Concept of Whole Brain Death

UK legislation defines brain death by the irreversible absence of brainstem reflexes. This is true to the clinical technique for brain death testing and rests on the idea that death of the brainstem includes death of the reticular activating system, the brainstem structure responsible for arousal and the maintenance of consciousness. The traditional argument here is that if the individual is permanently incapable of awareness at any level, they may be regarded as dead. Whether or not one accepts this argument, the definition is at least consistent with the tests that are done.

In Australia, the United States, and most other jurisdictions, death of the *whole brain* is legally required for brain death, and this is by no means universally the case when brain death is clinically diagnosed. Only around 50% of brain-dead patients have *diabetes insipidus*. Since vasopressin is produced by neurons in the hypothalamus and secreted in the posterior pituitary gland, it is clear that in around 50% of brain-dead patients, diagnosed clinically, at least this part of the brain is unequivocally working.

As to why the presence of *diabetes insipidus* is not one of the criteria for diagnosing brain death, this probably reflects the centrality of brainstem function in the original conception of brain death, which did not emphasise death of the entire brain in the same way as the subsequent legislation.

The gold standard for brain death testing, rarely used in 'routine' cases in most countries, is cerebral angiography, which typically shows absence of cerebral blood flow. Brain death meeting this criterion has been labelled 'medical decapitation', and it has been argued that this can be regarded as representing death in the same way as we would regard a physically decapitated person as dead. On this basis, legislation in Israel, France, Italy, Spain, and Singapore does not accept clinical testing, and requires demonstration of absent blood flow to establish brain death. However, a significant number of patients who unequivocally meet clinical criteria for brain death do not demonstrate the complete absence of flow on angiography. Because of this lack of sensitivity, it has not been more widely adopted.

Truog[5] and others have discussed the ethical difficulties of defining death by neurological criteria when integrated somatic function can be maintained for months or years, and this was also acknowledged by the President's Council on Bioethics in 2008.[6]

Miller, Truog, and Brock[7] argue that our current justifications of brain death and DCD use 'moral fictions'. These widely accepted rationalisations arise from the cognitive dissonance associated with reconciling the withdrawal of life support with the ethical norm that doctors must not intentionally kill patients. In their view, the DDR constitutes a similar moral fiction – removing vital organs from a live patient would be killing them, and therefore we must first ensure that the donor is dead, adjusting our conceptions of death appropriately to allow for organ donation. These and other authors argue that the DDR has led to new concepts of death, for the purposes of transplantation, which are not biologically, socially, or legally valid. In their view, organ donation is ethically justifiable without a declaration of death being mandatory, and the DDR should be abandoned. Supporters of the DDR rely mainly on slippery-slope arguments that the requirement for death to be declared protects the community from unscrupulous behaviour by transplant doctors.

In recent years, there have been legal challenges to the diagnosis of brain death on religious grounds, particularly in the United States. In the widely reported case of Jahi McMath, a 13-year-old girl who was declared brain dead from cerebral hypoxia following a post-tonsillectomy haemorrhage, the patient continued to be cared for at home by her family, with perhaps some features to suggest that she was minimally conscious, for almost five years before her family decided to 'let her go' after she developed liver failure and unexplained bleeding. As of 2019 Jahi had two death certificates, a Californian certificate indicating that she died on December 13, 2013, and a New Jersey certificate stating that she died on June 22, 2018.[8] This case, like many other cases where patients have survived for long periods of time following a diagnosis of brain death, challenged both the notion that brain death leads to the inevitable disintegration of the entire organism and the notion that brain death is irreversible – suggesting instead that brain injury is not static but that with time it may get better or worse.

Further legal challenges have also been made regarding the legitimacy of the apnoea test, in which the integrity of medullary respiratory centres is assessed in the context of brain death determination. Opponents argue that the test is dangerous and may worsen brain injury by raising pCO_2 and, consequently, intracranial pressure.

19.5 Consent for Organ Donation

Most Western countries follow the principle of required consent ('opt-in'), where the consent of the donor and/or next of kin is needed before peri-mortem organ donation can take place. In opt-in countries, there continues to be debate around whether families should have the power of veto over prior consent by a donor. In Australia, the National Health and Medical Research Council's policy supports this right of veto, and most doctors are reluctant to override family objections, even though Human Tissue Acts in most states empower them to do so where there is written consent.[9]

Proponents of family veto justify it on the basis that it is important for the maintenance of public trust in organ donation, for minimising family distress, and because family veto is rare in practice. Opponents argue that it violates the principle of autonomy and potentially harms several prospective organ recipients and their families – a factor that they claim outweighs any downside for donor families.

Several countries, including the United Kingdom, Belgium, Austria, Spain, Chile, Argentina, and Columbia, have accepted the principle of presumed ('opt-out') consent, where family consent is not required but donation can be overridden by evidence that the donor, during life, has indicated an objection. Experience in a number of countries suggests that this has the potential to double organ donation rates compared with opt-in systems, and many mainstream religious authorities see no objection to this, notably an authoritative Islamic group, who declared as far back as 1979 that 'permission of the family is not required since human organs belong to God and not to the family'.[10] However, some ethicists argue that this does not meet the fundamental principles of consent and even hints of coercion.

Something of a compromise between these alternatives is 'mandated request', where hospitals are required by law to refer all imminent deaths, meeting broad criteria, to 'trained requesters', who are typically intensive care physicians working in the same hospital.[11] Such legislation exists across most of North America and is promoted by transplant groups and others in Australia. This approach also has ethical problems, in particular the creation of conflicts of interest at various levels for the intensivists involved, who must balance the interests of the donor/patient, their family, the potential organ recipients, and the state.[9]

A final option that has been discussed is 'mandated choice', in which all adult citizens are legally required to stipulate whether they consent to organ donation in the future, should the situation arise.[12] In some models, a third alternative of 'let my family decide' is also included. This system was adopted in Texas for about five years, but was abandoned, due mainly to a very high refusal rate (around 80%).

19.6 Financial Incentives for Organ Donation

The sale of organs from poor, living donors in developing countries, often to wealthy foreigners, is common. It has been estimated that more than 2,000 kidneys per year are sold in India alone, and 'transplant tourism' is a substantial and profitable industry for brokers, private hospitals, and various other intermediaries. The practice has been condemned by many transplant societies and religious authorities worldwide, claiming that it promotes coercion, corruption, exploitation, and poor-quality medical care for both donors and recipients. It is illegal in most countries.

However, in Iran, a legal, regulated system allowing the sale of kidneys has operated for many years and has resulted in the reduction of waiting lists to zero. Proponents argue that organ sale may offer the only hope for the destitute, and its prohibition is an infringement of their autonomy. They claim that the negative aspects of organ sale are due to poverty and lack of education, and do not necessarily justify a ban in principle. A highly regulated market, which ensures screening, counselling, properly informed consent, and a high standard of medical care and follow-up for donors and recipients, could have a major impact on the organ shortage in most countries and would not necessarily be morally repugnant.[13] Whether this could be equitably achieved is perhaps doubtful.

Even in advanced countries, 'compensation' for organ donors or their families has been proposed. Suggestions have included contributions towards funeral costs, tax benefits, reimbursement of some medical expenses, and paid leave for living donors, which already exits under a Commonwealth Government program in Australia.[9] Pilot projects along these lines have previously been rejected by Congress in the United States. However, while opponents of such schemes voice slippery-slope concerns, proponents point out that donors are the only active participants in the transplantation process who are *not* compensated financially and should, at the very least, not suffer financial disadvantage as a result of their altruism.

19.7 Ante-mortem Interventions (A-MI)

DCD donation is technically more problematic than organ donation after brain death. This is because the relatively prolonged DCD process exposes transplantable organs to substantial periods of hypoxia and ischaemia, while ventilation and circulation are maintained in brain dead donors until the last possible moment. This limits the availability and quality of donated organs, and there is a higher incidence of delayed graft function in DCD recipients.

In recent years, there has been growing pressure from transplanters for various activities to be undertaken in potential DCD donors before death is declared. These include relatively benign interventions such as the administration of antibiotics, anticoagulants, and vasoactive drugs, but also may include more invasive activities such as femoral cannulation to permit the infusion of organ-preserving solutions immediately after death is declared, and coronary angiography to check suitability for cardiac transplantation. In many jurisdictions, legislative change would be required to permit A-MI.

These interventions are also ethically problematic because they potentially contradict the Kantian injunction against using people as a means to an end.[9] They are carried out without the potential donor's consent, and they primarily serve the interests of organ recipients rather than those of the potential donor. Substitute decision-makers cannot legally consent to these activities because they are also constrained to consent only to those actions that directly serve the donor's best interests.

Supporters of A-MI argue that the fact that the patient wished to be a donor indicates a legitimate interest in providing organs in the best possible condition and, by implication, an interest in accepting the interventions.

This argument assumes that all organ donors actively wished to donate. In fact, most donors express no particular view in their lifetime, but their families agree to donation as a gift or sacrifice, sometimes in response to varying levels of persuasion. As a result, some ethicists argue that A-MI should only be permissible in those who have registered their willingness to donate during their lifetime. Others insist that even in these cases, specific consent to A-MI should be required. As a result, specific consent for A-MI is increasingly being incorporated into organ donation registration websites and forms, and also appears in some pro-forma advance care directives.

19.8 Conflicts of Interest

Potential conflicts of interest and how these should be dealt with have received relatively little attention in the organ donation and transplantation literature.[9] In the current ethical practice guidelines for organ donation produced by the National Health and Medical Research Council in Australia, the only discussion of conflict of interest is in relation to commercial tissue banks, while the Australian & New Zealand Intensive Care Society's guidelines mention it only briefly.[14] Despite this, there are numerous potential conflicts for those clinicians involved in the end-of-life care, procurement, and selection of organ donors.

It is widely accepted that clinicians who have an active role in transplant procedures or organ allocation should not be involved in the donation process, especially the diagnosis of death and end-of-life care. Ideally the various clinical roles in transplantation and organ donation would be entirely separate, but this is not always possible, especially in hospitals where organ donation and transplantation take place side by side.

In this setting, intensivists, nurses, and others may be involved in the care of potential and actual donors, recipients, and those awaiting transplantation, sometimes simultaneously. This may give rise to real or perceived pressure to identify and recruit potential organ donors or to expedite end-of life care.

The advent of ante-mortem interventions (see above) creates further conflicts for intensivists, who must try to balance the interests of the dying patient and their family – which should always be the first priority – with those of potential organ recipients and the demands of transplanters. Designated organ donation physicians (most often intensivists) and donor coordinator nurses perhaps face the greatest ethical conflicts. They typically view their job as the facilitation of good decision-making through the provision of accurate information to families, and the provision of optimal end-of-life care for donors. However, they are directly or indirectly answerable to and sometimes paid by the transplant sector, which envisages their primary function as the maximisation of organ donation and the delivery of organs to transplanters in optimal condition. They may also have targets or key performance indicators that emphasise this and may be required to undergo specific training in how to request organs successfully.

19.9 Organ Donation and Euthanasia

While the legalisation of euthanasia and physician-assisted suicide provide no direct ethical conflict with organ donation, there are ethical questions about how the process should be undertaken. Currently, all jurisdictions require a form of DCD, in which, after euthanasia or suicide is carried out, a period of asystole and apnoea is mandated, in order to allow the dead donor rule to be fulfilled, before organ harvesting can commence. However, it has been proposed that in such cases there is no rational objection to death occurring as the direct result of organ removal, and that this would provide more organs, in better condition. There is also some evidence to suggest that a substantial proportion of the general public would support this view.

19.10 Future Directions

In the longer term, it is likely that transplantation will decline as in vitro techniques, artificial organs, and other, as yet unforeseen, technologies emerge. Meanwhile, it seems almost certain that the demand for transplantable organs will continue to outstrip supply. The pressure for innovative ways to expand the donor pool will inevitably involve ethical challenges.

While the DDR as a fundamental principle underpins organ donation, it provides an incentive to stretch the conceptual boundaries of our understanding of death. Brain death and, more particularly, DCD are examples of this, challenging not only social and biological ideas about death but also the legal definitions that apply. Legislative changes to the definitions of death have also been debated – for example, a change from 'irreversible' to 'permanent'. This would potentially have the effect of changing the legal concept of death as a biological fact to a matter of medical choice about whether to resuscitate or not.

DCD is becoming more ethically problematic as technology evolves. Cardiac transplantation, once excluded from DCD, is now regularly performed, with acceptable results, making the claim of circulatory death of the donor harder to justify. More recently, some centres have begun using extracorporeal membrane oxygenation (ECMO) to restore the circulation in DCD donors immediately after death has been declared. Various techniques can be used to ensure no restoration of blood flow to the brain occurs.

The newest idea for foiling the DDR is the Morrissey proposal, which has not yet been widely implemented.[15] Under this proposal, a patient in whom death within a few days is considered inevitable, but who has normal renal function, undergoes bilateral nephrectomy for donation (with appropriate consent), after which they are returned to the ICU for palliative care. Morrissey argues that since death from uraemia or electrolyte imbalance would take many days to develop, the patient will die from their underlying disease and its palliation, rather than as a direct result of the nephrectomies. In this way, the removal of vital organs has not resulted in death, and the intent of the DDR is not breached.

19.11 Conclusion

What then, have developments in neurosciences, intensive care, and transplantation taught us about death, dying, and brain death since the Harvard Ad-Hoc Committee (1968), President's Commission (1981), and President's Council on Bioethics (2008) statements on brain death?

- Brain death does not cause irreversible progression to cardio-circulatory death.
- With intensive support – particularly neuroendocrine support – it is now apparent that patients declared brain dead may be maintained for months to years (and in some cases may even gestate a pregnancy). Prominent cases, such as Jahi McMath, have provided clear and well-publicised examples where patients who satisfy brain death criteria may 'survive' for considerable periods of time. It is indisputable, however, that patients who satisfy brain death criteria never recover. In other words, it is an excellent marker of prognosis.
- Brain death does not consistently imply loss of physiological integration (e.g., < 50% of those who are brain dead have diabetes insipidus, and some young patients declared brain dead may enter puberty and begin to menstruate).
- Brain death does not imply death of the entire/whole brain – but a part of it.
- Death is a process not a single event – not biologically, not culturally, not socially, and not practically. This means both that the law may act to impose arbitrary boundaries between different states of dying and that at different points during this process, different obligations may be owed to the person.
- Death is also relevant to the tissue or organ in question, and the death of different tissues and organs may allow or require different medical, legal, or sociocultural responses – for example, dead foot (amputate foot), dead bone marrow (perform a transplant), dead tissue (excise or allow repair), and DCD (organ donation).
- A diagnosis of brain death does not, of itself, imply other forms of death or allow other practices (e.g., burial, reading of wills, insurance claims, cremation, donation of bodies for education). Rather, it enables only two things: organ donation or withdrawal of intensive care support to allow cardiocirculatory death to occur.
- It is only when the entire person is dead that disposal of the body (cremation, burial, or preservation in formalin for educational purposes) and burial rites proceed (which is true in all cultures and faith traditions). (None of which would be acceptable in a patient declared brain dead).
- It is not correct to equate brain death and cardio-circulatory death from a sociocultural perspective. Even though it is argued that these states are equivalent from a physiological or clinical perspective, there are many things that we do not do and would not tolerate in patients who are brain dead. For example, we would not cremate or bury a brain dead patient, and we would not perform a post-mortem on them – rather, we would wait until permanent cardio-circulatory standstill (i.e., we would wait for them to become cardio-circulatory dead). (And this is not simply a matter of the size or expense of ventilators, as even if a ventilator was worth $1, was the size of a coin, and could be implanted under the skin, we would still insist on the patient satisfying cardio-circulatory death before we buried them, cremated them, or used their body for educational or scientific purposes.)
- Points of the diagnosis of death are a function of necessity as well as biology and clinical context (i.e., the points of diagnosis of death have moved, in part, because of concerns to improve organ viability).

- Brain death criteria/testing is only *required* (and tested for) where organ donation is a possibility (i.e., brain death is inextricably linked to organ donation, both historically and clinically). (It is also true, however, that brain death testing may be done at other times – for example, where there is conflict regarding the appropriateness of continuing support for a person in the ICU in order to establish more clearly what is owed to the patient.)
- Different cultural groups, different families, and different individuals interpret death differently.
- There is ample empirical research demonstrating that many donor families do not believe that their loved one was not 'truly' dead until their heart permanently stopped but that this realisation would not have changed their decision to authorise organ donation (i.e., people appear willing to allow/support organ donation, even if they are sceptical about the notion that their loved one is 'truly dead' when they satisfy brain death criteria).
- Developments in brain science (e.g., neurogenesis and neuroplasticity) provide the possibility of brain repair and regeneration.

As a result of these insights, a small but growing number of clinicians, intensivists, and ethicists support the idea of abandoning the DDR. They suggest that organ donation in the context of the dying patient can be ethically justified, with appropriate regulatory safeguards and proper consent, without the prior requirement to establish that death has occurred. In this way, the potential organ pool could be expanded, and our conception of death as a truly irreversible biological state could remain intact. While it is unlikely that such proposals will find widespread support – at least in the short term – they remind us that death is not simply a medical phenomenon but a philosophical and sociocultural one, and they point to the need for further discussion and debate about what death means and how it may be shaped by political imperatives and transformed by science and technology.

References

1. A definition of irreversible coma. Report of the ad hoc committee of the Harvard Medical School to examine the definition of brain death. *JAMA* 1968; **205**: 337–40.

2. Diagnosis of brain death. Statement issued by the honorary secretary of the Conference of Medical Royal Colleges and their faculties in the United Kingdom on 11 October 1976. *BMJ* 1976; **2**: 1187–8.

3. AMA Judicial Council. Ethical guidelines for organ transplantation. *JAMA* 1968; **205**: 341–2.

4. National Health & Medical Research Foundation. Ethical guidelines for the care of people in post-coma unresponsiveness (vegetative state) or a minimally responsive state. Australian Government Publication, 2008. Available at: www.nhmrc.gov.au/abo ut-us/publications/ethical-guidelines-care-people-post-coma-unresponsiveness.

5. Truog R. D., Miller F. G. Brain death: justifications and critiques. *Clin. Ethics* 2012; 7: 128–32

6. Controversies in the determination of death: a white paper of the President's Council on Bioethics. 2008. Available at: http://bioethics .georgetown.edu/pcbe/reports/death/index .html.

7. Miller F. G., Truog R. D., Brock D. W. The DDR: Can it withstand critical scrutiny? *J. Med. Philos.* 2010; **35**: 299–312.

8. Truog R. D. Lessons from the case of Jahi McMath. Defining death; organ transplantation and the fifty-year legacy of the Harvard Report on Brain Death, special report. *Hastings Cent. Rep.* 2018; **48**: S70–3.

9. Australian Government, National Health and Medical Research Foundation. Organ and tissue donation after death, for transplantation. Guidelines for ethical practice for health professionals. 2007.

Available at: www.nhmrc.gov.au/_files_nh
mrc/publications/attachments/e75.pdf.

10. Abouma G. M. *Recent Pronouncements by
Two Major Religions on Organ
Transplantation: Current status of Clinical
Organ Transplantation*. The Hague,
Nijhoff, 1984, xi–xii.

11. Dodek P. Mandatory reporting of
'imminent' death to identify organ donors:
history, controversy, and potential
solutions. *Can. J. Anesth.* 2003; 50: 955–60.

12. Australian Government, Department of
Health. Supporting Living Organ Donors
Program. 2018. Available at: www
.health.gov.au/internet/main/publishing
.nsf/Content/Leave-for-living-organ-
donors.

13. Brown S. J. Autonomy, trust and
ante-mortem interventions to facilitate
organ donation. *Clin. Ethics* 2018; 13:
143–50.

14. Australian and New Zealand Intensive
Care Society. The ANZICS Statement on
Death and Organ Donation (Edition 3.2).
Melbourne, ANZICS, 2013. Available at:
https://csds.qld.edu.au/sdc/Provectus/ELI/
Module%202%20-%20Organ%20donation
%20after%20brain%20death/files/ANZICS
%20Statement%20on%20%20Death%20an
d%20Organ%20Donation%20Edition%20
3.2%20(3).pdf.

15. Morrissey P. E. The case for kidney
donation before end-of-life care. *Am.
J. Bioeth.* 2012; 12: 1–8.

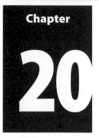

Ethical Aspects of Innovation in Neurosurgery

Mario Ammirati, Jeffrey V. Rosenfeld, Alexander Hulsbergen, and Marike Broekman

---

Key Points

Innovation in Neurosurgery

Innovations are fundamental to the continuous improvement of neurosurgery.

Neurosurgeons sponsors of innovations are by nature prone to overoptimistic assessment of their innovation.

This overoptimistic assessment is even more significant when there is potential for economic gains, enhancement of academic reputation, and an increase in patient referrals.

Institutional evaluation of the proposed innovation (IEB/IRB) and its responsiveness to a real clinical problem is important in order to exclude pseudo-innovations and put the proposed innovation on a robust footing.

Structured approaches like the IDEAL Framework could aid ethical introduction of novel procedures and/or devices in neurosurgery.

Detailed informed consent is required for any innovative procedure and should include disclosure of any conflicts of interest.

External outside (beyond the surgeon's institution) outcome evaluation of the innovative procedure strengthens ethical outcome reports.

At some point, the innovation process should be evaluated to confirm the proposed advantages of the innovation through RCT or equivalent trials so that the innovation may become the new standard of care or be discarded.

20.1 Introduction

Innovation is inherent in neurosurgery. Since its origins in the early twentieth century, the specialty has enjoyed a continuous tradition where clinical care and medical or technical innovation go hand in hand. The traditional twist drill and hand saw have been automated in most settings. Bipolar cautery devices are as much a staple of surgical equipment as tweezers or lancets. Surgical navigation has progressed from intraoperative ultrasound to sophisticated CT and MRI guidance. New technological adjuncts such as endoscopes and, more recently, exoscopes are continuously being proposed to surgeons as worthwhile innovations that are in turn marketed to patients as 'must-have tools' during their surgery. Indeed, neurosurgery would not be the state-of-the-art discipline it is today without innovation.

But what exactly constitutes innovation in neurosurgery? In the broadest sense, surgical innovation could refer to any procedure, device, or technique that is not standard of care. In neurosurgery, this encompasses a very large part of practice. Given the context-dependent (lack of) feasibility of randomized controlled trials (RCTs) in surgery,[1] the small sample sizes inherent to many neurosurgical diseases, and the rapid advance of medical technology, it is not surprising that most technical surgical improvements come from innovation rather than formalized research. However, this definition encompasses a very broad and unclearly delineated spectrum that leaves room for interpretation. On one end of this spectrum, one could find the use of a new type of suture that few would consider a significant deviation from standard practice. On the other end, there are procedures that are completely novel – for example, intratumoral delivery of an oncolytic herpes simplex virus for recurrent glioblastoma. Many cases in between these extremes are less obvious. For example, the use of pedicle screws in degenerative instrumented spinal fusion was embraced with relatively limited scrutiny; however, the benefits to patients can be questionable, and the impact of their use on healthcare costs has been considerable. Other examples include dural substitutes not previously tested in humans, the deployment of novel endovascular devices, and the application of deep brain stimulation for nonstandard indications for the use of thulium lasers in meningioma treatment.[2]

In short, while most would have an idea of what constitutes innovation in the broadest sense, there is no consensus on a precise definition. One important aspect to note, however, is that in contrast to research, the goal of innovation is often not to create generalizable knowledge but to improve individual patient care. An example is the recent case of a patient suffering from elevated intracranial pressure due to the rare Van Buchem disease leading to a thickening of the skull, who received cranioplasty of a complete 3D-printed cranium. Often, these personal adaptations will lead to generalizable knowledge in the longer term.[3]

This chapter will address the various ethical aspects of neurosurgical innovation, including those related to oversight, informed consent, vulnerable patient populations, conflicts of interest, the surgical learning curve, and the introduction of novel devices in surgery. Lastly, we will suggest directions for the future of innovation in neurosurgery.

20.2 Oversight

Because it is hard to pinpoint which adaptations are truly innovative, there has traditionally been little oversight for neurosurgical innovation. In contrast to the development of new drugs, the introduction of surgical innovation traditionally does not require Institutional Review Board (IRB) approval. In practice, this means that novel techniques have often been introduced into the scientific realm (and the associated IRB and peer-review oversight) after implementation in the clinical setting (i.e., through single-centre retrospective case series of complication rates).

Some would argue that innovation does not benefit from oversight and that the individual surgeon's discretion is sufficient to ensure ethical standards are upheld around innovative practices. Moreover, some features unique to surgery, such as the variability between surgeon's skills, patients' anatomical variation, or the difficulty of measuring and precisely reproducing surgical techniques, would make it almost impossible to subject all surgical innovation to oversight. This philosophy is usually referred to as *surgical exceptionalism*. While this approach maintains the surgeon's autonomy and encourages innovation, it may amplify the surgeon's biases and conflicts of interest. Moreover, it assumes rigorous ethical training, which is usually not incorporated into medical curricula or surgical residency. On the other hand, formal IRB oversight may not be ideal in all cases either. The process is time-intensive, which may hinder patient care. In addition, applications are usually assessed by people who are far removed from the patient and may not have relevant knowledge of the surgical intricacies of a particular innovation. Alternatives to surgical exceptionalism or IRB approval would be departmental, institutional, regional, or national oversight. Each of these comes with a set of benefits and drawbacks.[4]

Based on the degree of deviation from standard practice, different levels of oversight may therefore be appropriate.

- For small deviations, such as the use of new materials in otherwise standard procedures, surgical exceptionalism may suffice; additional oversight could make any minor adaptation unnecessarily burdensome.
- Some innovations have significant scientific ethical considerations but no human ethical risks. For example, say there is limited knowledge on the long-term risk-benefit ratio of a procedure but this is properly discussed with the patient, who is able to give informed consent. In this case, departmental oversight would be appropriate.
- Innovation in which there may be human ethical risks should have oversight managed through institutional ethics committees. These risks may emerge in the case of vulnerable patient populations, patients who may not be able to give fully informed consent, or potential conflicts of interest of the department or treating surgeon. Institutional ethics committees are multidisciplinary teams including physicians, ethicists, lawyers, and lay community members who are able to carefully assess the human risks and benefits of a situation, with special consideration for the medical ethical principle of justice. Many paediatric innovations would fall into this oversight category.
- Innovation in which there is an institutional conflict of interest would require centralized oversight (i.e., on a regional or national level). For example, consider the deployment of a novel endovascular device developed by a company with financial ties to the hospital. It must be acknowledged that individual institutions may be reluctant to cede to centralized oversight because it may be viewed as a loss of authority and independence; however, the institution carries legal responsibility in addition to the individual practitioner for procedures or new therapies carried out in the individual facility. IRB approval should be obtained if the primary goal of the innovation is obtaining new, generalizable knowledge or if there are major risks to patients, as is the case with any neurosurgical procedure. Many proposed innovations such as supra-total removal of low grade gliomas, oncolytic viruses therapy, or novel indications for functional neurosurgery are examples that fit this category.[4]
- A further check and balance that operates in some institutions is the Research Review Committee, which is a subcommittee of the Institutional Human Research Ethics Committee. The remit of this committee is to assess the innovative technology or new surgical procedures in detail and report back to the HREC. This committee is not concerned with minor variations on current practice. There are written and oral presentations from the practitioners, and the committee focusses on safety, cost, risk/benefit ratio, and the experience and credentialing of the practitioners. It recommends whether the practitioners require mentoring by a surgeon experienced in the procedure when they are doing the first few cases. Observing the procedure in another hospital or

attending a short cadaver or simulation course conducted by the manufacturer or by another institution may not be considered by the committee to be adequate preparation.

- Emergent cases form a special category that cannot be subjected to formal oversight. While these situations will vary on a case-by-case basis, post-hoc departmental oversight, including tracking and transparent discussion of outcomes, may be appropriate in cases where surgical exceptionalism does not suffice.[4]

Despite claims by some that ethical oversight only holds progress back, it may in fact empower innovation. A robust ethical framework has the potential to give neurosurgeons the ethical and medicolegal backing they need to keep innovating. The key driver of the ethical oversight is patient safety and well-being. Ethical oversight cannot be disjoined from the goal of providing 'generalizable knowledge' through IRB and proper design, at the appropriate stage of the innovation process, of clinical trials. The goal should be that of placing the 'generalizable knowledge' on robust grounds so that it can be available to all patients and become the new standard of care.

20.3 Conflicts of Interest

As in any specialty, conflicts of interest (COIs) play a role in neurosurgical research and innovation. These conflicts can be financial or non-financial. While financial COIs are generally subject to oversight and disclosure regulations, non-financial COIs are usually less overt and may not always be recognized as such. Examples of non-financial COIs of neurosurgeons include the incentive to publish papers or otherwise advance one's career, a strong personal belief or enthusiasm in a new procedure, or a desire to increase status among peers. Moreover, surgeons may often have a bias that favours operative treatment over a non-surgical alternative. On an institutional level, COIs may emerge from a hospital's desire to market novel or high-tech treatment options, such as Gamma Knife or intraoperative MRI technology.[5]

The medical device industry works closely with neurosurgeons, and this is usually a fruitful endeavour, as many innovations result from cooperation between surgeon and manufacturers. In fact, physicians are credited with inventing 20% of medical device patents.[5] Moreover, the industry enjoys consultancy from expert neurosurgeons. This co-dependency results in technological progress but can also create COIs in several ways. First, many neurosurgeons may have financial COIs through consultancy fees, stock, patents, or other financial gains from industry partnerships. Second, surgeons may be biased towards technologies or innovations that they themselves have contributed. Third, the device industry maintains a presence at conferences, provides guidance in operating rooms, and maintains cordial ties with physicians on an individual level, in addition to marketing their devices through courses. This may create goodwill that could bias physicians towards a certain manufacturer. Conflicts of interest, especially when non-financial, can be non-intentional or even subconscious, and a thorough reflection on potential conflicts is part of the critical attitude required for ethical practice.

The influence of the medical industry on shaping innovations cannot be underestimated; however, the primary goals of the industry are financial and not necessarily that of protecting patients. An example is represented by the widespread push for endoscopic surgery carried out by major endoscopic manufacturers who have, over the years, sponsored courses and used other marketing tools in a successful bid to create and expand a market for their products. However, evidence demonstrating the superiority of endoscopic versus non endoscopic surgery is limited, and large data evaluation points to endoscopic surgery being more costly and associated with more complications than non-endoscopic surgery.[6] There is also the more ominous issue of the often unreported complications associated with the steep learning curve required for these procedures, especially those of an isolated neurosurgeon practicing in a small setting.

This is another cogent reason why external evaluation of certain innovations should be carried out and individual performance and complication rates closely monitored.

When discussing innovative treatments with patients, financial and non-financial COIs on the individual and institutional level should be disclosed. However, it may be hard for patients to fully understand the severity of COIs and their implications for decision-making. Patients, too, may be subject to biases; for example, they may believe that novel is necessarily better or that trials should be expected to yield benefit for all involved patients. Patients who have a terminal condition may feel inclined to accept any innovative treatment no matter the risk, because they feel they have nothing to lose. Neurosurgeons have an ethical responsibility to honestly and openly discuss COIs with patients to ensure the best possible understanding.

In scientific reporting of innovation, COIs should be transparently disclosed. While most journals require financial and nonfinancial COI disclosure, reporting may be selective and inconsistent across journals. In addition, peer reviewers and editors should be subject to the same COI scrutiny as are those who submit research. Working towards a robust system of COI reporting should therefore be a specialty-wide priority. If a conflict of interest could hinder the objectivity or generalizability of reported outcomes of an innovation, one solution could be involving multiple neurosurgeons when performing a technique or implanting a device for the first time.[5] Presentations at scientific conferences should also include commercial disclosures.

To avoid conscious or unconscious bias, the post-operative assessment of patients who are part of a clinical trial of a new technology or innovation should be conducted by practitioners, independent of the neurosurgeon who did the surgery.

It has been suggested that 'declaration of interest' rather than COI would be a more accurate term for a mandatory and transparent disclosure of financial arrangements.[7] Working with industry is not necessarily a conflict or nefarious endeavour, but certainly financial arrangements should be disclosed, and one should have a clear understanding regarding the main stakeholders to whom the two parties are accountable: patients for the neurosurgeons and owners and shareholders for the industry.

20.4 Introducing New Surgical Devices

The introduction of surgical devices, as opposed to drugs, is relatively loosely regulated. In the United States, the Food and Drug Administration (FDA) distinguishes three classes of devices. Class I consists of non-invasive devices such as operative instruments. Class II includes surgical meshes, prostheses, or absorbable sutures. Class III devices generate or modulate biological signals (e.g., spinal stimulators or cochlear implants). Only Class III devices must provide pre-market-approval studies demonstrating safety and efficacy, but these studies are not necessarily RCTs that test a device against the golden standard. While the FDA can demand post-marketing studies, a device can only be retracted for lack of safety, not for lack of efficacy. In Europe, the Conformité Européene (CE) oversees device marketing. CE marketing is less rigorous than FDA marketing, as safety and efficacy studies are not always needed, even for Class III devices. Moreover, approval is decentralized and there is regional variance in strictness. As a result, manufacturers may approach a less strict approval authority to obtain CE certification for the entire European market.[8]

This system of introduction comes with some ethical risks. The FDA/CE approval process creates loopholes to introduce devices with an unknown risk/benefit ratio to the market. In Europe, this includes even Class III devices. Moreover, the discrepancy in strictness of regulation could incentivize device manufacturers to initially introduce new technology into the European market. This could result in innovative treatments being available in Europe before they are in the United States. On the one hand, this may give European patients earlier access to innovative treatment, potentially improving outcomes. On the other, Europeans may also be more exposed to the risks of unproven and potentially harmful devices. Both of these factors violate the medical ethical principle of justice. Lastly, as RCTs are not required for market approval, there is a responsibility in the medical community to conduct high-quality post-marketing research. Studies should compare novel devices to the golden standard and focus on long-term follow-up. Moreover, cost-benefit analyses are essential to assess whether the efficacy of new devices weighs up to the costs that are usually associated with them.

When discussing surgery involving innovative devices with patients, neurosurgeons should be aware of a number of factors. First, formal market approval of a device is not equivalent to proven efficacy, especially in Europe. Second, risk/benefit ratios may be unknown or hard to estimate, especially when RCTs are of poor quality or non-existent. Third, off-label use may come with unknown risk-benefit ratios, even if the off-label procedure is similar to the procedure for which the device was approved. Surgeons have the ethical responsibility to discuss the innovative nature and risk/benefit ratio of novel devices with patients, even when this is not legally required because of FDA/CE approval.[8]

20.5 Learning Curve

Adapting new operative techniques can be technically challenging, especially if they deviate significantly from standard procedures. While patient risks associated with this learning curve are inevitable at the very earliest stages of any innovation, it is important that the adaptation of new techniques across the neurosurgical specialty happens as safely as possible. The surgeon's learning curve can be stimulated by hands-on training (in cadavers or animal models), visiting workshops, and assisting surgeons who are already performing the novel procedure and being mentored by one or more experienced surgeons. While the ideal learning process will vary by procedure, experiences and outcomes should be shared with peers in all cases. Lastly, it may be beneficial to introduce an accreditation system for innovation. This may ensure that only sufficiently trained surgeons perform a new procedure, and it would allow outcomes to be systematically tracked.[3] The current trend of attending a course, often sponsored by the industry, and then becoming certified in a new procedure should be stigmatized as practically and ethically inadequate.

20.6 Informed Consent and the Vulnerable Patient

Informed consent has been a central *conditio sine qua non* (indispensable action) in medical research since the Nuremburg trials. In the context of neurosurgical innovation, it is essential that the surgeon discusses the novelty of a procedure, as well as the perceived risk/benefit ratio, knowledge (or lack thereof) of long-term outcomes, the surgeon's experience, potential conflicts of interest, the role of novel devices, and alternatives to the innovative procedure.

Due to the complexity of some novel procedures and the uncertainty of some risk/benefit ratios, informed consent procedures for innovative treatment warrant more time investment than standard preoperative discussions. It may be beneficial to have a third-party communicator present in the clinic. For example, when the neurosurgeon is also the researcher, this could be an independent physician or nurse who helps the patient understand the advantages and disadvantages of a procedure. Furthermore, multimedia presentations may help in improving understanding.

Within neurosurgery, several patient populations are especially vulnerable, and this should be taken into account when obtaining informed consent. Examples of vulnerable patient populations include paediatric patients, patients with a need for emergent surgery, patients with impaired cognitive functions, and patients with refractory disease. In children and patients whose cognitive abilities are impaired – for example, due to hydrocephalus, additional consent should be sought from relatives or caretakers. Patients with refractory disease, such as recurrent glioblastoma, may feel desperate and willing to accept any innovative treatment regardless of risk. In this case, 'informed consent' cannot be used as a permit to test any innovation no matter the expected risk/benefit ratio. In emergency cases, it may sometimes be impossible to obtain informed consent at all. In order to have innovation in traumatology at all, it may be inevitable to perform innovation without immediate informed consent. These innovations should always be subject to departmental oversight and post-procedure transparency regarding outcomes and follow-up.[3] Deferred consent may be applied in these cases by a HREC. Either the patient or their next of kin consents as soon as it is feasible to do so. This is often the case with innovative prehospital procedures. The POLAR study was an RCT that investigated efficacy of prophylactic hypothermia in severe traumatic brain injury. The innovation here was that the paramedics commenced hypothermia treatment in the ambulance prior to the patient arriving in the emergency room.[9]

Finally, it is important that patients should not have to pay for their treatment if they are part of a first-in-human study of a new innovation. Their long-term follow-up should also be included in the cost design for the study.

20.7 Future Directions

At the moment, innovations are introduced in neurosurgery in a rather unstructured way, with new procedures and devices being continuously proposed and introduced with little or no oversight and without any clear evidence that they benefit patients. When innovative procedures are marketed as 'minimally invasive' or 'no scar' surgery, they generate a demand in the public for that particular procedure obviously co-opting the practicing neurosurgeon to offer it to maintain their referral base and livelihood. This creates a vicious cycle not dissimilar from that used in marketing any non-medical product or service.

There is no doubt that innovation will continue to play a central role in the advancement of neurosurgery; however, it is important to ensure that this happens within a robust ethical framework in order to protect patients, stimulate or empower innovators, and ensure that the knowledge generated through innovations is generalizable. In this chapter, the most important aspects of such a framework have been outlined.

The question remains as to the future direction of neurosurgical innovation. A key aspect of ethical practice is continuous evaluation. For this purpose, the IDEAL (idea, development, exploration, assessment, long-term follow-up) system has been proposed. This evaluation distinguishes different phases of innovation with corresponding levels of oversight, sample sizes of patient populations, and methodologies of evaluation. Although this framework is not yet always followed when introducing new neurosurgical procedures or devices, it has the potential to be a future tool to guide innovation.[10]

An important element of the IDEAL concept is that the proposed innovation should answer a cogent clinical problem. Lastly, continuous and systematic analysis of surgical strategies and outcomes should be the norm rather than the exception. In an ideal health-care system, data from every patient's treatment would be recorded and contribute to new knowledge that can be applied to the next generation of patients. New advances in large-scale data storage and analysis may be able to facilitate these long-term goals.

Ultimately, individual surgeons play the central role in neurosurgical innovation. They have the ethical obligation to innovate sensibly, and developing and following sound ethical frameworks can give them the tools to do so, ultimately improving patient outcomes and advancing the field of neurosurgery.

20.8 Conclusions

Innovations are fundamental to the continuous improvement of neurosurgery. However, neurosurgical innovators are, by nature, prone to make overly optimistic assessments of their innovation, new product, or technique. This assessment is likely to be even more significant when the potential exists for economic gains and enhancement of academic reputational. Institutional evaluation of the proposed innovation and its responsiveness to a real clinical problem is important in order to establish clinical efficacy, and external evaluations of the outcome strengthen the surgeon's ethical position.

Funding: National Institutes of Health (NIH) T32 CA009001 (DJC).

References

1. Martin E., Muskens I. S., Senders J. T., et al. Randomized controlled trials comparing surgery to non-operative management in neurosurgery: a systematic review. *Acta Neurochir (Wien)* 2019; **161**: 627–34.

2. Zaki M. M., Cote D. J., Muskens I. S., et al. Defining innovation in neurosurgery: results from an international survey. *World Neurosurg.* 2018; **114**: e1038–48.

3. Broekman M. L., Carriere M. E., Bredenoord A. L. Surgical innovation: the ethical agenda: a systematic review. *Medicine (Baltimore).* 2016; **95**: e3790.

4. Gupta S., Muskens I. S., Fandino L. B. et al. Oversight in surgical innovation: a response to ethical challenges. *World J. Surg.* 2018; **42**: 2773–80.

5. DiRisio A. C., Muskens I. S., Cote D. J., et al. Oversight and ethical regulation of conflicts of interest in neurosurgery in the United States. *Neurosurgery* 2019; **84**: 305–12.

6. Ammirati M., Lai W., Ciric I. Short term outcome of endoscopic versus microscopic pituitary adenoma surgery. A systematic review and meta-analysis. *J. Neurol. Neurosurg. Psychiatry* 2013; **84**: 843–49.

7. Bernards R. When a conflict of interest is not a conflict. *Nature* 2019; **568**: 458.

8. Muskens I. S., Gupta S., Hulsbergen A., et al. Introduction of novel medical devices in surgery: ethical challenges of current oversight and regulation. *J. Am. Coll. Surg.* 2017; **225**: 558–65.

9. Cooper D. J., Nichol A. D., Bailey M., et al. POLAR trial investigators and the ANZICS clinical trials group. Effect of early sustained

prophylactic hypothermia on neurologic outcomes among patients with severe traumatic brain injury: the POLAR randomized clinical trial. *JAMA* 2018; **320**: 2211–20.

10. Muskens I. S., Diederen S. J. H., Senders J. T., et al. Innovation in neurosurgery: less than IDEAL? A systematic review. *Acta Neurochir (Wien)* 2017; **159**: 1957–66.

Chapter 2

Stem Cells and Brain Repair: Ethical Considerations

Ivar Mendez

21.1 Introduction

The rapid advance of research in stem cells has opened the door for their potential use in cell-based therapies to treat neurological conditions, some of which are currently incurable. Encouraging studies in animal models are moving into early phase clinical trials that hold realistic promise for the future. However, important ethical challenges remain as stem cells are translated from preclinical research to the clinical realm.

Stem cells have captured the imagination of the public and the media, and have generated substantial expectations for patients and their families. The legitimate needs and hopes of individuals suffering from devastating neurological diseases have, in some cases, been exploited by the administration of commercially available unproven 'stem cell' interventions.

As the field advances and clinical trials in stem cell therapies are conducted for neurological conditions, neurosurgeons will become key members of stem cell research teams. Accurate and safe delivery of stem cells to brain and spinal cord targets will require neurosurgical procedures. The neurosurgeon's roles will expand as stem cells move from clinical trials to effective potential therapies in the future. This chapter will review selected stem cell ethical issues that may inform and guide the practicing neurosurgeon in a rapidly moving field of great scientific promise as well as ethical challenges.

21.1.1 Stem Cells

Stem cells are cells that have the unique capacity of self-renewal, which is the ability to undergo multiple divisions while maintaining an undifferentiated state. Stem cells also have the ability to differentiate into different cell lineages.[1] They can be classified in embryonic stem cells and non-embryonic stem cells – the latter are also called adult or somatic stem cells.

Embryonic stem cells (ESCs) can self-renew and be differentiated into all embryonic germ layers. The first human embryonic stem cells (hESCs) were isolated from the late blastocyst of human embryos produced by in vitro fertilization (IVF).[2] These cells are also called *pluripotent*, as they have an extraordinary capacity to differentiate into many cell lineages and are responsible in the adult organism for tissue growth, repair, and maintenance. The ability of hESCs to maintain their undifferentiated state during cell division and to be directed into any cell lineage of the body make them ideal candidates for cell-based therapies. However, ethical and moral considerations on their origin and methods of isolation have made their use controversial and influenced their translation to clinical applications.

Non-embryonic stem cells are undifferentiated cells that are also referred to as adult/somatic stem cells, as they are found in post-natal tissues. These cells have a limited ability of self-renew and differentiate preferentially to committed lineages dictated by their tissue of origin.[3] They are often referred to according to their tissue source – that is, bone marrow stem cells (BMSCs) or hematopoietic stem cells (HSCs). Clinical applications of HSCs for the treatment of certain cancers of the blood or bone marrow, such as multiple myeloma or leukaemia, have being going on for years, and thousands of patients have been treated. Other promising clinical applications of these adult/somatic stem cells are in skin grafts and corneal regeneration.

In 2006 the exciting discovery of induced pluripotential stem cells (iPSCs), created a pathway that may avoid the ethical issues and moral conflicts related to the clinical applications of hESCs.[4] These cells are generated by the 'reprograming' of somatic cells such as fibroblasts into cells that have the capacity for self-renewal and differentiate into multiple phenotypic lineages. They also hold great therapeutic promise, as they can be produced in unlimited quantities, under controlled standardized conditions, without the ethical and moral limitations of hESCs. Furthermore, iPSCs can generate autologous cell-restorative strategies because they can be produced from donor cells, from the same individual receiving the cell-therapy. Autologous cell therapies may decrease the possibility of immune rejection or transmission of external pathogens and open the possibility of creating 'personalized cell lines' for central nervous system (CNS) repair.

Although iPSCs hold great promise for clinical translation, several issues related to the reprograming techniques need to be resolved before they can be used in clinical practice. Introduction of viral vectors to the host genome for reprograming could produce interference with gene transcription, causing mutagenesis, genome instability, or malignant transformation. Several reprograming techniques that do not use viral vectors are currently being developed to avoid these issues.

21.1.2 Stem Cell Ethics

Regenerative medicine is one of the most promising and rapidly moving fields of biomedical research. The public expectation for the development of treatments and cures using stem cells is enormous. Although general principles of bioethical research must be applied to stem cell research, a wide range of ethical issues particular to stem cells and their translation to the clinical arena must be considered.

The use of stem cells derived from human embryos or hESCs is a topic of strong ethical debate and controversy. The reprograming techniques used to generate iPSCs and their potential effects on the human genome, as well as the possibility of tumorgenicity, raise ethical issues that need to be considered when contemplating their clinical application. Recent advances in gene-editing technology, mitochondrial transfer, and human-animal generation of chimeras raise serious ethical concerns.

Complex informed consent issues are present in stem cell research, as informed consent is not only focused on recipients of stem cell–based therapies but also on the donors of cellular products for the generation of clinical cell lines. The intense public and media attention to the potential of stem cell–based therapies has promoted the emergence of a market of unproven 'stem cell' interventions, which has created a thriving global industry of stem cell tourism. This is presently the major ethical challenge for the practicing neurosurgeon, who is confronted with the responsibility of guiding the genuine needs and hopes of patients afflicted with devastating incurable neurological conditions, rightfully seeking treatment.

Navigation of the ethical challenges and complexities of stem cell research and its clinical translation has been facilitated by the publication of guidelines for stem cell research by the International Society for Stem Cell Research (ISSCR). The ISSCR guidelines focus on hESCs research, clinical translation, and major innovations in the field, as well as new ethical challenges,[5–7] constituting a useful and practical road map for the ethics of stem cell research and its progress in clinical practice.

21.2 Ethical Issues in Clinical Translation

Successful studies in animal models of neurological conditions hold promise for the translation of stem cells into clinical trials. Clinical translation of stem cell–based therapies must be framed within a rigorous scientific and ethical process. This framework extends to the continuum of preclinical work in the laboratory and with animal models, through to the execution of early- and late-phase clinical trials. This section will discuss the ethical issues related to research on human embryonic tissue, cell preparation and manufacturing, preclinical animal models, and clinical trials.

21.2.1 Research with Human Embryonic Tissue

There is a consensus in the scientific community and major international organizations[8,9] that research on pre-implantation-stage human embryos, human embryonic stem cells, foetal cells, and other types of research involving human embryonic cells must be performed under a rigorous scientific and ethical oversight process. A formal impartial process of review, approval, and ongoing monitoring of human embryo research (EMRO) must be in place in any institution conducting this type of research. Specialized committees in some countries, such as the US Embryonic Stem Cell Research Oversight (ESCRO) committee, are already in place to ensure that the scientific and ethical aspects of the research are rigorously assessed and monitored. Committees conducting the EMRO process are usually composed of scientists and clinicians with the relevant expertise, ethicists, legal advisors, and representatives of the community.

There is also consensus that research in stablished hESCs cell lines and iPCSs that are not produced to create embryos or totipotent cells are exempt from the EMRO process. There is broad international agreement that research in human embryos in culture beyond 14 days of age, embryos produced by nuclear reprogramming, and embryos with modified nuclear genomes, along with the production of human-animal chimeras, are prohibited activities. No consensus has yet been reached in emerging areas of research such a gene editing and mitochondrial transfer technologies.

21.2.2 Stem Cell Processing and Manufacturing

All the stages of processing and preparation of stem cells (manufacturing) for clinical trials must adhere to robust scientific and ethical processes. Even the minimal manipulation of cells could introduce risks. Contamination with potential pathogens and changes in genome stability that may modify cell behaviour are risks of cell processing, cell culture, storage, or other manipulations.

Procurement of human biomaterials for both hESCs and iPSCs must be obtained with appropriate informed consent. Screening of donor material for potential infectious agents and a comprehensive genetic and epigenetic assessment are mandatory for the clinical use of stem cells. Genetic mutations or karyotype instability can lead to inappropriate phenotypes or malignant transformation.

Manufacturing of stem cells should follow good manufacturing practice (GMP) standards. Biomaterials used in cell culture and storage processes should be screened for infectious agents. Components of animal origin should, if possible, be avoided and replaced with human biomaterials, as they carry the risk of transferring animal pathogens to the host. Helpful guidelines for the manufacturing process and screening of clinical-grade stem cells have been elaborated by regulatory agencies such as the US Food and Drug Administration (FDA) and the European Medicines Agency (EMA).

21.2.3 Animal Models and Preclinical Studies

Preclinical studies demonstrating the safety and efficacy of stem cell interventions are required, prior to conducting any clinical trials. Careful stem cell characterization, in both in vitro and in vivo conditions, must be established. Long-term toxicity studies determining the biodistribution and tumorgenicity of stem cells must be part of the safety profile of candidate stem cells for clinical trials. The irreversibility of transplantation of stem cells into the human CNS must be considered, as differentiation to unwanted phenotypes, migration to areas not targeted by the therapy, and tumour formation are major risks.

Efficacy studies in small and large animal models must be relevant to the clinical conditions considered for stem cell therapies. Robust and reproducible preclinical research aimed at establishing the mechanism(s) of action of the intervention, in addition to demonstration of clinically meaningful efficacy, are needed before proceeding to clinical trials. Dose-escalation studies, under the same conditions to be used in clinical trials, should be conducted to optimize reproducibility and scaling-up to the human realm. The use of non-human primate models that better emulate the human illnesses to be treated may be required. These studies in non-human primates are particularly relevant for clinical trials that have higher risk or to obtain preclinical information not possible using other animal models.

21.2.4 Clinical Trials

The successful translation of potential stem cell therapies to clinical applications is only possible by performing clinical trials under the most rigorous scientific and ethical parameters. All clinical trials must be conducted under established ethical principles that protect the human subject.[10] Review, approval, and monitoring of clinical trials must adhere to accredited local, national, or international regulatory frameworks. Assessment of the scientific and ethical validity of a proposed trial requires the participation of independent committees with the necessary expertise in the preclinical, clinical, and ethical aspects of the proposed trial. A rigorous assessment of the risk/benefit balance of the trial must be conducted to minimize the risks and optimize the potential benefits to trial participants and society, understanding that although society may benefit from the production of generalizable knowledge, most of the risk is taken by the participant. Accepted ethical and legal standards for obtaining informed consent must be followed. Clear information must be given to the trial participants that stem cells may not be removable, once implanted into the host CNS. This irreversibility of stem cell implantation challenges the accepted right of the patient to withdraw from the clinical trial at any given point. Careful consideration should be given to the legal and ethical implications of obtaining consent in cases involving children or vulnerable individuals with diminished mental capacities due to neurological conditions.

Early-phase clinical trials are aimed at establishing safety and feasibility of unproven interventions. These trials pose potentially high risk to the enrolled subjects and should only be conducted in individuals who have exhausted standard treatments for the condition studied. Although efficacy is not the principal aim of early phase trials, there must be robust preclinical evidence of the potential benefits of the intervention to be tested. These trials aim at evaluating safety, validating and refining techniques, and should be designed to minimize risk in order to avoid catastrophic adverse events. Monitoring of early and long-term adverse events is mandatory, as stem cells can change their phenotype, migrate to unwanted locations, be rejected by the host, or generate tumours. Autopsy consent from trial participants and their next of kin is necessary to evaluate the effects of the stem cell therapy in the host CNS and must be part of any stem cell trial protocol.

Late-phase trials seek to answer the question of efficacy of the stem cell intervention and must be adequately powered to yield meaningful clinical results. Late-phase trials should compare the efficacy of the intervention against current medical or surgical therapeutic approaches for the condition studied. Blinded randomized controlled trials are particularly challenging for interventions where stem cells have to be surgically implanted into the brain or spinal cord. Placebo controls or sham operations must be carefully considered, and the ethical implications of surgical procedures that do not have benefits to the participants should be contemplated when designing the comparator arm. Independent oversight and monitoring of the trial is paramount. Early and late adverse events should be communicated in a timely fashion. Transparency in data sharing is crucial in both early and late phase trials, and may be facilitated by national and international regulatory oversight by entities such as the FDA. Open public communication is essential, as trials must be prospectively registered in public databases (such as https://clinical trials.gov/).

21.2.5 Unproven 'Stem Cell' Interventions

The clinical application of stem cell therapies outside the framework of scientifically and ethically sound clinical trials is fraught with peril. A valid ethical argument could be made for the use of an innovative stem cell intervention that has demonstrated robust potential benefits in preclinical studies. Such an intervention could be accepted as a life-saving measure in a limited number of seriously ill patients. This exceptional circumstance must be rigorously reviewed, ethically and scientifically, by an independent oversight committee with appropriate expertise, before being approved to proceed without a formal clinical trial.

Perhaps the most common challenge that the practicing neurosurgeon could face at present regarding stem cell therapies is the request of his or her patients for guidance in relationship to a commercially available 'stem cell' intervention that promises major benefit, or even a cure, for their condition. A thriving market of unproven 'stem cell' interventions has proliferated across the globe. This 'stem cell' industry, which aggressively promotes stem cell tourism, preys on the genuine hopes of patients suffering devastating and often incurable conditions. Treatments and cures for a vast array of neurological conditions, ranging from chronic pain to Alzheimer's disease, are advertised on the Internet and through social media networks worldwide. Patient testimonials that are misleading as to the benefits of these interventions are used as effective marketing tools to attract clients. Deceiving tactics like the registration of bogus trials in public databases such as clinicaltrials.gov does not guarantee their legitimacy. Stem cell trials, sponsored and paid for by individual patients or patients' advocacy groups, raise serious ethical concerns about conflicts of interest and pressure for researchers and clinicians to engage in the scientifically unsound stem cell interventions in the clinic. Infusion of a 'stem cell' preparation, either intravenously or intrathecally, is the most frequently marketed intervention for neurological conditions. The nature of the 'stem cells' or their short- or long-term benefits are largely undetermined. The safety of these treatments is questionable, and serious adverse events have been reported.[11]

Neurosurgeons have a responsibility to guide patients in a sensitive, non-judgemental manner, warning them about the risks of 'stem cell' interventions that are ethically dubious and have no scientific evidence of clinical benefits. Vulnerable patients in desperate situations are often willing to undergo unproven treatments and at times can pressure their physicians for 'approval or permission' to proceed. It is necessary to maintain open and frank discussions with these patients about available standard-of-care therapies and the risks of commercially driven, unproven interventions that are often invasive and can cause harm.

Numerous scientific stem cell international organizations have denounced these unethical and potentially harmful unproven 'stem cell' interventions.[7] In addition to commercially exploiting patients, who often spend considerable financial resources to travel and be treated with unproven 'stem cell' interventions, these clinics can erode public trust and cause confusion as to the current state of stem cell research. This confusion and disinformation to the public is detrimental to the reputation of the legitimate field of stem cell research and may interfere with its advancement.

Regulatory oversight of stem cell–based therapies by accredited institutions and governments is essential to ensure public safety and facilitate timely access of scientifically proven therapies to appropriate patients. Transparency in reporting adverse events and the benefits of stem cell trials to regulatory bodies and timely public communication to the scientific community, the public, and other stakeholders must be a guiding principle of clinical stem cell research.

21.3 Short-Term Neurosurgical Applications

One of the most attractive targets of stem cell–based therapies is the CNS. Neurological conditions affecting the brain and the spinal cord are often severe and disabling. The lack of effective therapies make disorders of the CNS ideal for the application of cell-restorative strategies aimed at brain and spinal cord repair, although at present no randomized clinical trials have conclusively demonstrated the efficacy of stem cells in the treatment of neurological diseases or injury. Promising studies in animal models have reported efficacy in several CNS conditions,[12,13] increasing the expectations of effective therapies. The development of iPSCs and the possibility of generating specific neuronal and glial phenotypes from autologous sources and the production of 'personalized cell lines' is exciting. Autologous stem cell implantation into the CNS may prevent rejection and avoid the necessity of immunosuppressive therapy or the transmission of infectious agents.

Neurosurgeons will be key members of research teams, conducting clinical trials of stem cell implantation in the brain and spinal cord. The delivery of stem cells to specific targets in the CNS will require neurosurgical techniques such as minimally invasive stereotactic approaches. The development of surgical instruments capable of delivering precise volumes of stem cells to discrete brain or spinal cord targets while minimizing injury will be necessary.[14] Understanding stem cell biology and processes of cell manufacturing, storage, and cell preparation will also be necessary. Management of surgical complications such as haemorrhage or neurological injury, as well as the risks inherent to stem cells, such as unwanted phenotypic differentiation, migration outside the intendent target, or tumour formation, will be required.

There is currently a great deal of research on the use of stem cells for several neurological diseases. However, there are relatively few CNS conditions that have a realistic chance of being amendable to stem cell–based therapies, at least in the short-term. Neurodegenerative diseases that are amendable for cell restoration of a single neuronal phenotype, such as Parkinson's disease (PD) or Huntington's disease (HD), are likely to be the first to be tackled. Similarly, glial and myelin disorders that could potentially be treated by stem cell–derived astrocytes and oligodendrocytes or their precursors are good candidates for short-term clinical trials. Stem cell–based treatment of conditions that affect multiple neuronal and glial phenotypes such as stroke, spinal cord injury, or Alzheimer's disease will require more complex approaches and are considered long-term applications.

Parkinson's disease is likely to be the first neurological disorder that has a realistic chance to be successfully treated or even cured by stem cell therapy. The following section will discuss the issues to be considered and the reasons why PD can be thought of as the 'low-hanging fruit' for brain repair. Although other potential applications of stem cells are in the horizon, PD will likely provide the benchmark and a road map for the development of stem cell–based CNS therapies in the future.

21.3.1 Stem Cell Brain Repair in Parkinson's Disease

There is good understanding of the pathophysiology of PD, which is caused by the progressive degeneration of a specific neuronal phenotype – the dopaminergic neuron of the substantia nigra. There is currently no treatment that alters the natural history of the disease. Medical therapy, although very effective in controlling symptoms early in the disease, loses its efficacy with time and often produces disabling side effects. Deep brain stimulation (DBS) is also effective in controlling some of the motor symptoms in PD, but does not prevent the loss of dopaminergic neurons and the progression of the disease.

There is robust scientific evidence in animal models of PD of the efficacy of cell-replacement strategies.[15] Clinical trials of implantation of foetal dopaminergic cells into PD patients, more than two decades ago, demonstrated that cell-restoration is feasible in the human brain. Although the results of these trials showed that clinical efficacy was variable, there was clear clinical benefit in some patients.[16,17] Long-term survival of transplanted dopaminergic neurons was also documented.[18] In addition, a great deal was learned about the development of side effects, such as transplant-induced dyskinesias that were not predicted by animal models.

However, at the time, clinical implantation of foetal dopaminergic neurons in PD was impractical because of the ethical issues associated with the use of foetal tissue and its procurement. However, this experience with foetal cells provided the scientific platform for the use of stem cells in PD and remains the gold standard that stem cells must emulate. Currently, an attractive approach is the use of autologous iPSCs obtained from the patient's own bone marrow and directed to a dopaminergic phenotype. This approach has the advantage of decreasing the possibility of rejection and preventing the necessity of immunosuppressive therapy.

Even if autologous clinical-grade dopaminergic cells conforming to all the scientific and ethical requirements were available, several important issues must be considered before proceeding to clinical trials. Defining the criteria of patient selection is paramount. When is the best time to intervene in the progression of the disease? This is a complex issue, as there is significant variability in the rate of progression of PD. The patient's responsiveness to drug therapy and the availability of a validated surgical alternative such as DBS also needs to be carefully assessed. The existence of standardized assessment tools that were developed for the clinical studies using foetal cells should provide a solid reference for stem cell studies. It was clear during those studies that responsiveness to L-dopa was a crucial criterion for patient selection.

Neurosurgical issues,[19] such as selecting the appropriate surgical target, will also need to be determined. The putamen was the main target in the foetal cell trials. However, the putamen is not the homotopic location of nigral dopaminergic cells, which reside normally in the substantia nigra. Choosing the appropriate anatomical target is important when considering the risks of potential neurological injury and its clinical consequences.

The choice of minimally invasive neurosurgical techniques to optimize accurate stem cell delivery and minimize brain injury will be the responsibility of the neurosurgical team. Standardization of stem cell delivery by programmable cell injectors capable of reliably controlling implantation parameters, such as the number of cells, volume of the deposits, or rate of infusion, will be needed. These delivery systems will likely be used in combination with neurosurgical navigation and intraoperative imaging.

Imaging of stem cell transplants, by PET and MRI modalities aimed at ensuring the accurate placement of the stem cells in the intended target, as well as cell survival after implantation, will be also be required. Monitoring the potential risks inherent to stem cell therapy, such as unwanted migration, infection, or tumour formation using post-operative imaging, will also be necessary. It is highly unlikely that the stem cells could be removed after implantation, and the management of short- and long-term complications of stem cell behaviour will need to be an integral part of the neurosurgical management.

21.4 Last Words

As stem cell technologies move into from the laboratory into clinical trials for neurological conditions, a rigorous scientific and ethical oversight process must be followed. The potential risks of moving too rapidly to the clinic without robust and reproducible pre-clinical evidence of safety and efficacy can cause harm to patients and negatively impact the advance of the entire field.

Helpful guidelines for stem cell research have been published by international scientific societies, and regulatory oversight by local, national, and international bodies is required to proceed with clinical trials. Stem cells generate complex ethical challenges, but their potential for the treatment of devastating neurological diseases or injury is enormous.

Neurosurgery will play a fundamental role in the stem cell therapies of the future. New neurosurgical techniques and instruments will be developed for the delivery of stem cells to

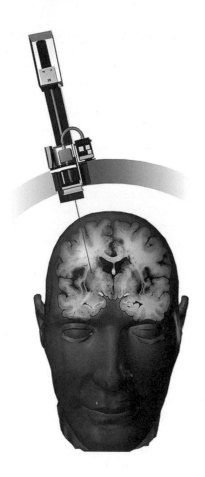

Figure 21.1 Illustration of a computerized stem cell injector. Implantation parameters such as cell numbers, volume of deposits, number of deposits, and rate of injection could be programmed to standardize the neurosurgical procedure.

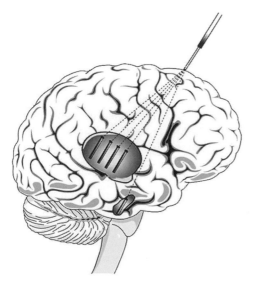

Figure 21.2 Illustration of a multitarget neurosurgical strategy to repair the dopaminergic circuitry in Parkinson's disease. Note that four stem cell deposits are planned in the putamen and one in the substantia nigra, in order to restitute dopaminergic input to both the nigra and striatal systems.

single or multiple targets within the CNS. New stem cell imaging technology for the monitoring of stem cell function and potential complications will emerge. The stem cell neurosurgeon of the future will be well versed on the fundamentals of stem cells and their capacity for brain and spinal cord repair. As clinical trials demonstrate efficacy and are scaled up to standard-of-care therapies, a new neurosurgical field will emerge: reconstructive neurosurgery.

References

1. Evans M. J., Kaufman M. H. Establishment in culture of pluripotential cells from mouse embryos. *Nature* 1981; **292**: 154–6.

2. Thomson J. A., Itskovitz-Eldor J., Shapiro S. S., et al. Embryonic stem cell lines derived from human blastocysts. *Science* 1998; **282**: 1145–7.

3. Mendez-Ferrer S., Scadden D. T., Sanchez-Aguilera A. Bone marrow stem cells: current and emerging concepts. *Ann. NY Acad. Sci.* 2015; **1335**: 32–44.

4. Takahashi K., Yamanaka S. Induction of pluripotent stem cells from mouse embryonic and adult fibroblast cultures by defined factors. *Cell* 2006; **126**: 663–76.

5. International Society for Stem Cell Research (ISSCR). Guidelines for the conduct of human embryonic stem cell research. 2006. Available at: www.isscr.org/docs/default-source/hesc-guidelines/isscr hescguidelines2006.pdf.

6. International Society for Stem Cell Research (ISSCR). Guidelines for the clinical translation of stem cells. 2008. Available at: www.isscr.docs/default-source/clin-trans-guidelines/isscrglclinicaltrans.pdf.

7. International Society for Stem Cell Research (ISSCR). Guidelines for stem cell research and clinical translation. 2016. Available at: www.isscr.org/guidelines2016.

8. ESHRE Taskforce on ethics and law. The moral status of the pre-implantation embryo. *Hum. Reprod.* 2001; **17**: 1409–19.

9. Ethics Committee of American Society for Reproductive Medicine. Donating embryos for human embryonic stem cell (hESC) research: a committee opinion. *Fertil. Steril.* 2013; **100**: 935–9.

10. Department of Health, and Education and Welfare. Report of the National Commission for the Protection of Human Subjects of Biomedical and Behavioral Research (The Belmont Report). *Fed. Reg.* 1979; **23**: 192.

11. Berkowitz A. L., Miller M. B., Mir S. A., et al. Glioproliferative lesion of the spinal cord as a complication of 'stem-cell tourism'. *N. Engl. J. Med.* 2016; **375**: 196–8.

12. Goldman S. A., Nedergaard M., Windrem M. S. Glial progenitor cell-based treatment and modeling of neurological disease. *Science* 2012; **338**: 491–5.

13. Thompson L. H., Bjorklund A. Reconstruction of brain circuitry by neural transplants generated from pluripotent stem cells. *Neurobiol. Dis.* 2015; **79**: 28–40.

14. Mendez I., Hong M., Smith S., et al. A neural transplantation cannula and microinjector system: experimental and clinical experience. *J. Neurosurg.* 2000; **92**: 493–9.

15. Lindvall O. Dopaminergic neurons for Parkinson's therapy. *Nat. Biotechnol.* 2012; **30**: 56–8.

16. Barker R. A., Barret J., Mason S. L., et al. Fetal dopaminergic transplantation trials and the future of neural grafting in Parkinson's disease. *Lancet. Neurol.* 2013; **12**: 84–91.

17. Mendez I., Sanchez-Pernaute R., Vinuela A., et al. Cell type analysis of fetal dopamine cell suspension transplants in striatum and substantia nigra of patients with Parkinson's disease. *Brain* 2005; **128**: 1498–1510.

18. Mendez I., Vinuela A., Astradsson A., et al. Dopamine neurons implanted into people with Parkinson's disease survive without pathology for 14 years. *Nat. Med.* 2008; **14**: 507–9.

19. Master Z., McLeod M., Mendez I. Benefits, risks and ethical considerations in translation of stem cell research to clinical applications in Parkinson's disease. *J. Med. Ethics.* 2007; **33**: 169–73.

Chapter 22

Brain-Machine Interface Technology in Neurosurgery

Jeffrey V. Rosenfeld and Marike Broekman

"The future has arrived - it's just not evenly distributed yet." (William Gibson, 1999)

22.1 Introduction

Diseases of the nervous system impose an immense burden on patients and society. Brain-computer interfaces aim to improve or even eliminate the handicaps associated with these diseases.

A *brain-computer interface* (BCI) is an electronic linkage between the brain and a computer via scalp, subdural, or intracortical electrodes. Neurobionics is the science of brain (or nervous system)/electronic interfaces. The therapeutic goal of the BCI is to replace, restore, enhance, supplement, or improve neurological disability. Advances in microelectronics, electrode interfaces, and wireless technology are enabling the rapid transfer of large volumes of data with higher spatial resolution to and from the brain. Human applications are rapidly advancing. What might be regarded by many as science fiction in BCI capability is rapidly becoming reality.

Neuroprosthetic devices are implanted BCIs. Signals from the cerebral cortex are first acquired through the electrode recording interface, then features are extracted using signal processing and finally features are decoded or translated by a computer to create 'commands' or instructions that operate an assistive device. Recordings from the primary motor cortex or from the parietal cortex are used in neuroprosthetic devices for the control of prosthetic limbs, robotic limbs, robot assistants, wheelchairs, exoskeletons, and paralysed limbs[1] and from language areas of cortex to decode speech.[2] Applications for BCIs include spinal cord injury, amyotrophic sclerosis, and stroke. Epilepsy surgeons have the opportunity to explore experimental aspects of BCIs for patients who are having electrodes placed during investigation for intractable epilepsy.[2] These opportunistic studies can inform the future design of BCIs.

Transmission of electronic signals from a computer into the cerebral cortex via microelectrodes is being developed for sensory substitution (hearing, vision, cutaneous sensation/proprioception), memory replacement or enhancement, and to abort epileptic seizures following early detection based on subdural strip electrode recordings.[1]

Scalp EEG recording–based BCIs and transcranial direct current stimulation of the cerebral cortex BCIs are non-invasive, and the neurosurgeon should be aware of these alternate technologies. Non-invasive BCIs are clearly more attractive to potential users than implanted devices, but the choice will depend on their purpose, functionality, and reliability compared with implanted devices.

The BCI may enhance the independence and confidence of the recipient. For example, consider the ability of a quadriplegic individual to execute manual tasks such as grasping a cup of coffee by BCI robotic arm or the generation of pixelated vision for a totally blind individual from a retinal or cortical neuroprosthesis. However, there are numerous ethical, social, and legal challenges in this regard, which have recently been reviewed and discussed.[3-6] It is imperative that engineers and physicians/neurosurgeons maintain the highest ethical standards when they introduce new neuroprosthetics.

22.2 Background

22.2.1 History

Vidal posed the concept and challenges of BCI in 1973 and proceeded to demonstrate a human EEG/BCI interface in 1977.[7] Following this, there was considerable developmental BCI research with implanted electrodes in non-human primates. The first human implanted with a bionic vision device was Dobelle's first prototype, which was implanted into a blind man in 1978. This was one of the earliest commercial BCI devices (for which the patients paid!). Wireless bionic vision neuroprostheses will soon be ready for human implantation.[8]

The first motor prosthetic was implanted in 1997 in a man with locked-in syndrome, who could subsequently move a cursor on a computer screen. In 2005 the Cyberkinetics Braingate 96 electrode array was implanted in the motor cortex of a tetraplegic man who could operate a robotic arm.[9] Deadwyler et al. showed in 2013 that electrical patterns of activity in the hippocampus of a donor rat could enhance the memory in a naïve rat via a BCI[10] and developed a memory neuroprosthesis in the non-human primate.[11]

22.2.2 Current Evidence

The more invasive the technology and the finer the electrode interfaces, the higher the fidelity or signal to noise ratio of the information being transmitted. Although the quality of signal recording is progressively improving for scalp electrode BCI interfaces, the fidelity is still poor compared with intracortical microelectrodes. This is because the intracortical micro-electrodes have a more direct interface with smaller groups of neurons.

An alternative to these types of electrodes is the 'Stentrode'. This is an electrode array embedded in a stent, which is placed by an interventional radiologist in the sagittal sinus. The electrodes become embedded in the wall of the sinus. The 'Stentrode' can then be used for thought control of assist devices for paralysed individuals. This device creates a BCI interface with motor cortex, without the need to place electrodes directly into the motor cortex.[12]

22.3 Ethical Issues

22.3.1 Agency and Identity

An *agent* is an autonomous actor persisting through time who can be held responsible (causally, and potentially legally and morally) for his/her/its actions.[13] Humans are moral agents. The autonomy of the individual could be violated by a BCI. As BCIs evolve, the concept of 'self' may yield to the communal sense of identity. Artificial intelligence of computers may equal or exceed that of humans, and so could also affect individual human autonomy if a person is connected to a BCI.

Unexpected effects of the BCI on agency and identity can also occur. Gilbert et al. reported six patients with medically intractable epilepsy implanted with first-in-human 'BCI advisory devices' for seizure prediction. Although BCIs can positively increase a sense of self, confidence, and control, one patient had distress, feelings of loss of control, and a 'rupture' of patient identity or self-estrangement.[14] Psychological preparation of potential patients to build resilience and prepare them for the likely effects on self-image should be developed for future recipients of BCIs. Gilbert et al. recommend that the BCIs not be implanted in those with self-image issues in relation to their pathology.[14]

22.3.1.1 Neural Privacy

Questions of agency relate to the privacy of neural data. Who owns the thoughts generated in the networks? Who is responsible for actions? What is the authenticity of the output. What is the computer contributing to the input/output? Agency and identity are human rights and must be protected, for example by specific laws as for genetic data. Discussion on agency and identity should be part of the consent process for the implantation of neuroprosthetics.

22.3.1.2 Humanity and Personhood

Some philosophical questions arise. Does the functioning BCI become part of the human mind or is it just a tool? Does the BCI make the recipient more a cyborg and less a human? Does the body schema change with machine extensions? Could the BCI induce changes in the brain through neural plasticity, resulting in changes in personhood such that behaviour or character are altered? Feelings of loss of identity have been reported with deep brain stimulation.[6]

22.3.1.3 Stigma and Normality

The goals of a BCI are to improve neurological function and the quality of life. However, the situation is more complex and nuanced. Would disabled people choose to have a BCI in order to reduce disease stigma or reduce their perceived burden on society? Conversely, some users may feel an increased stigma using the device and would then choose to restrict its use. Some disabled people do not see themselves as disabled, so the BCI would be an enhancement to them rather than a treatment.

22.3.1.4 Autonomy

Autonomy is undermined by severe neurological disability. The BCI could on one hand empower the individual by giving them more independence and thus improving their autonomy and dignity. On the other hand, a BCI having a causal role in the decision-making of the individual may further affect autonomy.

22.3.1.5 Responsibility

Is the user entirely responsible for the BCI output? The law has not kept pace with BCI advances, so the attribution of responsibility is not clear. Where does the legal and moral responsibility of the behavioural effects of the BCI lie? One view is that the individual should be held responsible for any unintended consequences. Passing thoughts could trigger an unwanted response. Others would say the unwanted effects could be due to the device itself, and hence the manufacturer bears some responsibility. This is a complex interrelationship and depends on the situation. A third party possibly hacking into the control of the BCI adds further complexity.

What if the robotic arm connected to an individual's brain by BCI injures a bystander? Was it the unconscious thought of the individual that triggered the action, was it their conscious malicious thought, or was it the semi-independent robot? The BCI user should be able to cancel the action of the robot by a 'veto switch' activated by eye movements. Clausen et al. suggest that all-new BCI systems should include a veto control.[5] Inappropriate use of the device by the individual may make them liable for causing harm. The medical team and the manufacturer also have a responsibility to train the user in the correct and safe use of the device.

22.3.2 Privacy and Security

The individual's thoughts and emotions are sensitive and private, and should not be accessible to an external agent. Therefore, privacy is a very important issue for users of BCI devices. However, a person with a BCI may not be aware of the information that is being obtained from their brain. The algorithms derived from an individual's brain that are used in a BCI may be used as a template for other individuals in turn, but who owns or controls this information? Who has access to the data? Could the future BCI be used to read thoughts, gather information on the neural underpinnings of decision-making, or become the ultimate lie detector? Could psychological traits, motivations, intentions, mental states, and attitudes towards other people also be accessed? Recordings of neural information should be held securely by the coordinating physicians and any commercial entity involved. The patient should understand what is being stored and for how long, how it will be used, and that it will be protected from unauthorized use. They will need to give consent for the data to be shared.

Hacking into the information would also breach privacy. Wireless transmission of the BCI could render the system vulnerable to hacking. Hackers could potentially alter the settings of the device (integrity), alter the activity or availability of the device, and breach confidentiality of the data. The encryption of transmitted data may offer some protection and should be incorporated into all BCIs (Table 22.1).

22.3.3 Informed Consent

The invasiveness of the neuroprosthesis raises safety and ethical issues. Performing a craniotomy to implant electrodes is a major undertaking and must be outweighed by the potential benefits of the direct BCI as opposed to a scalp electrode or even skull electrode interfaces, which have less

Table 22.1 Unacceptable outcomes of a brain-computer interface (BCI)

1.	The data collected from the individual brain is used for commercial purposes without consent.
2.	Coercion of action: an external agent coercing the individual for political mind control or incitement to unwanted or criminal behaviour. This has been labelled 'brainjacking'.
3.	The artificial intelligence residing in the device may also initiate certain actions. Who is responsible for untoward consequences of the BCI – the user, the designer, or manufacturer of the BCI, or the device itself?
4.	Blocking the thoughts/speech of the host while 'shadowing' the BCI communications.
5.	A malevolent actor hacking into the BCI and retrieving thoughts or thought patterns of the individual.
6.	The BCI interface may have untoward effects on other parts of the brain.
7.	The BCI induces mental illness by interfering with thought patterns.

risk but at the expense of a poorer quality of BCI. Competing technology and less-invasive options should be fully disclosed to the potential recipient and their family.

22.3.3.1 Managing Expectations

A realistic explanation of what is involved with the screening, selection, surgery, and its risks, along with the post-insertion assessment, rehabilitation, and care, is essential. Researchers and manufacturers have a responsibility to accurately portray the BCI, its effects, and potential in media articles and releases to the general public and to a vulnerable audience of the disabled and their families. Hyperbole and exaggeration are unethical. Media stories about BCIs tend to be very optimistic and should not use emotive words like 'cure'. The use of selected videos of patients performing impressive actions with their BCI is a powerful tool for raising expectations. The issue of voluntariness may arise because of the unrealistic expectations of family members who could also exert undue influence on the potential recipient. If the BCI reduces demands on their care, this could reduce family burden and put pressure on the patient to agree to proceed with the BCI. BCI subjects may also fear disappointing the researchers.

Informed consent should include a discussion of the possible effects of the device on mood, personality, or sense of self.[6] Therapeutic misconception is a belief by patients that they will only benefit from the intervention. This may not be the case with a BCI, which will not always be effective.

22.3.3.2 Balance of Risks and Benefits

Extensive discussion of risks versus benefits with the participant and their family is mandatory, particularly for a new experimental device. There should be full disclosure of all the available information, the patient should have the capacity to understand the information that is presented in an appropriate manner, and the patient should be free from any coercion or undue influence in making a decision to proceed. Consent must be voluntary. The consent process should involve extensive exploration of all the issues. The participant also has the right to withdraw participation at any time (but preferably prior to implantation). It is important that the physician provides the patient with hope in the discussions, but it should be based on 'realism' not 'idealism' and placed in perspective.

The psychological and physical condition of the patient must be considered, and psychologists, psychiatrists, and physicians should be involved in the screening of potential recipients. Cognitive or affective impairment would be contraindications to having an implantable BCI, except if in the future it were being used specifically to boost cognitive function such as a memory prosthesis. BCIs may become less reliable in the presence of cognitive impairment or may result in aberrant communication with the device.

Locked-in syndrome (LIS) could be considered a perpetual torture for the individual who has been unable to move or communicate for years. The individual may be desperate to communicate and have social access but is not able to provide informed consent. Can consent be presumed until the BCI is in place and communication is possible? The BCI links for LIS are likely to be non-invasive. Locked-in patients may also have impaired cognitive function, rendering the BCI ineffective. Perhaps the individual does not wish to connect to BCI, or alternatively they may want to die and wish to communicate this. Patients in the minimally conscious state (MCS) have severely impaired neurological function, and their cognitive abilities are usually severely affected, so using a BCI becomes an even greater ethical challenge. The amyotrophic lateral sclerosis (ALS) patient who is becoming progressively disabled may wish to have a BCI device to improve their quality of life before they die.

Researchers implanting a new device into a patient have a duty of care to that individual for the long term, and the neurosurgeon should be prepared to manage complications whenever they might occur and also be prepared to deactivate or remove the device if requested by the recipient.

22.3.3.3 User Safety

Short-term risks of implantation, including infection, haemorrhage, and epilepsy, must be fully explained. The likely functional longevity of the device must also be explained. The long-term risks of the implanted device include device failure due to gliosis around the electrodes or loss of the hermetic sealing exposing the internal electronics to fluid damage, and the potential leaking of toxic materials such as heavy metals from the device into the circulation around the electronics must also be explained. Epilepsy and infection are also longer-term risks. It would also be useful to have patient registries established so that all implanted BCI neuroprostheses can be tracked over time.

22.3.3.4 Inappropriate Expectations

The potential benefits need to be put into perspective and explained in terms of likely quantum of improvement in neurological function and activities of daily living if the device performs according to expectation. The patient also needs to be told what the chance is that the device will not work for them or may completely fail at some time. The participants in a first in human trial should not be expected to pay for any aspect of the study or the device. Alternative assistive devices should be explained to the participant.

Lane et al. has surveyed potential recipients of bionic vision devices and reports that they may see themselves as pioneers, trailblazers, adventurers, and explorers, and could be welcomed as integral members of the research, as there are usually very small numbers in a first in human BCI trial.[15] However, the desire of the recipient to be involved in cutting-edge research should not outweigh the need for improvements in neurological function, which is of course the purpose of the research. Psychological maladjustment to blindness or other neurological disability, feelings of guilt, and the desire for atonement or punishment are all contraindications to implantation of these devices.[15]

A BCI neuroprosthesis may be relatively soon superseded by newer technology. If it is a newly developed neuroprosthesis and is being implanted by craniotomy as a once-off procedure, the investigators will need to explain to the recipient what benefit they are likely to derive but also could explain that that they are a pioneer and will be helping the investigators understand the device function and capabilities, even if it may be superseded in the future.

The rehabilitation of BCI users may be arduous and extensive and include scientific research conducted by the investigators. This may have physical, emotional, and financial burdens for the individual and their families, which need to be explained to the potential recipient. A slow pace of improvement may result in frustration, lack of motivation of the patient to cooperate with the investigators, and possibly depression. Failure of the device could have a serious emotional effect on the user, particularly if they are dependent on the technology. A range of 15–30% of recipients fail to use their BCI effectively, which has been called 'BCI illiteracy'.[4] However, this is a pejorative term and has been criticised because there is a range of ability to use BCIs, a variable time for acquisition of skills, intrinsic system design factors, a variable quality of training instructions, and variable human anatomy and physiology.[16]

Independent assessment of engineering and manufacturing quality control is necessary prior to human application. Permission to perform an implantation of neuroprostheses will need to be obtained from the institution's human research ethics committee. This hospital will also need to credential the neurosurgeons performing the procedure.

22.4 Placebo Effect and the Establishment of Efficacy

Placebo effects may occur following a new device implantation, which inflate outcome results. Increased therapist/physician support of a disabled patient following implantation of a neuroprosthesis may also have a positive effect on the patient's performance. Having controls in a BCI device trial is not feasible. However, the patient can to some degree act as their own control when the device is turned off. Although 'sham surgery' has been used to investigate the efficacy of a surgical procedure, this is not feasible for the disabled patient having a BCI neuroprosthesis.[1]

22.5 Justice and Equity of Access

BCIs are expensive devices and will not have a large market unless medical insurance or government covers of the cost. It would be inequitable and patently unjust if only the wealthy could afford this technology. Relatively few paralysed individuals will probably benefit from implanted BCIs. Some would argue that considerable sums spent on developing advanced technologies such as BCIs could be better directed to more common diseases. The contrary argument is that the relief of individual disability and suffering is also a worthy endeavour.

Is developing a BCI implant for an ALS patient the fairest or most just way to spend money in healthcare when there are so many other worthy competing priorities for the health dollar? When does individual right trump that of society at large? These are difficult ethical challenges for any society, but perhaps one could argue that the quality of a just society is how it cares for its sick, vulnerable, and disabled citizens.

22.6 Enhancement

Enhancement or augmentation moves the BCI beyond therapeutic assist devices. Augmentation of normal mental, cognitive, or physical function to enhance physical endurance or sensory or mental capacity creates inequities. The resultant competitive advantage could create new forms of discrimination in society. Would this be akin to drug cheats in sports, or are there milder versions of enhancement that are acceptable? Acquiring new skills more easily, such as music, additional language, or sporting moves, could be construed as a good outcome. There also may be therapeutic benefit to using a BCI. The repeated use of the BCI may enhance or stimulate neural recovery. Conversely, it is also possible that BCI use could adversely affect neural plasticity.

A *cyborg* is a technically enhanced human. Could the BCI be used to give the soldier or jet pilot a more direct thought link to a computer/weapon interface to produce a 'supersoldier' with heightened reflexes and reduced decision and action time frames? This cyborg could be perceived as the ultimate killing machine. What if the human brain could be supplemented with additional senses? Would it be ethical to achieve this? This has already been achieved in rats using a BCI. The rats can perceive infrared information when it is transmitted to their sensory cortex.[17]

Table 22.2 Illustrative cases of possible future ethical issues

1. A patient who had an expressive aphasia due to a stroke has a speech-recognition device implanted, which is able to read 'covert' speech (inner private thoughts) as well as 'overt' speech.

2. A hacker reprograms a BCI in a patient who uses the BCI to control a wheelchair. The wheelchair goes too fast and tips over and injures the patient.

3. A patient who has advanced amyotrophic lateral sclerosis (ALS) and cannot move his limbs or speak requests an implanted neuroprosthesis to communicate and control a robotic helper. But the surgeon is reluctant to do it because of the risks of surgery and the short lifespan of the patient.

4. A BCI is used as a lie detector in a criminal trial. This could make the difference between a verdict of innocent or guilty. How reliable is it? Could the individual have control of the responses and suppress lies?

Many would regard the enhancement of the capabilities of a soldier as immoral and unethical, but militaries always aim for competitive advantage. There clearly should be strict regulation of these technologies, such as the regulations that exist for various weapons systems via the Geneva Conventions (Table 22.2).

22.7 Future Directions

Alternative energy sources could be used for BCIs, such as transcranial magnetic stimulation, magneto-encephalography, light activation (optogenetic techniques), near infrared spectroscopy (NIRS), and focused ultrasound.

In the future, it may be possible to use thousands or millions of nanoscale devices ('nanobots') to connect individual neurons to 'the cloud'. Large amounts of data could potentially be transferred, such that thoughts and memories could be downloaded. Could humans communicate via BCI by thought alone? Perhaps unwanted thoughts of depression or schizophrenia could be suppressed or eliminated using BCIs.

'Brain nets' are networks of animal brains connected via BCIs. This could be thought of as an 'organic computer'. Information is enhanced in real time through direct brain-to-brain interfaces. Cortical activity is recorded, analysed, and delivered to the somatosensory cortex of other animals, enabling them to solve computational tasks. A four-rat-brain net was found to perform at a higher level than a single rat.[18] A brain net has been created between three monkeys operating an avatar arm.[19] As the human BCI develops, will it be possible to enhance the function of one individual through the extant knowledge of others using a brain net? This clearly raises ethical issues of autonomy, agency, and identity, consent, and enhancement. Conscious transfer of information between human brains at a distance is 'hyperinteraction'.[20] Cross-species neural coupling has been achieved, with a human controlling rat tail movement with a non-invasive link to an anaesthetised rat's motor cortex. This creates further ethical challenges if this type of interface develops further.[21]

22.8 Conclusion

The capability of BCIs is advancing rapidly, but the long-term effects of these new technologies are unknown. At this time, the number of individuals who have had implanted BCIs is limited, and those having a wired Braingate electrode array are 'tethered' to the laboratory.

Unless these devices are wireless, there will not be much uptake in the technology beyond the laboratory.

Existing ethics guidelines do not address all the issues and challenges presented in this chapter. It is time for world bodies such as the United Nations to address these challenges and for governments to develop new policies and legislation.[6] Protection of the individual with respect to agency (autonomy), identity, privacy, and security is mandatory. However, the neurosurgeon also takes responsibility to provide informed consent without bias, a duty of care to achieve beneficence and justice, and ongoing care of the patient. Ethical, psychological, and legal studies should be conducted in parallel with scientific and technical studies.

References

1. Rosenfeld J. V., Wong Y. T. Neurobionics and the brain-computer interface: current applications and future horizons. *Med. J. Aust.* 2017; **206**: 363–8.

2. Martin S., Iturrate I., Millan J. D. R., et al. Decoding inner speech using electrocorticography: progress and challenges toward a speech prosthesis. *Front Neurosci.* 2018; **12**: 422.

3. Burwell S. M., Sample M., Racine E. Ethical aspects of brain computer interfaces: a scoping review. *BMC Med. Ethics* 2017; **18**: 60.

4. Klein E. Informed consent in implantable BCI research: identifying risks and exploring meaning. *Sci. Eng. Ethics* 2016; **22**: 1299–1317.

5. Clausen J., Fetz E., Donoghue J., et al. Help, hope, and hype: ethical dimensions of neuroprosthetics. *Science* 2017; **356**: 1338–9.

6. Yuste R., Goering S., Arcas B. A. Y., et al. Four ethical priorities for neurotechnologies and AI. *Nature* 2017; **551**: 159–63.

7. Vidal J. Real-time detection of brain events in EEG. *IEEE Proceedings* 1977; **65**: 633–44.

8. Lewis P. M., Ayton L. N., Guymer R. H., et al. Advances in implantable bionic devices for blindness: a review. *ANZ J. Surg.* 2016; **86**: 654–9.

9. Hochberg L. R., Serruya M. D., Friehs G. M., et al. Neuronal ensemble control of prosthetic devices by a human with tetraplegia. *Nature* 2006; **442**: 164–71.

10. Deadwyler S. A., Berger T. W., Sweatt A. J., et al. Donor/recipient enhancement of memory in rat hippocampus. *Front Syst. Neurosci.* 2013; **7**: 120.

11. Deadwyler S. A., Hampson R. E., Song D., et al. A cognitive prosthesis for memory facilitation by closed-loop functional ensemble stimulation of hippocampal neurons in primate brain. *Exp. Neurol.* 2017; **287**: 452–60.

12. Oxley T. J., Opie N. L., John S. E., et al. Minimally invasive endovascular stent-electrode array for high-fidelity, chronic recordings of cortical neural activity. *Nature Biotech.* 2016; **34**: 320–7.

13. Roskies A. L., Agency and intervention. *Philos. Trans. R. Soc. Lond. B. Biol. Sci.* 2015 **370**: 20140215.

14. Gilbert F., Cook M., OBrien T., et al. Embodiment and estrangement: results from a first-in-human intelligent BCI trial. *Sci. Eng. Ethics* 2019; **25**(1): 83–96.

15. Lane F. J., Huyck M., Troyk P., et al. Responses of potential users to the intracortical visual prosthesis: final themes from the analysis of focus group data. *Disabil. Rehabil. Assist. Technol.* 2012; **7**: 304–13.

16. Thompson M. C. Critiquing the concept of BCI illiteracy. *Sci. Eng. Ethics* 2019; **25**(4): 1217–33.

17. Thomson E. E., Carra R., Nicolelis M. A. Perceiving invisible light through a somatosensory cortical prosthesis. *Nat. Commun.* 2013; **4**: 1482.

18. Pais-Vieira M., Chiuffa G., Lebedev M., et al. Building an organic computing device with multiple interconnected brains. *Sci. Rep.* 2015; **5**: 11869.

19. Ramakrishnan A., Ifft P. J., Pais-Vieira M., et al. Computing arm movements with a monkey brainet. *Sci. Rep.* 2015; **5**: 10767.

20. Grau C., Ginhoux R., Riera A., et al. Conscious brain-to-brain communication in humans using non-invasive technologies. *PLoS One* 2014; **9**: e105225.

21. Yoo S. S., Kim H., Filandrianos E., et al. Non-invasive brain-to-brain interface (BBI): establishing functional links between two brains. *PLoS One* 2103; **8**: e60410.

International Neurosurgery

23

Ann Mansur and Mark Bernstein

23.1 Introduction

The world has been plagued with gross inequities in the delivery of medical care, including the provision of neurosurgical and surgical care at large. The poorest third of the world receives only 3.5% of surgical aid yet it represents more than 10% of the world's disease burden.[1–2] An estimated two billion people worldwide lack adequate access to surgical care, and that number is much more staggering for neurosurgical care.[3] There are even nations with no neurosurgical services and some with staggering ratios of patients to neurosurgeons,[4] indicating the need for improved global neurosurgical capacity and education.

It is of no surprise that there is growing interest in making contributions to neurosurgical care and its capacity building in low- to middle-income countries (LMICs) through missions, remote teaching, and charitable donations. While these initiatives stem from virtuosity and benevolence, the reality of their provision is one coloured by unique ethical challenges and opportunities for inadvertent harm. Hence it is of paramount importance to reflect upon and discuss the ethical issues that arise in these global health venues.

23.2 Background

Despite the commendable efforts and generosity of those surgeons and organizations that aim to level the playing field in neurosurgical care, there are numerous ethical dilemmas that arise from both the providers and recipients of these exchanges. These dilemmas can arise in the planning of a neurosurgical initiative, such as how to deliver sustainable and locally relevant education/resources, which stakeholders to engage, and how to ensure that the initiative does not place undue burden on the host country.

Throughout these initiatives, surgeons can encounter situations that challenge their moral compass, such as being asked to provide care that is outside the scope of their practice, being placed in situations with suboptimal resources for the type of work planned, lack of ethical practice in the host nation, or issues surrounding informed consent. Lastly, upon the conclusion of the initiative, the question arises: 'Now what?' What happens to the people in the host nation that must now try to implement new information/techniques within the context of their limited environment? Ethical challenges arise in ensuring that the invested efforts are sustainable, that appropriate follow-up is arranged, and that the local neurosurgeons are provided with appropriate mentorship and continual support.

These ethical concerns have been only briefly discussed in the literature in isolated papers and anecdotal references. We would be doing our global neurosurgical community a disservice by not attending to and furthering exploration of these pertinent issues. The aim of this chapter is to explore the various types of ethical challenges that international neurosurgeons might encounter in their charitable work through a review of the literature as well as highlighting personal experience in the field. While it will become apparent through this chapter that there is often no clear right or wrong way of conducting international initiatives, we hope that in exploring these issues, neurosurgeons and their collaborators will at least become more conscientious of the ethical implications of their work. We start by highlighting some relevant issues as they pertain to the planning, implementation, and follow-up of neurosurgical initiatives. We then focus on the core ethical principles that are in play in these situations and demonstrate how they apply to specific cases.

23.3 Current Evidence and Examples

23.3.1 Pre-intervention

23.3.1.1 Reflection on Motives

Prior to initiating a global health initiative, the first step towards a moral high road is to reflect upon the intention behind the initiative. Neurosurgeons can easily fall into the trap of visiting LMICs and attending to tough cases without enabling the locals to conduct the operation; upon departure, the visiting neurosurgeon is praised for his/her good work and the locals are pleased with the outcomes but will not be able to do the subsequent case when the surgeon leaves. This is colloquially known as 'white knight' syndrome,[5] in which the neurosurgeon is seen as an altruistic white knight that comes to the rescue of those in need. It is a paternalistic view of global health; superficially, it is altruistic, but a deeper look will show that the only person who benefits from this interaction in the long run is the visiting neurosurgeon. His/her status is elevated in the LMIC through local praise or even press releases, and upon return home, he/she is applauded by his/her academic community.

In order to mitigate these consequences, surgeons must reflect upon their intentions and goals for international aid. There is no such thing as 100% altruism; however, honesty in this exercise can distinguish between those surgeons who would make the local community thrive and those whose résumés and egos would be the greatest beneficiaries. There is nothing wrong with reaching the latter realization, but the ethical thing to do in that situation is to refrain from proceeding with the initiative for personal gain.

This reflection is not a singular exercise but one of iteration throughout the initiative. In doing so, the neurosurgeon and his/her team can continuously remind themselves of the basic intentions driving their efforts, and this moral compass can help them navigate through some difficult situations.

23.3.1.2 Surgery versus Primary Care

The next step in developing a global health initiative is to choose a health disparity to address. At the inception of 'global health' as a recognized entity in medicine, the focus of international efforts was on maternal and child health, vaccination strategies, communicable diseases such as HIV/AIDS, and the development of infrastructure such as access to clean water. Efforts invested in these initiatives have positively affected millions of individuals worldwide, and their effects have transcended generations. Hence, one might think, 'Is it just to invest capital in neurosurgical missions when they are potentially more expensive and are subspecialty-specific?'

In response to this commonly posed ethical dilemma, surgical specialties such as neurosurgery can be seen as a neglected area of medicine in global health efforts. The lack of access to basic surgical care is known to cause three times as many deaths as communicable diseases such as HIV/AIDS, tuberculosis, and malaria combined.[2] This disparity in access to surgical care also has economic implications, with a projected burden of $20.3 trillion between 2015 and 2030.[2] In an attempt to address this alarming concern, the Lancet Commission on Global Surgery defined safe and affordable surgical care as a global priority back in 2015. Since then, there have been a growing number of surgical initiatives in LMICs and assessments on optimal ways to enhance workforce capacity in these underserved regions. Choosing a neurosurgical focus is in line with these concerted efforts and morally sound if the need is significant and the host nation desires investments in neurosurgical care.

23.3.1.3 Choosing the Initiative Model

Upon choosing a focus of the initiative, the subsequent step is to decide how best to deliver the resources. Fundamentally, the provision of resources is most ethical when it is allocated justly and sustainably; hence, 'surgical tourism', whereby neurosurgeons visit LMICs to perform isolated surgeries and return home, is obviously not the best option.

Sustainability is not just skill transfer but also resource transfer and mentorship. There have been other models discussed in the literature that address these multifaceted components of sustainability. Ibrahim and colleagues explored these models of international aid and categorized them based on depth of commitment and breadth of applications, as follows:

> Narrow breadth, low commitment: benevolent donation
> Narrow breadth, high commitment: focused teaching
> Wide breadth, low commitment: philanthropic travel
> Wide breadth, wide commitment: committed partnership[3]

While committed partnerships are the most ideal, each of these models has its unique benefits and challenges. For example, benevolent donation implies a donation of material goods such as equipment, which can help LMICs gain access to resources. However, these donations can have unintended consequences: they are often too costly to repair and end up collecting dust in a storage room, or their use is prohibitively expensive.

Focused teaching, on the other hand, entails teaching on a specific procedure, such as an awake craniotomy or endoscopic third ventriculostomy (ETV), which can rapidly build capacity in that singular procedure, yet may neglect the need for more generalized care. In order to mitigate this challenge, a thorough understanding is needed on the utility and sustainability of the intended procedure. For example, a prospective database of outcomes from an ETV teaching mission in Uganda showed that the intervention was indeed beneficial and resulted in a greater propensity towards ETV in Africa.[6]

23.3.1.4 Choosing a Location

In looking at the literature, there are no specific data on the method of selecting the appropriate host nation for a surgical mission; however, anecdotally, many visiting surgeons choose their host nation on simple parameters such as having an established connection with a local surgeon, choosing a nation that is safe and is easily accessible, and ensuring that there is already an established infrastructure upon which to build. Is it ethical to choose city A where a colleague invited you while cities B and C also have a need for your services?

Inevitably, surgeons cannot be in all places at once; one must choose a location, but this choice must be ethically made so that efforts benefit the greatest number of people. This can be achieved by choosing a central location where trainees from more distant towns rotate through, or organizing a conference type venue where surgeons and trainees from a larger diaspora convene for educational purposes. The choice of location should not reinforce existing disparities in access to surgical care in rural areas but, rather, try to assuage them. For example, more complex procedures can be taught at tertiary centres, whereas procedures that address the most common pathologies, such as trauma, can be taught to the rural centres that deal with the greatest burden of these conditions.[4]

The next step would involve establishing a connection with a local medical professional to ensure that the presence of foreign surgeons is desired and lastly to conduct a needs assessment to determine the degree of need. These steps help ensure fairness in resource allocation among LMICs and that visitors are going where they are both needed and wanted.

23.3.1.5 Coordinating Efforts

Communication is often poor between medical agencies involved in the provision of neurosurgical care in LMICs; hence, it is not uncommon to arrive at your host hospital and find that another visiting surgeon is there conducting his/her own surgical mission. This not only causes a disjointed educational experience, but also is an example of poor utilization of limited resources. The waste of fiscal and human capital is unethical when there is such a striking need for neurosurgical care worldwide. This calls for the development of a repository of global surgical initiatives, including past successes and failures and current efforts being invested.[2,5] Such a repository would allow interested surgeons to either coordinate efforts with each other or divert their efforts elsewhere.

23.3.1.6 Choosing the Team

Neurosurgeons do not work in isolation in developed countries, nor should they work in isolation in global health initiatives. The assembly of a team requires thought on which members and stakeholders are most appropriate to ensure the greatest overall potential for good. The team can involve other healthcare providers such as anaesthesiologists or neurologists, allied health members (nursing, physiotherapy, occupational therapy), engineers to teach locals how to maintain equipment or databases, research assistants to enhance local research capacity, and organizational stakeholders. It would be undesirable to provide surgery without the ability to augment the capacity for care, such as the provision of adjuvant therapies, rehabilitative services, or conservative treatments.

Lastly, there may be conflicts of interest that arise when neurosurgical initiatives are sponsored by organizations that have financial or political interests. Despite their baggage, these organizations can provide great benefit, such as the needed financial support material donations, or human capacity to ensure widespread impact. A balance is struck in this tale of two intentions by having a direct conversation at the outset highlighting the expectations of both parties, their level of involvement throughout the initiative, as well as the potential conflicts of interest for all involved members and the local beneficiaries.

23.3.1.7 Cultural Sensitivity

Cultural sensitivity refers to the principle of respect for all persons, irrespective of differences in cultural beliefs or backgrounds. It may seem be to an obvious and inherent attribute of all humans, but issues surrounding cultural sensitivity arise all the time in global health settings, even if they are inadvertent. Situational insensitivities or faux pas can be prevented through appropriate pre-departure training of all team members on global cultural sensitivity and some targeted education around local cultural nuances. This can centre on specific topics such as the nature of the local patient-doctor relationship or the role of spirituality in medical decision-making. It can also focus more broadly around social skills such as being malleable to different social situations or reinforcing the notion that the initiative is not a paternalistic one, but a true partnership.

23.3.1.8 International Research

As more attention is paid to the benefit of international neurosurgery in building capacity and education worldwide, there is an equally growing focus on the role of international research in either learning more about neurosurgical cases that occur worldwide or the impact of education or initiatives in dealing with these cases. Venturing in these research endeavours can be equally if not more challenging than setting up an educational mission, as it is laced with complex interactions, biases, contexts, and unique ethical dilemmas.

Principally, one must appreciate that the host country may be the most vulnerable in this interaction because of the following factors: (1) the host staff and their patients might view researchers as superior beings who should be trusted, leading to an unequal dynamic and inadequate attention to potential risks; (2) a lack of formal ethical training and practice in the host nation can lead to inadvertently unethical local research practices; (3) a lack of research training in host nations can place locals at a disadvantage in leading their own studies; and lastly, (4) a lack of health literacy can place human subjects in a more vulnerable position when obtaining informed consent for research.

There are several ways to mitigate some of these challenges in order to facilitate a more ethical research practice in global settings. First of all, just as in the development of educational missions, the design and implementation of a research project must engage both visiting and host members. Documents can be appropriately translated and written in a way that academic institutions and their research subjects can best understand and appreciate the intended benefits and risks of the study in question.

Collaboration extends beyond research members to academic institutions and research ethic review committees (RECs). There is great variability in the international experience with RECs, with some nations having no committees and others having RECs with formal training from organizations such as the UN, WHO, or the US Department of Health and Human Services Office for Human Research Protections. About 92% of researchers from LMICs believe their national research guidelines meet a high standard of ethical training; nevertheless, many visiting researchers can attest to the various challenges with RECs, both from home and host institutions[7]. The REB process can be a huge bottleneck in the development of global surgical research, in that some review processes are carried sequentially, where one review board will only approve a project pending the approval from the other institution. There are often great delays in the formal review of research ethics from host nations; it is not uncommon to arrive in the host nation and find out that the research proposal has not even been reviewed yet. This quickly leads to both unethical as well as unsafe research practices. There is an obvious need for the development of more RECs with formal training and greater collaboration between RECs. The collaboration can be in the form of case-by-case email communication, a central review board between long-term relationships, or designating one REC (preferably the host nation) as the primary one that coordinates the review and communication with researchers.[7]

With the development of RECs in LMICs, a focus should be made on developing local research capacity by teaching local members about scientific principles, data acquisition/storage, standards of research ethics, and steps of scientific writing. It would only seem ethical that publications from these collaborations should include researchers from host nations as equally recognized authors.

23.3.2 Intervention

23.3.2.1 Misrepresentation and False Advertising

While the visiting neurosurgeon might have a specific intended teaching focus, they might encounter situations where they are asked to perform surgeries in LMICs that are outside their scope of expertise. Patients may be promised that the visiting surgeon will do the entire procedure, or the visiting team might be given false information about available resources.[5,8] These dilemmas occur when hosts view the visiting neurosurgeon as an outright authority, as opposed to a partner with his/her own set of strengths and weaknesses. These situations can be avoided by formulating clear expectations and criteria for patient selection prior to the intervention; both the visiting and host teams should be involved in this planning, to ensure everyone is on the same page. Nevertheless, some situations might still arise where neurosurgeons are challenged with this dilemma and then the surgeon is tasked with the responsibility of self-reflection and honesty about the limitations of his/her skill.

23.3.2.2 Settling for Second Best

This scenario focuses on the provision of care with less-than-ideal resources or circumstances. For example, in developed nations we can agree that it would be unethical to perform a procedure such as an excision of an intramedullary spinal tumour without a microscope or resection of a left frontal speech-area brain tumour without neuromonitoring.[5,8] On the other hand, in global health settings the circumstances might be different. We consider it malpractice at home since there are alternatives that can reduce risk of harm, such as the use of certain equipment or resources. However, in LMICs there may be no alternatives. So, would performing these procedures without a functioning microscope be unethical if the option is to do nothing? Would doing a glioma surgery be futile if there are no adjuvant therapies, including radiation or chemotherapy? If the alternative is mortality or undue suffering, then maybe settling for 'second best' is the most a surgeon can do in that limited construct.

23.3.2.3 Local Ethics

Even if the visiting team equips itself with all the skills and armamentarium to provide the most ethical care and training, a bottleneck can be the lack of equivalent ethical practices in the host community. For example, neurosurgery programs in LMICs may not be accustomed to ethical standards of developed nations, including proper informed consent practices, appropriate patient follow-up and monitoring, structured morbidity and mortality discussions, and a commitment to elective surgery schedules. In order to ensure the best provision of neurosurgical care around the world, visiting neurosurgeons and their teams must make it a priority to not only engage host teams in surgical training but also increase ethical capacity. Studies in LMICs have shown that locals appreciate the dedication, passion, and ethical standards espoused by developed nations and value opportunities to grow in these facets as well.[1]

23.3.3 Post-intervention

23.3.3.1 Inappropriate Application of Teaching

Upon completion of an international neurosurgical initiative, some teams end up never knowing what happens to the host nation, and others maintain contact and follow-up. Of the latter, some may find out that the host nation is employing a technique in an unintended manner. To what extent is the visiting neurosurgeon ethically responsible for the actions of fully autonomous and capable host neurosurgeons after departure? This stresses the importance of determining morality based on a combination of both intentions (pre-intervention and intervention) and outcomes (post-intervention). To that effect, neurosurgeons and their teams must maintain regular contact with host teams and ensure that they have an infrastructure to monitor outcomes that can be shared between both parties. In doing so, everyone is held accountable for the potential benefits and ramifications of the intervention. Negotiations need to be made about the applicability of techniques taught in order to prevent unintended harm while recognizing the unique opportunity to facilitate surgical innovation through improvisation and creativity in local contexts.

23.3.3.2 When Is 'Enough' Enough

Various longitudinal models of education have been employed, including repeated visits to LMICs (visiting model), twinning between developed nations and LMICs,[9] and even electronic-based platforms for the provision of continued education and mentorship.[10] Each of these models provides excellent opportunities for longitudinal partnerships to ensure sustainability of efforts invested; however, they come at an expense of financial and human capital. In a world of finite resources, one must determine when it is appropriate to signal the completion of a project. This can be difficult to do when the host team requests further support and close relationships have been built between the two teams. However, an end-point is needed in order to divert efforts to places with the greatest need. Determining a priori end-points between the two teams is the best way of achieving global justice, fairness, and accountability.

23.4 Ethical Analysis

Ethics is the systematic analysis of morality based on formal philosophical principles and theories. While this chapter explores neuro-ethics in the global context, it is not that far removed from the concepts explored in other chapters, in that it is based on the same general ethical principles and theories that govern medical practice. Bioethics can provide physicians and surgeons with the framework needed to navigate ethical ambiguities that colour their day-to-day practices.

23.4.1 Ethical Principles

Principalism is a simplistic yet effective ethical system based on the fundamental four pillars of ethics, including autonomy (free will), beneficence (do good), non-maleficence (do no harm), and justice (just distribution of resources). These four principles are of equal importance and are designed to each contribute to ethical decision-making. They are the initial 'go-to' framework, but sometimes the principles are too broad and it can be difficult to govern sound decision-making in complex situations. Hence, further theories and philosophies can be explored to complement principalism.

23.4.2 Ethical Theories

There are various theories based on moral philosophies that can be applied to bioethical dilemmas. These include utilitarianism, Kantian deontology, contractarianism, rights-based theory, communitarianism, and casuistry, to name a few.

Philosophers Jeremy Bentham and John Stuart Mill derived utilitarian theory whereby good is measured by the greatest amount of happiness conferred to the largest number of people.[5] It is 'outcomes based' in that one does not concern oneself with intentions or means just by the greatest outcome of happiness. It is useful when applying it to resource allocation, such as choosing a host location where the most patients frequent at the expense of some isolated rural hospitals that might also desire the help.

John Rawl's contractarianism also focused on the good of the group instead of the individual.[5] His theory was that we are all equal individuals that would best function if we follow the 'golden rule: do unto others as one wants to be done unto himself'. Our society thereby works as a social contract between beings that all actions must be done in the light of fairness and justice for all. In slight contrast with utilitarianism, contractarianism does rely on people's good intentions to help others and see the benefit of others as also a benefit to oneself; however, the outcome is the same. It too can be applied to resource allocation and decisions around community or societal medical issues.

Immanuel Kant was a philosopher who believed that morality was a categorical and absolute imperative that is based on neither intention nor sentiments such as happiness. Instead, Kantian deontology dictates that humans are autonomous beings that do not rely on group-based thinking, as in contractarianism, but rely on morality as a strict duty based on reason; it implies that one must do 'the right thing' irrespective of intention or outcome, in contrast to utilitarianism[5]. While this theory aims at freeing people of outside influences and of self-interest, purity of reason is challenging to practice since the concept of 'doing the right thing' is not well defined; it in essence just relies on the pillars of beneficence and autonomy, which can be applied to various medical contexts, including informed consent.

There are many philosophies arguing that the sense of morality, the determination of what is 'right and wrong', can also be based on tradition. For example, religion is an organization of actions and beliefs based on spirituality; it in itself is an attempt at implementing morality in practice. It is not necessarily governed by any of the philosophical camps and can lend itself to very specific and sometimes peculiar ways of thinking or practicing morality. This is of paramount importance to the physician who may encounter patients of diverse religious backgrounds in a multicultural urban centre or a hospital in a developing nation that is richly embedded in a religious school of thought. Making ethical decisions in these contexts relies on a certain balance of one's moral background and a respect for diversity and religious sensitivity.

Similarly, cultural norms such as communitarianism (the community values trump individual rights) or feminism/paternalism (where values are based in the context of either a matriarchal or patriarchal society, respectively) can be the foundation for a society's moral views. This is of particular importance in global neurosurgery, whereby a visiting surgeon and his/her team must negotiate their cultural and ethical backgrounds with that governing the host nation in order to truly provide a sustainable educational service while maintaining moral integrity.

23.5 Case Example

Illustrative Clinical Case 1

You are a senior neurosurgeon in a developed nation. A colleague of yours in LMIC 'A' calls you and invites you to prepare some talks on awake craniotomies and perform some cases at the local hospital. You have not seen your colleague in a while and think it would be a good way to reconnect in a nice climate and a fun way to reinvent yourself in your stage of practice. You agree and assemble a team of nurses and residents to join you on this mission. You bring some OR tools and medications that promptly get confiscated at the airport. You arrive at the hospital and are already presented with a busy itinerary of cases, some of which include complex aneurysms and spinal tumours. A patient and his family comes to you excited to finally get his tumour resected and refuses to have the local surgeons involved in the case since it is a 'complex tumour'. You reluctantly agree and then find yourself in an OR with multiple observers taking videos with their phones and a TV crew without OR attire. You successfully resect the tumour (a high-grade meningioma) without a microscope, neuromonitoring, or blood on demand (Figure 23.1), but there is no radiation treatment or physiotherapy in the local community to supplement your efforts. You wonder if it was worth it. Your stay is over and you return home, feeling content with your efforts and applauded by your academic community. You make one subsequent visit two years later and find out that there are still no working microscopes available and only two awake craniotomies have been performed since you left. Your local practice picks up and you forget about the LMIC for years on end.

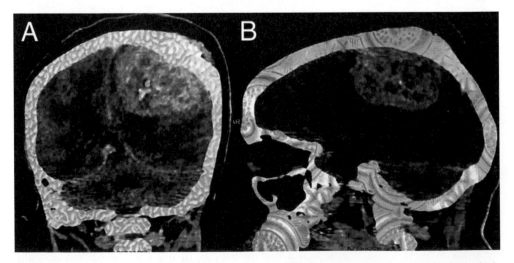

Figure 23.1 CT of large meningioma in coronal (a) and sagittal (b) views, operated on in an LMIC without a high-speed drill, neuronavigation, or ultrasonic aspirator, and with only one unit of blood available

This case illustrates many of the challenges already highlighted in this chapter and the ethical principles that apply to them. For example, the case starts with a concern about personal gain. This scenario is governed by the pillar of benevolence where we must always do what is best for other others, not for ourselves; it is also based in Kantian deontology to just do the morally right thing. Choosing a location for the mission is largely driven by justice and the concepts of utilitarianism and contractarianism. Cases that are outside of the scope of the mission or that involve operating fully on a patient without the inclusion of local surgeons raise the need to balance benevolence and non-maleficence. Lastly, lack of appropriate follow-up is a common issue that stresses the importance for just allocation of time and resources as well as non-maleficence.

23.6 Future Directions

While fundamentally based in goodwill and virtuosity, there are clearly complex layers of motives, risks, and benefits that underlie international surgical aid. These complexities require further attention and exploration in order to ensure that neurosurgeons and their teams have the greatest potential to empower the sustainable growth of global neurosurgical capacity in an ethically sound manner. It is as C. S. Lewis once said: 'Education without values, as useful as it is, seems rather to make man a more clever devil.' We must share attention to both education and the values that govern its implementation in day-to-day life decisions in order to advance equality in healthcare for all.

References

1. Cadotte D. W., Sedney C., Djimbaye H., Bernstein M. A qualitative assessment of the benefits and challenges of international neurosurgical teaching collaboration in Ethiopia. *World Neurosurgery* 2014, **82**(6): 980–6.

2. Fallah P. N., Bernstein M. Unifying a fragmented effort: a qualitative framework for improving international surgical teaching collaborations. *Globalization and Health* 2017, **13**: 70.

3. Ibrahim G. M., Bernstein M. Models of neurosurgery international aid and their potential ethical pitfalls. *Virtual Mentor, American Medical Association Journal of Ethics* 2015, **17**(1): 49–55.

4. Dewan M. C., Rattani A., Fieggen G., et al. Global neurosurgery: the current capacity and deficit in the provision of essential neurosurgical care. Executive summary of the Global Neurosurgery Initiative and the Program in Global Surgery and Social Change. *Journal of Neurosurgery* 2017, doi:10.3171/2017.11. JNS171500.

5. Ammar A., Bernstein M. *Neurosurgical Ethics in Practice: Value-Based Medicine.* Berlin, Springer, 2014.

6. Kulkarni A. V., Riva-Cambrin J., Browd S. R., et al. Endoscopic third ventriculostomy and choroid plexus cauterization in infants with hydrocephalus: a retrospective Hydrocephalus Clinical Research Network study. *J. Neurosurg. Pediatr.* 2014, **14**(3): 224–9.

7. Ng L. C., Hanlon C., Yimer G., Henderson D. C., Fekadu A. Ethics in global health research: the need for balance. *Lancet Glob. Health* 2015, **3**(9): e516–17.

8. Howe K. L., Malomo A. O., Bernstein M. A. Ethical challenges in international surgical education. *World Neurosurgery* 2013, **80**(6): 751–8.

9. Branch C. L., Boop F., Haglund M. M., Dempsey R. J. Introduction. Neurosurgical

opportunities in global health inequities. *Neurosurgical Focus* 2018; **45**(4): E1.

10. Blankstein U., Dakurah T., Bagan M., Hodaie M. Structured online neurosurgical education as a novel method of education delivery in the developing world. *World Neurosurgery* 2011, **76**: 224–30.

Chapter 24

Live Televised Surgery

Eiichi Ishikawa, Nobuyuki Sakai, Stephen Honeybul, and Akira Matsumura

24.1 Introduction

Instructing trainees during the course of an operative procedure has formed the cornerstone of surgical training since the inception of surgical practice as it is known today. Indeed, the term 'theatre' originates from the early days of surgery when the operative facilities were constructed in such a way as to accommodate a large number of spectators, ranging from surgical trainees through to paying members of the public. The relatively recent advent of television bought with it the ability to broadcast surgery to millions of households, and this led to documentary series such as *Your Life in Their Hands* (produced by the BBC in London).

More recently, surgical procedures have been televised and broadcast live to audiences at surgical conferences as an educational adjunct in order to demonstrate a surgical technique, innovative instrumentation, or implanted device.[1-3] There have been several formats utilized for these so-called live televised surgeries (LTS), the most common of which is to have an invited expert in the field perform surgery at a hospital local to the conference, with the surgery being broadcast live to conference delegates. Proponents of these live demonstrations argue that the real-life nature of these broadcasts provides educational insight into surgical techniques and decisions in a real-time fashion that cannot be obtained from edited tapes or textbook descriptions. In addition, observers can obtain valuable experience regarding the management of unexpected surgical complications as and when they occur. Finally, developments in audio-visual technology, combined with the introduction and refinement of endoscopic techniques, has enabled acquisition of high-quality footage with minimal encroachment on the operative environment, especially in fields such as cardiovascular and urological surgery.

However, notwithstanding the potential educational benefits, there has been an increasing awareness that surgery performed under these conditions presents a number of unique ethical considerations that have caused considerable controversy in recent years.[4-6] First, there are patient-centred issues such as privacy, consent, and possible benefits or harms that may occur when being part of a live televised event (Table 24.1). Second, there may be surgeon-related issues that need to be considered, given that they may be operating in an unfamiliar environment with the possible added stress of being watched by a large number of well-informed and possibly critical colleagues (Table 24.2). Finally, there are participant-related issues regarding the advantages or disadvantages of this type of medical education compared with other types of medical education (Table 24.3).

Over the past two decades, as use of this type of educational format has increased, the intensity of debate has grown in parallel, and this has led in certain circumstances to some

Table 24.1 Patient-centred issues when performing LTS

	Potential patient-centred problems	Possible solutions
Privacy	Privacy must always be guaranteed. A patient's medical and social history are often relevant to the surgical procedure and are often presented to the audience.	Patients faces should never be shown unless specifically stated in the consent. All information must be de-identified.
Consent	Consent is required, but there is an obvious power imbalance between the surgeon and the patient (who may be reluctant to refuse to be part of the event). Have there been any financial incentives to participation (such as waiver of fees)?	A clear explanation of what is involved in an LTS, including who will perform the surgery and the size and type of audience. A detailed explanation of an alternative to live surgery that does not compromise patient care should be provided, and a patient advocate may be appointed to act as a third-party counsellor. If financial incentives have been offered, the surgeon should probably refrain from participation.
Safety	There may in certain circumstances be added risk to the patient if the surgeon becomes distracted due to audience questions. Delays in surgery can occur due to scheduling surgery for an event that may be some months away.	A moderator should be appointed (Table 24.2). Delays that may lead to disease progression should not occur.

surgical societies either banning these events or issuing guidelines to restrict their usage. A good example of the evolution that has occurred comes from the practice of LTS in Japan.

24.2 The History of LTS in Japan

One of the first cases of LTS was performed in Nagoya, Japan, in 2003, at the 33rd Japanese Conference on Surgery for Cerebral Stroke. In this LTS, a 48-year-old man with an unruptured middle cerebral artery aneurysm underwent a craniotomy and clipping of the aneurysm. The surgery went well, and there were no intraoperative or post-operative complications.[7,8] At the time, there appeared to be obvious advantages, given that the audience comprised more than 1,300 observers. However, even at that time, it was acknowledged that there were no specific guidelines for this type of surgical presentation, and this could present logistical and ethical problems for future cases. Following this initial success, the use of LTS became more widespread; however; it became increasingly apparent that the aforementioned issues were leading, in certain cases, to compromise in patient care due to the unique and unfamiliar circumstances in which the surgery was being carried out. This was brought to a head following a fatality that occurred during a live televised cardiothoracic procedure.

Table 24.2 Surgeon-centred issues when performing LTS

	Potential surgeon-centred problems	Possible solutions
Surgical environment	A surgeon may have travelled considerable distances to work in an unfamiliar theatre environment, possibly with unfamiliar staff.	The surgeon must arrive well before the surgical date to familiarize themselves with the working environment, surgical and nursing staff, surgical instruments, the patient, and all investigations. In certain cases, the surgeon can bring their own instruments and staff, or they can operate from their own institution. Language barriers must be identified and addressed well in advance of the procedure.
Surgical procedure	Performing surgery in front of a live audience may provide added stress, especially if complications occur or if the surgeon is distracted by questions from the audience. It has previously been noted that live broadcasting may involve additional personnel within the theatre, which may compromise movement within the working environment.	The use of moderators is recommended, with one in the theatre and one in the auditorium. This can reduce pressure placed on the surgeon, especially during difficult steps in the procedure where the theatre moderator is well placed to assess the surgical thermostat. This may be a historical issue, given the advances in audio-visual technology (as discussed later).
Surgical decision-making	Surgeons may be influenced by the fact that they are operating in front of peers and may not want to have their reputation tarnished if they have a surgical complication or if they have to significantly change or even abandon a procedure, especially if they are demonstrating a new technique or instrument for which they may have been sponsored.	Surgeon selection is important. They must obviously be competent but their commitment must be to education rather than advancement of their career or reputation. Appropriate choice of surgeon is one of the most important tasks of a local conference director. The moderator must have the capacity to ask that either the broadcast be terminated or the procedure be abandoned if significant complications occur.

This occurred in 2006 following surgery conducted at Toyohashi Heart Center in Toyohashi, Aichi Prefecture, and transmitted live to a training session in Hyogo Prefecture.[9] The surgery involved a 63-year-old man who died soon after the surgical repair of a dissecting aortic aneurysm, and a subsequent investigation highlighted a number of significant problems. First, the case was high risk, with a mortality rate in the region of 20%.

Table 24.3 Participant-centred issues when performing LTS

	Potential participant-centred problems	Possible solutions
Surgical environment	Participants may be drawn to an event more out of curiosity rather than from an educational perspective. A voyeuristic approach to see a surgical catastrophe is certainly not in the best interests of the patient.	Participants must be limited to medical practitioners who attend with the explicit intention of learning. Attendees must pre-register for the event and be part of the surgical society that is hosting the event. Surgeons form other societies may attend at the discretion of the event director. Members of the public should not be allowed to attend.
Surgical procedure	Complications may occur that may place the patient at risk of an unfavourable outcome, especially if the surgeon's performance is compromised because of audience participation.	The use of moderators is recommended (Table 24.2), with one in the theatre and one in the auditorium. This can reduce the pressure placed on the surgeon, especially during difficult steps in the procedure where the theatre moderator is well placed to assess the surgical thermostat.
Surgical decision-making	Audience members may disagree with certain aspects of the surgical procedure, whether it be clinical indications, surgical technique, or management of surgical complications.	It is important that any audience involvement does not affect the performance of the surgeon. The use of moderators must allow timely and appropriate discussion of the surgery, and the moderators must be allowed to filter and limit interactions with the surgeon at all times.

The surgeon was from outside of the region and was unfamiliar with the operative environment. Just prior to the surgery, there was some debate regarding surgical indications, and during the surgery there were frequent questions, discussions, and comments, with some of the participants voicing criticism of the surgeon's technique. This led to the procedure being repeatedly interrupted.

The case, in conjunction with some similar cases worldwide, prompted several national surgical associations such as the American College of Obstetricians and Gynecologists and the American College of Surgeons to actually ban LTS and warned surgeons that they would face disciplinary action if they continued to participate in these events. In 2007 the Japanese Society for Cardiovascular Surgery (JSCVS) issued guidelines for live presentations of thoracic and cardiovascular surgery (Table 24.4).[10] While these recommendations would appear very reasonable, they did in many ways serve to highlight how problematic the use of LTS had become. For example, having a guideline that advises against ostentatious behaviour would seem to imply that this was a regular occurrence.

One of the stipulations of the guidelines was that reports be submitted to the JSCVS regarding each case of LTS, outlining the degree to which the guidelines had been followed. A subsequent review of these reports demonstrated some ongoing problems.

Table 24.4 Some of the key points in the Japanese guidelines to live presentations of thoracic and cardiovascular surgery[8]

Key issues	Highlighted recommendations
Aims of live surgery	Live surgery is NOT intended to provide highly technical information or to teach rarely used surgical techniques.
Ethical matters	Informed consent must be obtained from the patient AND from the ethics committee of the institution where the operation is to be conducted. Consent must be obtained from the surgeon, and the patient must be informed that surgery in these circumstances provides no benefit and may result in harm due to surgeon distraction.
Selection of patients	Patients with common ailments and low-risk surgery are ideal.
Selection of operative procedure	Difficult operative techniques requiring high technical skills are NOT ideal. Ethical approval for all techniques is required.
Selection of faculty	All medical practitioners must be highly experienced.
Selection of surgeon	The surgeon must have a good understanding of the purposes of live surgery and avoid ostentatious behaviour.
Surgeon and facility	Ideally, the surgeon will perform surgery in the institution to which they belong.
Relationships with private companies	Use of new equipment must be limited, even if no monetary exchange is involved.
Audience conditions	Restricted to members of the relevant academic and research societies. Practice restraint in timing of their questions.
Recording procedures	The surgeon must not allow the efficiency to deteriorate for the sake of superior imaging.
Final assessment	The surgeon must report on the post-operative course of the patient at an organized society or research meeting.

Between the years 2007 to 2012, there were 33 cases of live surgery, and while it was acknowledged that surgeons had made considerable efforts, there remained significant deficiencies. Among the 33 reports,

➤ 14 reports were submitted less than 2 weeks before the scheduled date of live surgery or had no specified date;
➤ 7 reports had no printed program;
➤ 5 programs did not obtain local ethics committee approval;
➤ 30 programs did not include reports of the meeting of the local program committee; and
➤ 16 programs failed to provide a post-operative follow-up.

In addition, there was a further death in 2012. The case involved a 77-year-old man with an aortic aneurysm who underwent stent grafting. During this procedure, the surgeon acted as a moderator and presenter simultaneously, and this appeared to distract his attention. Despite being told by the anesthesiologist that the blood pressure was falling, he continued to present to the audience, ignoring his responsibilities to the patient. The patient suffered a cardiac arrest two minutes after the initial alert, and unfortunately the live broadcast continued for a further nine minutes after the cardiac arrest. A subsequent investigation revealed that no ethical committee approval had been obtained prior to the procedure, and the ethical committee approval was only sought retrospectively.

In the light of these findings, the guidelines for live surgery in JSCVS were revised in 2014, to reflect the increasingly acknowledged limitations and possible dangers of LTS.[11] In these guidelines, the 'pros and cons' of live surgery were described as follows:

> In cardiovascular surgery, unexpected circumstances may arise intraoperatively that challenge the operative surgeon's judgement and management skills. The ability of the surgeon to manage those scenarios is the key to good clinical outcomes. Live surgery has the potential to instruct audiences on such management, and can provide marked educational impact, consequently contributing to the improvement of the quality of surgery for future patients. Live surgery imparts additional stress to the operating surgeon and may interfere with the surgeon's ability to use his/her skills as effectively as they usually do. This may endanger the patient, and for this reason, it is crucial to give priority to the patient's safety and to ensure sufficient educational benefit during cases of live cardiovascular surgery.

In addition, the objectives of live surgery were also clarified:

> Live surgery aims to provide opportunities to learn diverse operative techniques related to cardiovascular surgery, rather than serve as a display of a masterful surgical performance or to satisfy an audience's voyeuristic desires. Therefore, its scope should be limited to typical surgical procedures in which advanced operative techniques are used. Ideally, the surgical procedures should be performed in a standardized fashion familiar to both the operating surgeon and the host operative team. In addition to demonstration of surgical techniques, the educational program should include appropriate strategies, such as indications, surgical equipment and instruments, and support systems, such as anesthesia.[11]

Overall, the revised guidelines reflect the increasing recognized limitations of LTS and the need to be ever mindful of the possible harms that can come to patients when they are submitted to surgical procedures in circumstances where the surgeon's performance may be compromised. What remains to be established is the role of this type of educational format in the context of neurosurgery.

24.3 The Role of LTS in Neurosurgery

The vast majority of LTS has been performed by general surgeons, cardiothoracic surgeons, and urological surgeons, and there have been relatively few instances of its use in neurosurgery. A good example of where its use appears appropriate has been at the Brush-Up Seminar of Neuro-Endovascular Therapy (BSNET) organized by the Society of Neuro-Endovascular Techniques and Tools, which has been held since 2011.[12] These yearly events and accompanying LTS take place at Kobe City Medical Center General Hospital with careful preparation and performance consideration by several organizers and about 40 participants.[12] In 2018, 7 cases of intracranial aneurysm were treated with stent coiling with or without stent and flow-diversion. A case of intracranial atherosclerotic disease was treated with angioplasty and stenting, and a dural arteriovenous fistula was treated with Onyx transarterial embolization. These cases were all performed uneventfully and were ethically approved by the local ethics committee. This type of format demonstrates the educational benefit that can be obtained by performing real-time procedures of relatively new technology with minimal risk of harm to the patient. The World Federation of Neurosurgical Societies (WFNS) is also currently providing live surgery demonstrations within several training courses, which again serves to emphasize that this type of format does have a place in surgical education if organized appropriately and recognizes the lessons learned from previous LTS events.

The role of LTS outside of this carefully controlled educational format remains controversial, and this was clearly demonstrated by a case in 2015.

24.4 Live Televised Public Neurosurgery

On Sunday, 25 October 2015, Greg Grindley, a 49-year-old retired naval electrician, underwent live deep brain stimulation (DBS) surgery at University Hospital's Cleveland Medical Center.[13] The surgical procedure was performed for Parkinson's disease, and it was broadcast live on the *National Geographic* channel. It was also rebroadcast on Sunday, November 1, at 10:00 a.m., in 171 countries and in 45 languages.

Overall, the context in which the surgery was performed appeared reasonable, and the patient appeared fully informed regarding what was involved. The surgery was completed uneventfully, and the patient made a good recovery. However, notwithstanding the intended public educational benefits, the case attracted a considerable amount of criticism, mainly because it appeared to ignore a number of lessons learnt from similar LTS events in other surgical specialties.[14,15]

In the first instance, the stated intention of the broadcast was to raise awareness of DBS surgery among the general population.[13] However, these techniques are by no means new, and most general practitioners will either be aware of their capabilities or be aware of an appropriate specialist to whom patients with Parkinson's disease can be referred.

Second, the involvement of the television crew certainly appeared to have the potential to interfere with surgery, given that the broadcast involved more than a dozen cameras in and around the theatre complex and a 60-foot-long television production truck, like those used for major sporting events, which served as the hub for a crew of 100 coordinating the show.

Finally, and perhaps most telling, is the fact that despite innumerable videos of surgical procedures being available on the Internet, there has not been a repeat of such a live public broadcast of neurosurgical surgery anywhere in the world. This is probably a reflection of opinion among the neurosurgical community regarding the appropriateness or otherwise of these types of event from the perspective of patient safely, surgical career advancement, and institutional advertisement.

Overall, the use of LTS has come a long way in the past 20 years. There would certainly appear to be a role for this type of broadcast in the controlled and ethically scrutinized environment of a surgical society educational program. However, it is clear that unregulated use of these types of events raise ethical concerns regarding patient consent, safety, and confidentiality. It also clear that if motivation for surgeons becoming involved in these types of events moves beyond pure education, then there is potential for significant conflicts of interest that can involve personal, financial, industrial, and institutional issues.

Table 24.5 Some of the comments regarding the live broadcast of the deep brain stimulation surgery[13-15]

Source	Comments
Boston Globe	The Society of Thoracic Surgeons instructs its members worldwide not to participate in live surgery broadcasts to the public and warns that violating its guidelines could lead to disciplinary action. (While the chest cavity is not the cranium, the advice is just as applicable)
Dr Lawrence B Schlachter[13]	The telecast was little more than voyeuristic reality TV. Otherwise, why not just tape the long, arduous and even tedious procedure and edit it for telecast at a later date? The 'live' angle to it, with the inherent possibility that something could go wrong – maybe even terribly wrong – was surely intended to give it a 'Flying Wallendas' or 'Evel Knievel' (i.e., minus the safety net) aspect that NatGeo was no doubt counting on to draw in viewers.
	That is not to question the expertise of the surgeons at Case Medical Center. They are no doubt highly skilled and working for the best outcome for their patient. But whether by design or not, is it possible the bigger beneficiaries were in fact the doctors; the medical center; and Medtronics, the manufacturer of the electrodes inserted into Grindley's brain? After all, it could be argued that 'Brain Surgery Live' could be seen as little more than a two-hour infomercial for them.
Washington Post	While the procedure is no longer considered experimental, 'Apparently, it's not super helpful to have tons of cameras around while doctors are trying to perform a six-hour surgical procedure.'
David Armstrong	The event will showcase University Hospitals, which has a much lower national profile than the neighbouring Cleveland Clinic. It will also feature equipment and devices made by companies that have financial relationships with neurosurgeons at the medical center. That information will not be disclosed during the telecast.
	The surgical team will implant a neurostimulator from Medtronic LLC. One of the neurosurgeons received $42,769 in payments from the company during 2013–14, according to filings made with the federal government. A little more than half of that amount was for promotional speaking. The rest was for consulting work, travel, and food. The surgeon's relationship with Medtronic was not reported under industry relationships on his hospital biography.
	The show also features a 3D simulator from Surgical Theatre LLC that creates a model of the patient's brain. The technology was developed at University Hospitals, and the medical centre's chairman of neurological surgery, Warren Selman, is listed as Surgical Theatre's medical director on the company's website. He also reported owning stock options in the company in a 2013 medical article.
	His relationship with the company is not disclosed in his official biography on the hospital website, which promises 'transparency in our interactions with industry partners'. The hospital said his biography will be updated.
Richard Huxtable	If the broadcast is being beamed beyond doctors, we might then ask whether the standards of 'good' television will lead to pressure being placed on the surgeons to depart from the standards of good medicine.

24.5 Conclusion

The role of LTS remains controversial. On initial examination, it would appear to provide an ideal opportunity to enhance the traditional model of a surgical trainee observing a procedure performed by a more senior practitioner, with a view to eventually performing that procedure themselves. LTS allows many participants to observe that same procedure, thereby enlarging the surgical audience and therefore the educational experience. However, notwithstanding these benefits, previous experience has clearly demonstrated that this type of format can affect a surgeon's performance and decision-making, thereby compromising patient's safety.

It is now evident that clear guidelines are required in order to minimize harm to the patient and maintain maximal educational benefit to participants for whom the event is relevant. There are currently no such guidelines in neurosurgery; however, if the use of this educational format is to continue, the time may have come for an authoritative society such as WFNS to perhaps adapt existing guidelines from other surgical societies.

References

1. Shimizu S., Han H. S., Okamura K., et al. Live demonstration of surgery across international borders with uncompressed high-definition quality. *HPB (Oxford)*. 2007; **9**: 398–9.

2. Shimizu S., Ohtsuka T., Takahata S., et al. Remote transmission of live endoscopy over the Internet: Report from the 87th Congress of the Japan Gastroenterological Endoscopy Society. *Dig. Endosc.* 2016; **28**: 92–7.

3. Roser F., Pfister G., Tatagiba M., et al. Live surgery in neurosurgical training courses: essential infrastructure and technical set-up. *Acta Neurochir (Wien)* 2013; **155**: 541–5.

4. Philip-Watson J., Khan S. A., Hadjipavlou M., et al. Live surgery at conferences - Clinical benefits and ethical dilemmas. *Arab. J. Urol.* 2014; **12**: 183–6.

5. Williams J. B., Mathews R., D'Amico T. A. 'Reality surgery' – a research ethics perspective on the live broadcast of surgical procedures. *J. Surg. Educ.* 2011; **68**: 58–61.

6. Dikkers F. G., Klussmann J. P., Bernal-Sprekelsen M., et al. Live surgery broadcast: who is benefiting? *Eur. Arch. Otorhinolaryngol.* 2016; **273**: 1331–3.

7. Nagata K. Live surgery at the 33rd Japanese Conference on Surgery for Cerebral Stroke. *Surgery for Cerebral Stroke* 2005; **33**: 58. *(Translated from Japanese)*

8. Live surgery at the 33rd Japanese Conference on Surgery for Cerebral Stroke. Available at: http://knagata.kt.fc2.com/ron bun.htm. *(Translated from Japanese)*

9. Patient in 'live' surgery showing died soon after. 2007. Available at: www.japantimes .co.jp/news/2007/06/07/national/patient-in-live-surgery-showing-died-soon-after/.

10. Misaki T., Takamoto S., Matsuda H., et al. Guidelines to live presentations of thoracic and cardiovascular surgery. 2007. Available at: http://square.umin.ac.jp/jscvs/eng/live .html.

11. Miyamoto Y., Ueda Y., Sakata R., et al. Guidelines for live presentations of cardiovascular surgery (revised). Available at: http://square.umin.ac.jp/jscvs/english/li ve.html.

12. Brush-up seminar of neuroendovascular therapy. Available at: www.bsnet.umin.net/.

13. Why this doctor is performing brain surgery on live TV – latest stories. 2015. Available at: https://www.nationalgeographic.com/news/ 2015/10/151022-brain-surgery-live-deep-bra in-stimulation-parkinsons/.

14. Brain surgery on live TV – helpful or exploitative? STAT. 2015. Available at: www.statnews.com/2015/10/21/brain-surgery-on-live-tv-helpful-or-exploitive/.

15. Schlachter L. B. Brain surgery on live TV – first do no harm. 2015. Available at: www .cleveland.com/opinion/index.ssf/2015/11/p ost_140.html.

Index